VOGUE® MODEL

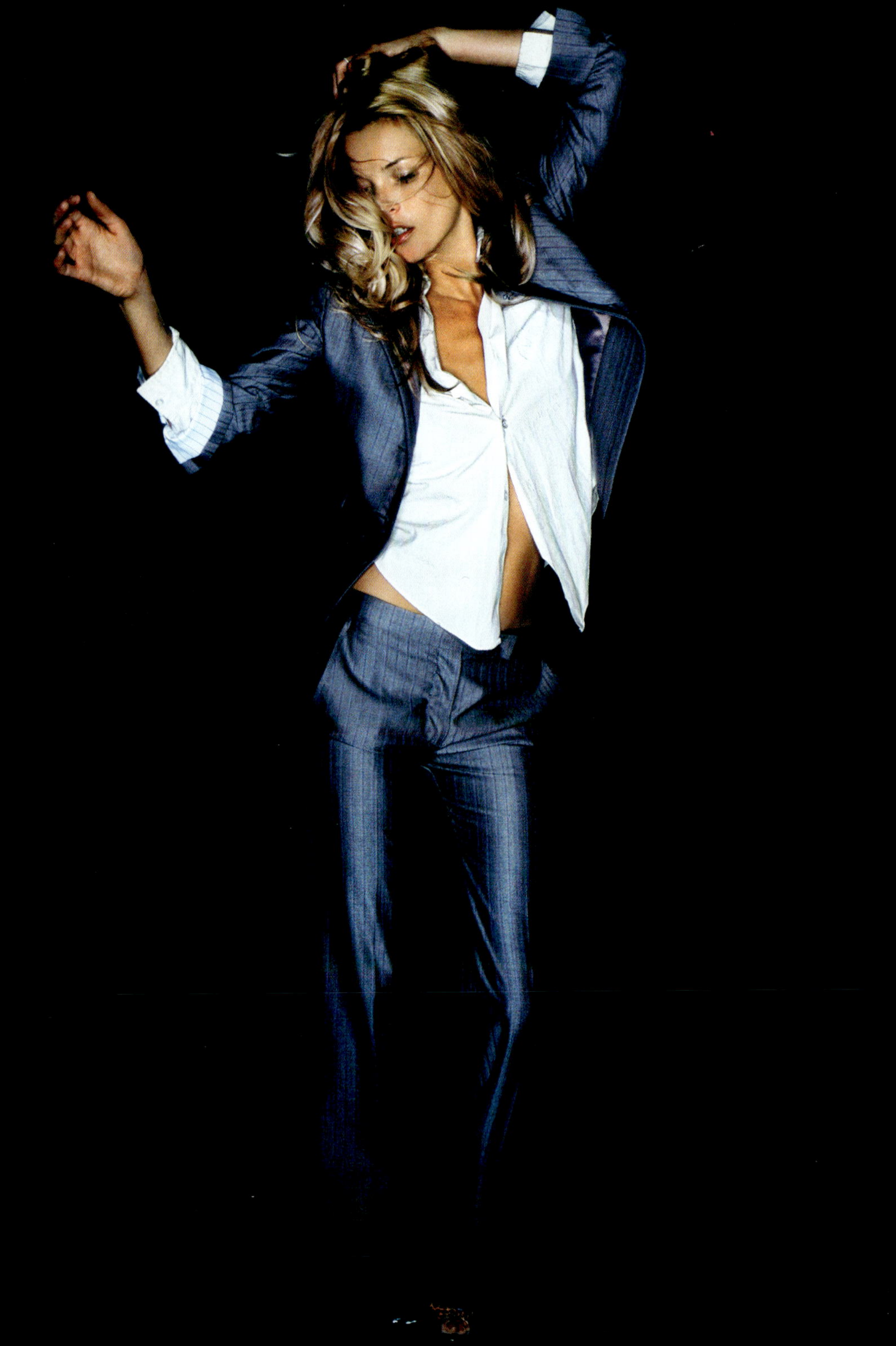

The Faces of Fashion

VOGUE MODEL

Edited by Robin Derrick and Robin Muir

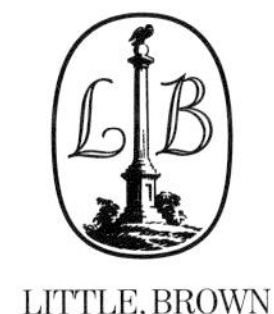

LITTLE, BROWN

LITTLE, BROWN

First published in Great Britain in 2010 by Little, Brown
This paperback edition published in 2013 by Little, Brown

Design: Rebecca Mason
Picture research: Michael Donkin
Sub-editing: Stephen Patience
Picture co-ordination: Lucy Cox
The Condé Nast Library: Brett Croft

A CIP catalogue record for this book is available from the British Library.

ISBN 978-1-4087-0254-3

Printed and bound in China

Little, Brown
An imprint of
Little, Brown Book Group
100 Victoria Embankment
London EC4Y 0DY

An Hachette UK Company
www.hachette.co.uk

www.littlebrown.co.uk

Frontispiece
'A Piece of Kate', April 2007,
by Nick Knight.
Fashion by Kate Moss Topshop

Contents

Foreword
by Alexandra Shulman

About a year ago, a reader of *Vogue* sent me a photocopy of a page from the *Western Gazette*, a Somerset local newspaper, dated Friday September 14, 1888. Under the headline 'General News', there was an item flagged 'A New Occupation for Girls'. The paragraph describes how a 'beautiful girl' in New York had been engaged by a firm of milliners to be photographed, 'adorned in the various costumes with which they appeal to the taste of New York young ladies'. It continues that she was hired to address complaints of the 'woodenness' of fashion-plate illustrations, and concludes that she 'would seem to be having what young ladies of her nationality call "a good time" and to be well paid for it'.

The first fashion model? Perhaps. What we do know is that when *Vogue* launched in America in 1892, fashion in the magazine was illustrated solely by drawings – line sketches of utterly unrealistic mannequins and simple outlines of the clothes. It was not until the 1920s that photography was employed and the clothes began to be photographed on flesh and blood. It took until 1932 for the first *Vogue* cover to feature a real woman.

Interestingly, the earliest people to wear fashion in the pages of *Vogue* were actually the it-girls of the time rather than professional models – society women like Paula Gellibrand and Daisy Fellowes, who would be photographed in the glamorous outfits of the day. Robin Muir describes here how *Vogue* first realised that a model girl had her own worth when Marion Morehouse became a popular figure in the States: 'She was not an actress, a music-hall star or a society figure, but something new entirely – a model girl. *Vogue* began to use her name in credit lines.'

The concept of a fashion model appears, on the surface, a simple notion. Take one beautiful woman (or man), dress them in whatever you want them to wear, photograph them, and there you have it – a fashion shot. But the reality is somewhat more complex. A successful model has to be of their time, and to be able to embody something about the era that people respond to positively. That may be how they look naturally, or it may be in their ability to be transformed and become whatever they need to be – a scrubbed-clean beauty, a sultry vamp, a techno-babe.

As this book clearly demonstrates, many of the models with the greatest impact have achieved that through collaboration with a particular photographer, who has been able to convey something totemic about them. Models need photographers. Without photographers, they are simply (or even not so simply) beautiful girls. In these pages you see the immaculate, haughty perfection of Dorian Leigh captured by Irving Penn, sculptured and distant – a series of lines and shapes rather than a woman. Then there is the groundbreaking modernity of David Bailey and Jean Shrimpton in the 1960s, where Bailey falls in love with 'a democratic kind of beauty', as he puts it – a shift away from the stylised, aristocratic appearance of the Fiona Campbell-Walters and Barbara Goalens of the previous decade. And in another shift in the late 1970s, partnerships such as those of Chris von Wangenheim with Janice Dickinson and the tragic Gia Carangi reacted against the dreamy hippiedom of previous years with high-voltage shots of aggressive glamour.

And that collaboration, the product of the model and the photographer, needs to be seen. No great model, nor great fashion photographer, has reached that status in total privacy. The essential ingredient is that their work must be viewed by others, to be on display. Their careers are heightened by the exposure of fame.

Vogue has unarguably been the most influential creator of famous models and famous photographers. The magazine has not only provided a forum whereby they can work together, it has also been involved (via generations of talented editors, art directors and fashion editors) in forming the memorable images that are the great models' legacy.

This encyclopaedia of the greatest models not only shows us who the faces and bodies of the age have been, but also documents their relationship with the magazine. Tellingly, it is structured not in chronological, but in alphabetical order. And the emphasis is on the Christian name – starting with Agyness Deyn and ending with Yasmin Le Bon. It seems an appropriate acknowledgement of their modern kind of fame, recognising the feeling of intimacy we like to have about our celebrities. By featuring them in order of name, *Vogue Model* celebrates the rise of the model as personality – a big move away from that anonymous New York clotheshorse of 1888. In some cases, their name has become a vital part of their iconic status – Twiggy, Shrimpton, Naomi, Kate.

At first this will seem a curious choice, meaning that as the pages turn you are flipped from a Liz Collins picture of Jessica Stam in 2007 to a Bob Richardson image of the British model Jill Kennington in 1966, and then back again to a Nick Knight headshot of flame-haired Karen Elson in 2008. But by ordering it in this way, each model occupies her own space, rather than being an exemplar of a time or particular style.

It's tempting to group models in tribes: fresh-faced sexpots like Bridget Hall, Patti Hansen and Claudia Schiffer; mavericks, such as Peggy Moffitt, Erin O'Connor, Lily Cole; the aristocrats – Anne Gunning, Lisa Fonssagrives, Carla Bruni. But *Vogue Model* resists. Instead, the book allows each to be viewed independently, and in doing so shows them for what they are: the most beautiful girls in the world, each with an individual story that has contributed to the collective history of *Vogue*.

Alexandra Shulman is editor of British Vogue

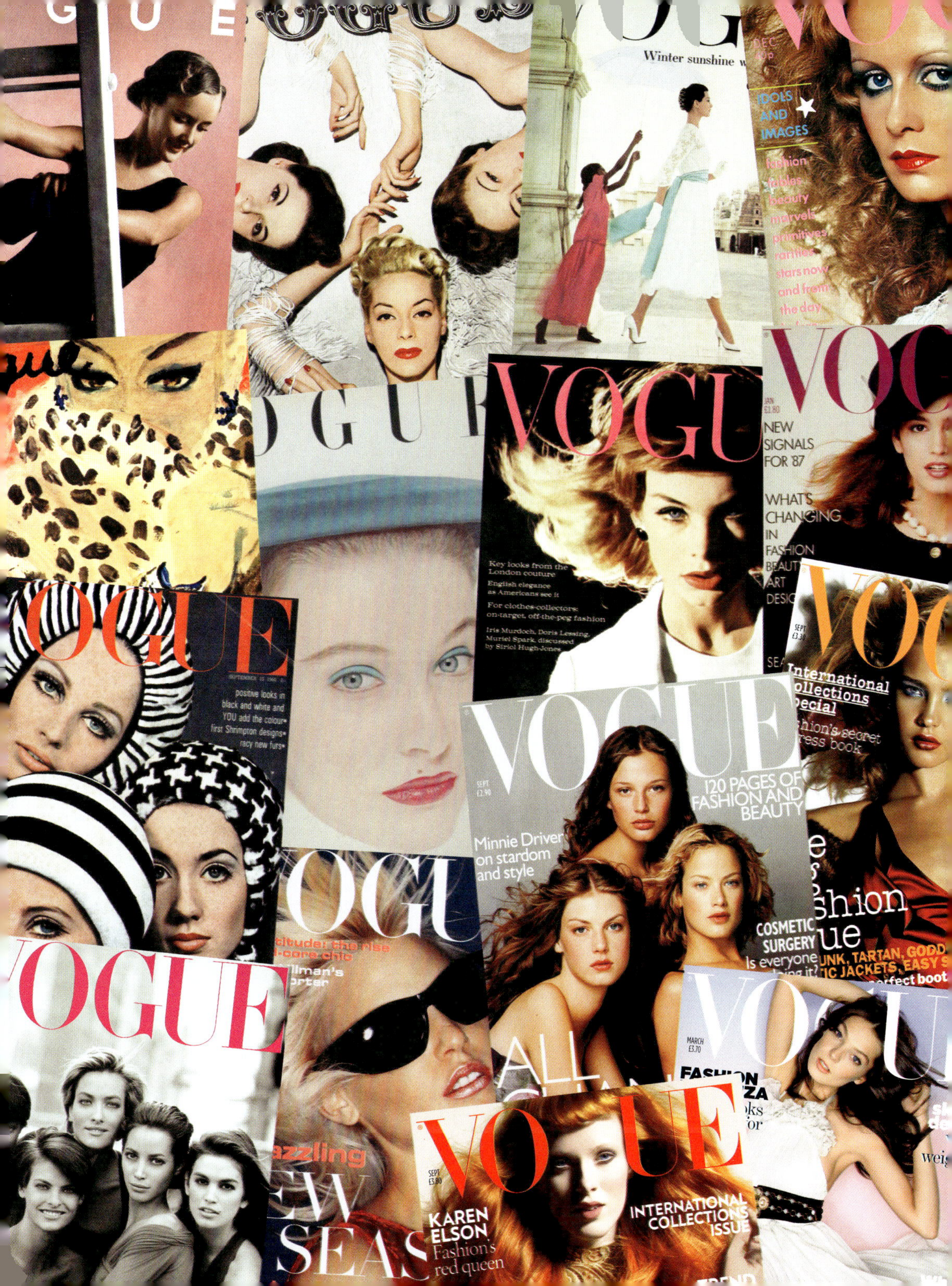
VOGUE
Winter sunshine
IDOLS AND IMAGES
fashion
fables
beauty
marvels
primitives
rarities
stars now
and from
the day
VOGUE
VOGUE
NEW SIGNALS FOR '87
WHAT'S CHANGING IN FASHION
Key looks from the London couture
English elegance as Americans see it
For clothes-collectors: on-target, off-the-peg fashion
Iris Murdoch, Doris Lessing, Muriel Spark, discussed by Siriol Hugh-Jones
VOGUE
positive looks in black and white and YOU add the colour•
first Shrimpton designs•
racy new furs•
VOGUE
120 PAGES OF FASHION AND BEAUTY
Minnie Driver on stardom and style
COSMETIC SURGERY
VOGUE
VOGUE
VOGUE
KAREN ELSON
Fashion's red queen
INTERNATIONAL COLLECTIONS ISSUE

Agyness Deyn

The story seems so unlikely it can only be true. Childhood friends from the north of England, Henry Holland and Laura Hollins, think that one day they might make it big in London, though they are not entirely sure at what. He's a fledgling designer, then making T-shirts; she's been working part-time in a chip shop back home. The T-shirt business begins to take off, because he's funny and his shirts bear rhyming slogans poking fun at the industry he's fast becoming a part of. She, meanwhile, has changed her name to something almost unpronounceable, possibly Scandinavian. This is, apparently, on the advice of a numerologist, a friend of her mother's. Mrs Hollins had always wanted to call Laura 'Agnes' anyway, and the inventive spelling would bring the recipient much good fortune. The new surname is potentially lucky too. Down in London on a trip to see Henry, she is spotted by a talent scout. Did she want to be a model? 'It sounded like a laugh,' she told *Vogue*, 'so why not?' And guess what: written in the stars or not, it worked out.

Within a year or two, Agyness went positively global. The most exciting new English face; the most newsworthy model since Kate Moss; a tabloid personality; the face of Burberry with a propensity for handsome indie-band members; an effervescent distributor of goodwill with the common touch, who does not mind at all if she's recognised; a style icon (favourite party get-up: 'My fast-food dress by Jeremy Scott, a pair of Mickey Mouse ears and electric-pink lips'). She's the star she always dreamt she could be.

'[Modelling] is hard,' she told *Vogue*, 'and you have to be dedicated to it, but not too much, otherwise you take it too seriously. You just have to give it your best shot.' Agyness's bleached blonde boy-crop, down-to-earth demeanour, cheery homespun disposition and distinctive personal aesthetic set her apart from her peers and that, of course, has been her calling card. Compared to what else is on offer out there, none of it should really work – she's almost *too* idiosyncratic – but it does. Moreover, the sparkiness and the casual manner belie a fierce drive. 'The minute she turned up for a casting, I knew Agyness had it,' the designer Michael Kors told US *Vogue*. 'There's a freshness to her, but that sounds a little too… wholesome. She's hard-edged fresh. It's a strange dichotomy I know, but it's so new and exciting to see.'

It also appears to be great fun (if a little exhausting) being Agyness, being young with boundless energy and in thrall to it all. This is Agyness on her debut *Vogue* shoot with David Bailey: 'After the show I hop on a motorbike with a driver and we race to the East End. David Bailey really gets my northern humour – we hit it off immediately… Bailey finds an old sofa which he makes me jump up and down on for our first shot. Modelling is a bit like being an actress – you have to get into character. It's so much fun, especially when I start singing "Chim-chim-cheree" while holding an old broom…'

English through and through (according to *Vogue*, she likes the Clash and collecting royal memorabilia), she's refreshingly real-life, winningly grounded and fiercely loyal. And if it all ended tomorrow, then so what? Her style mantra: 'Just have fun. Me and Henry always have a ball…' It's probably apocryphal that most of the model-formerly-known-as-Laura's family have gone for the lucky Deyn as a surname. But quite understandable.

Agyness Deyn (b. Laura Hollins, 1983, UK)

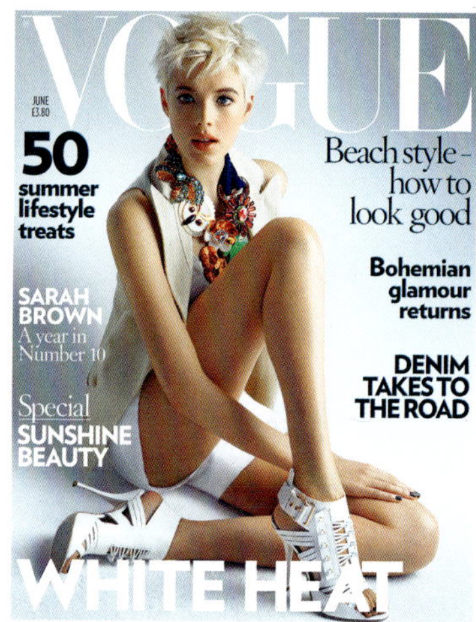

Above: 'White Heat', June 2008, by Patrick Demarchelier. Fashion by Ann Demeulemeester

Opposite: 'Light and Shade', October 2007, by Nick Knight. Fashion by Alexandre Herchcovitch

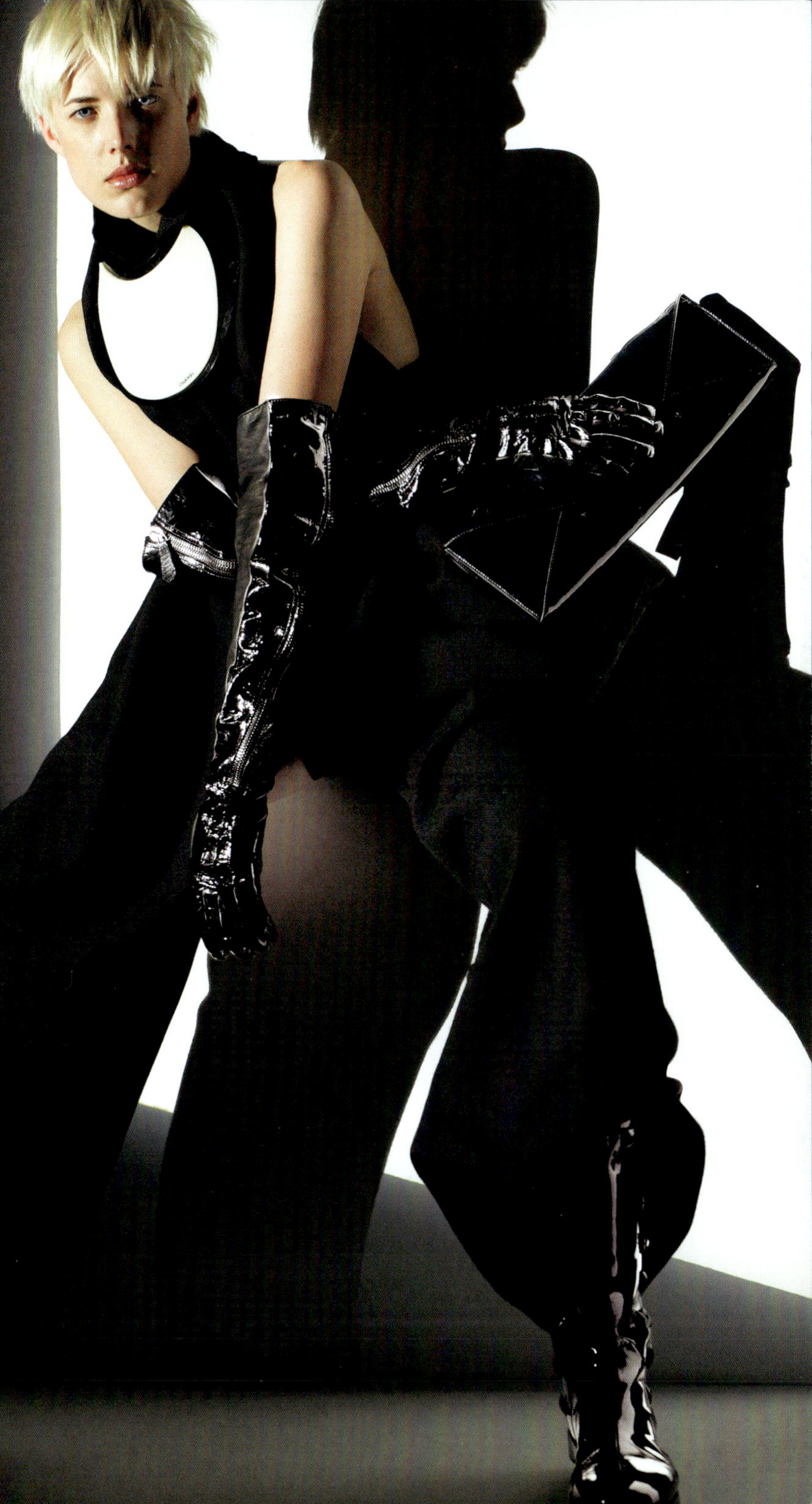
CHANEL

Amber Valletta

In tandem with her modelling career – and at the height of her earning power – Amber Valletta channelled her considerable energies into environmental causes. Taking ecology classes at NYU, she spent the summer of 2000 in India doing voluntary aid work. 'Not that Amber has completely turned her back on favourite modelling pastimes,' reported *Vogue*, 'she turned up at [a *Vogue* shoot] after an extensive shopping spree in Manhattan, with a Tibetan singing bowl and a string of fairy lights in the shape of rosebuds…'

And that earning power was significant and exponential, though she wore it lightly and treated it with nonchalance: 'I don't really care if I die with a million dollars,' the languid, delicate face of Prada told American *Vogue*. 'I'd rather die with a nice life and nice memories and lots of people around me who I love and love me.' Riffing on Linda Evangelista's famous and occasionally misquoted aperçu, she added sagely: 'I've gotten out of bed a lot these days for a *lot* less than $10,000.'

Born in Phoenix, Arizona in 1974, she and her family relocated to Tulsa, where at 15 she took a modelling course. She told *Vogue* she found the notion 'goofy', but it worked. It really took off for her in Paris when her previously mid-length cut was cropped in a gamine style to reveal vulnerability, character and mesmeric eyes. By the mid-1990s she, Shalom Harlow and a handful of others were hailed as a new breed of supermodel, the immediate follow-on to the first wave, determined not to let stardom cloud their judgement and dog their every move. 'These girls are weightless,' said Karl Lagerfeld, 'not in the physical sense, but they give the impression that nothing is serious. They are not obsessed with fame… [they] are free, modern, giving girls and this, I think, is divine'.

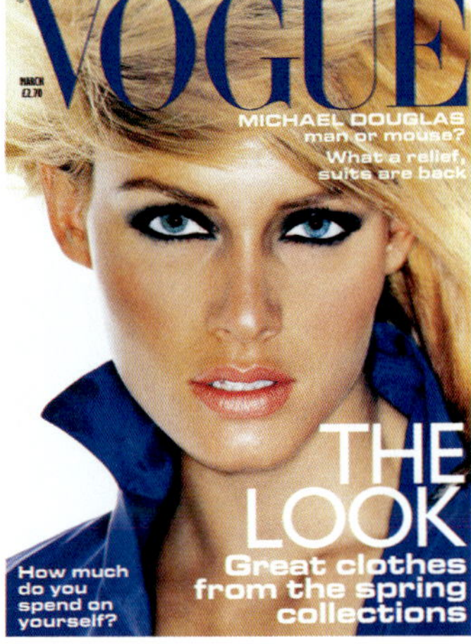

Their close-knitness was remarked upon as a something of an industry departure. Amber's friendship with Shalom was well documented (they were co-hosts of MTV's *House of Style*), and a shared interest in spirituality and esotericism cemented it. 'We've both had our past lives read,' Amber told *Vogue*, and they discovered in the process that in a former life they had crossed paths as men. 'We had horrible, tortured deaths,' she concluded.

Almost alone in her generation, Amber successfully made the transition to films with popular appeal, ranging from 2000's *Hitch* with Will Smith to *The Spy Next Door* (2010) with Jackie Chan. She still models occasionally. With her late thirties looming on the horizon, she told *Love* magazine: 'I can't stop the decay,' adding with equanimity, 'but I'm coming to accept that.'

Amber Valletta (b. 1974, USA)

Above:
'The Look', March 1995,
by Nick Knight.
Fashion by Jil Sander

Opposite:
'Rocket Girl', August 1994,
by Mikael Jansson.
Fashion by Edina Ronay

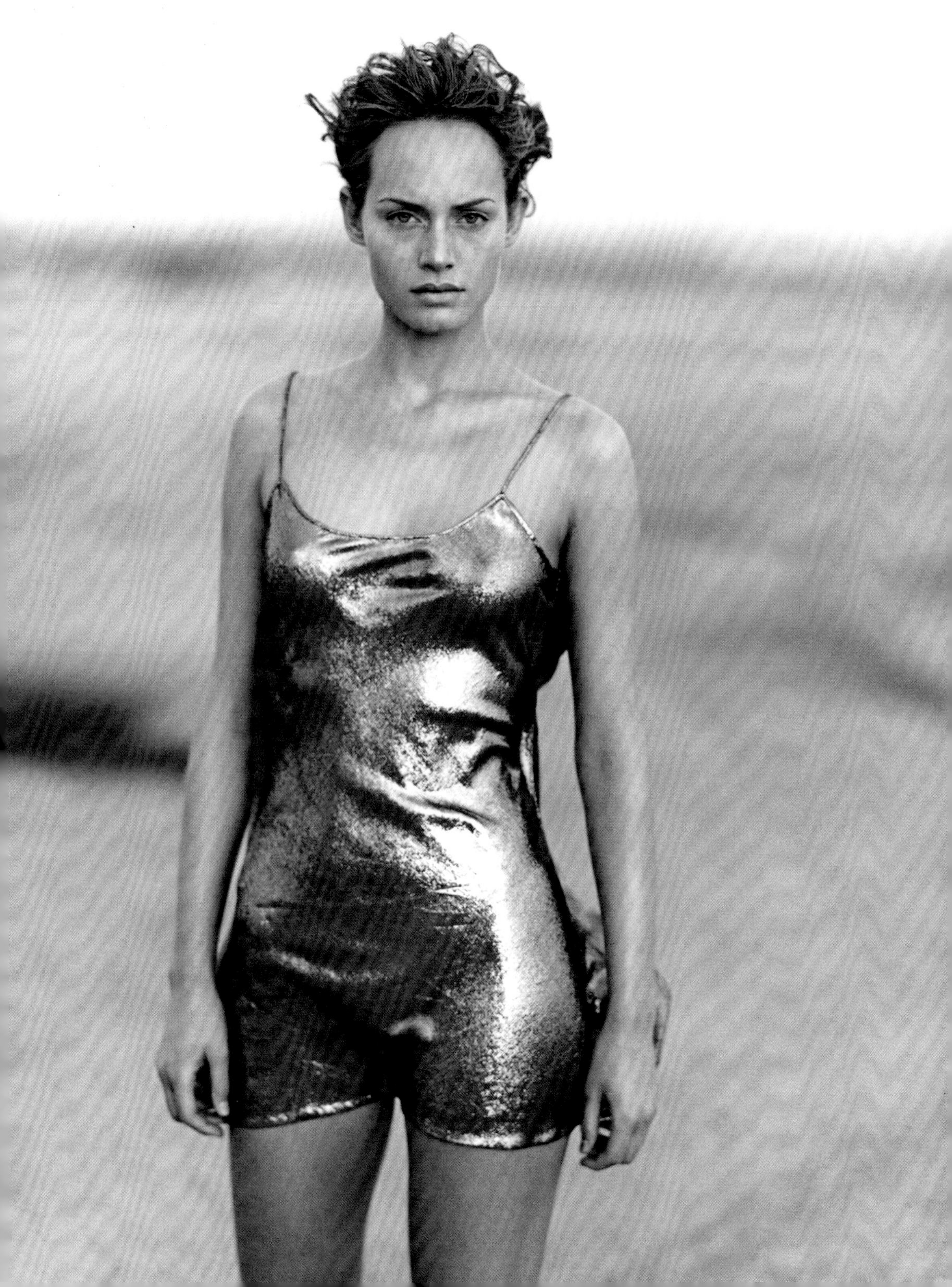

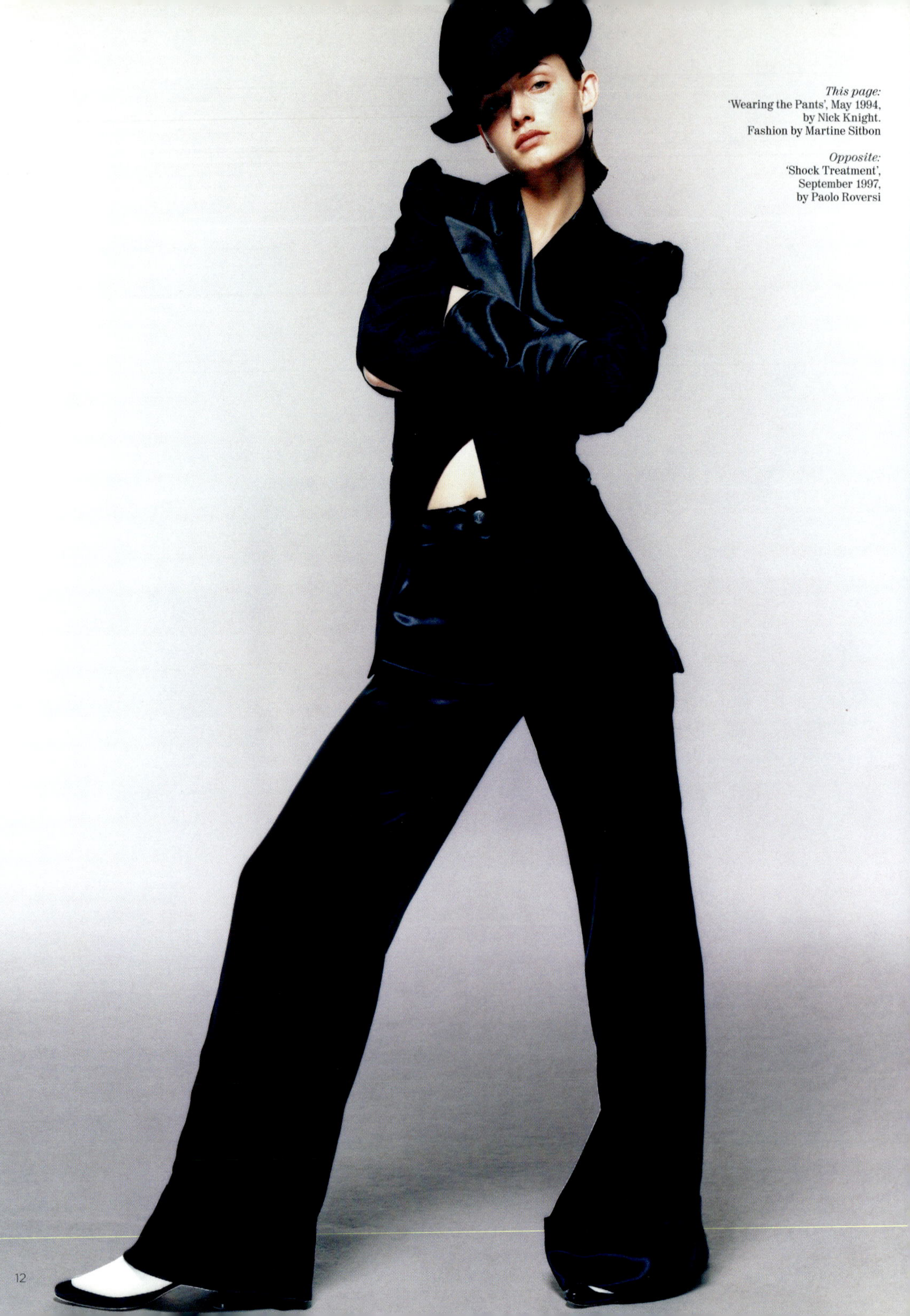

This page:
'Wearing the Pants', May 1994,
by Nick Knight.
Fashion by Martine Sitbon

Opposite:
'Shock Treatment',
September 1997,
by Paolo Roversi

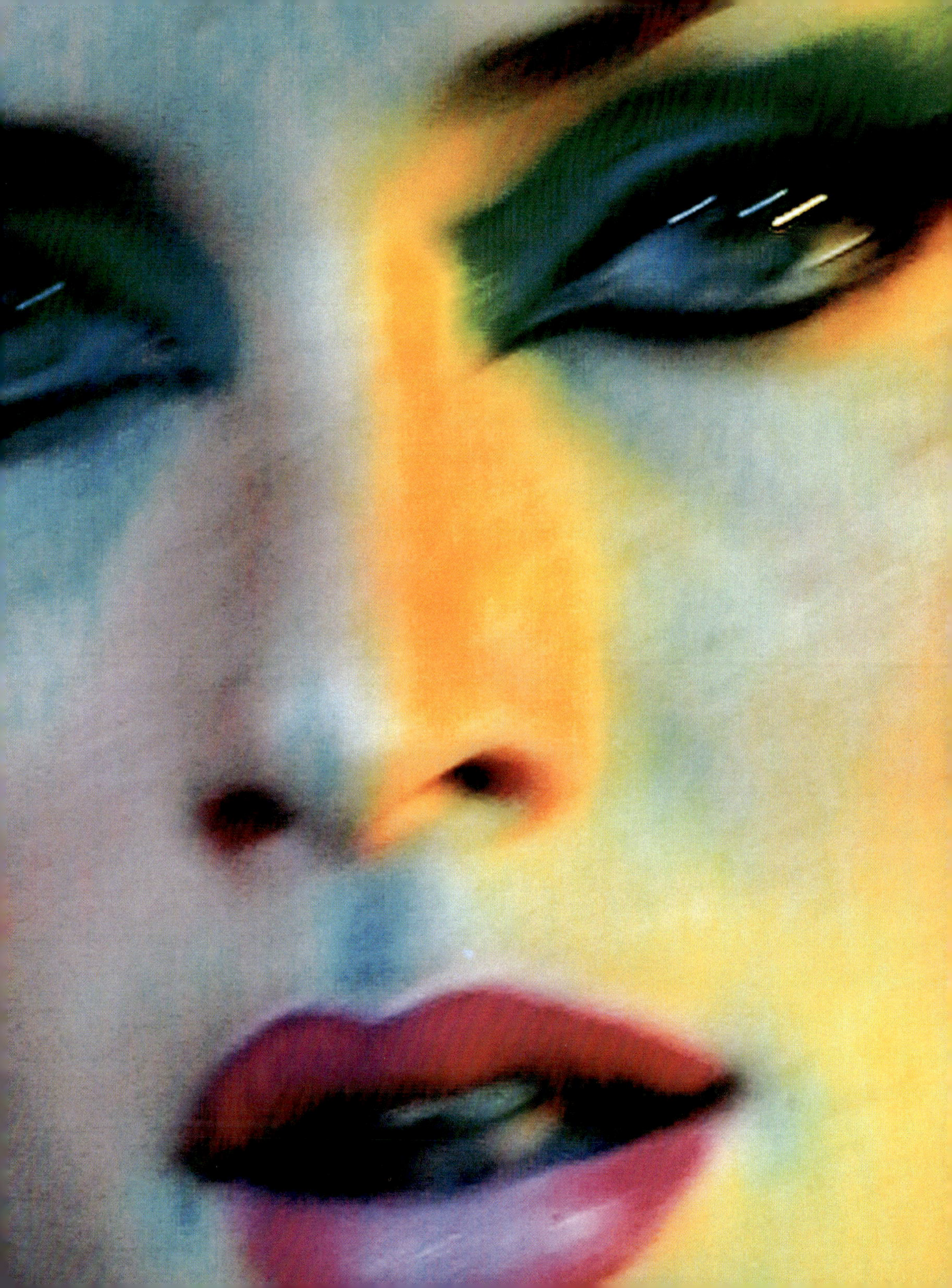

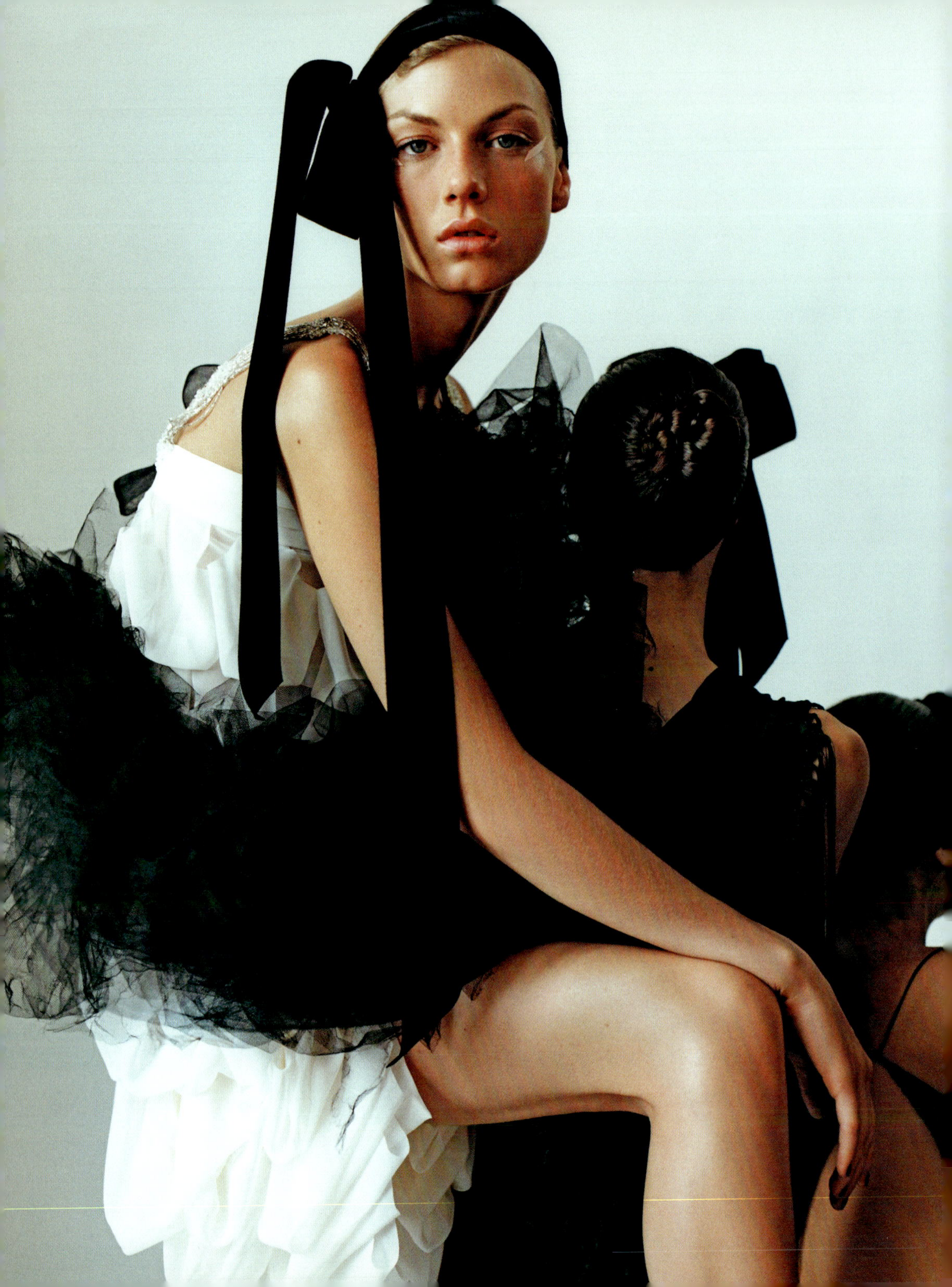

Angela Lindvall

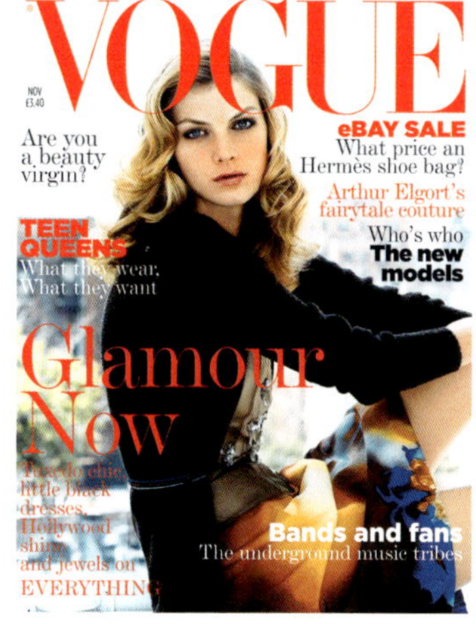

Whatever the current trend, British *Vogue* marvelled in 1997, there is an almost ceaseless supply of freckle-faced, apple-pie all-American girls. The latest on its radar, following a line that included Patti Hansen and Christie Brinkley in its recent history, was Angela Lindvall. The magazine also noted that Lindvall's life story appeared to be straight out of a John Steinbeck dustbowl-era novel: born into a large family in Oklahoma, raised in Missouri, spending endless days in Kansas just strumming her guitar and recently driving her entire family cross-country to Florida.

On modelling, she remarked 'How could I not like it? I'm seeing the world!' And in truth she was not in Kansas any more, or indeed the Midwest – as *Vogue* discovered in 2009, her life begins and ends out of seven acres in Topanga, California, north-northwest of Los Angeles. The magazine devoted 12 pages to her enviably low-key, bohemian approach to family life, marvelling at Topanga and its environs: frozen, it appeared, sometime in the mid-1970s. Equestrianism lives side by side with Malibu surf culture, and both rub along with remnants of the first wave of West Coast hippydom. An ideal place for 2005's Best Dressed Environmentalist (as awarded by the Sustainable Style Foundation) to raise her sons William Dakota and Sebastian, whom *Vogue* also liked enormously.

Environmental issues engage Lindvall greatly: 'It drives me crazy,' she told one visitor, 'to think that when I run my kitchen taps it goes down the same drain as my septic,' so she has replumbed her house to enable most waste liquids to flow into the garden. More evidence of an old head on young shoulders: her Collage Foundation, which promotes awareness of environmental issues in young people, to inform the choices they make.

Without her being the well-rounded, two-feet-on-the-ground person that she is, it is likely that her career might have been even bigger – but fame and fortune do not drive her in the slightest. Nor have they ever. Born in 1979, Lindvall did not remotely consider herself model-girl material until the age of 13, when she ended up in a Kansas City modelling pageant. There she was spotted by a scout for the IMG agency and after a false start and a retrenchment, the yellow brick road took her to a familiar final destination: Italian *Vogue* and Steven Meisel.

Her modelling curriculum vitae is impressive, including campaigns for Dior, Prada, Valentino, Jil Sander and Louis Vuitton, among many others. Lindvall's youth is worn lightly: 'It's great fun wearing clothes,' she told American *Vogue*, 'but you have to sell to those older, more reserved women too.' She says she sacrificed the best years of her teenage life to the fashion industry, but harbours few regrets, seeing it as an investment which has richly paid off.

Angela Lindvall (b. 1979, USA)

Opposite:
'Black Gold',
December 2000,
by Mario Testino.
Fashion by Chanel

Above:
'Glamour Now',
November 2004,
by Patrick Demarchelier.
Fashion by Prada

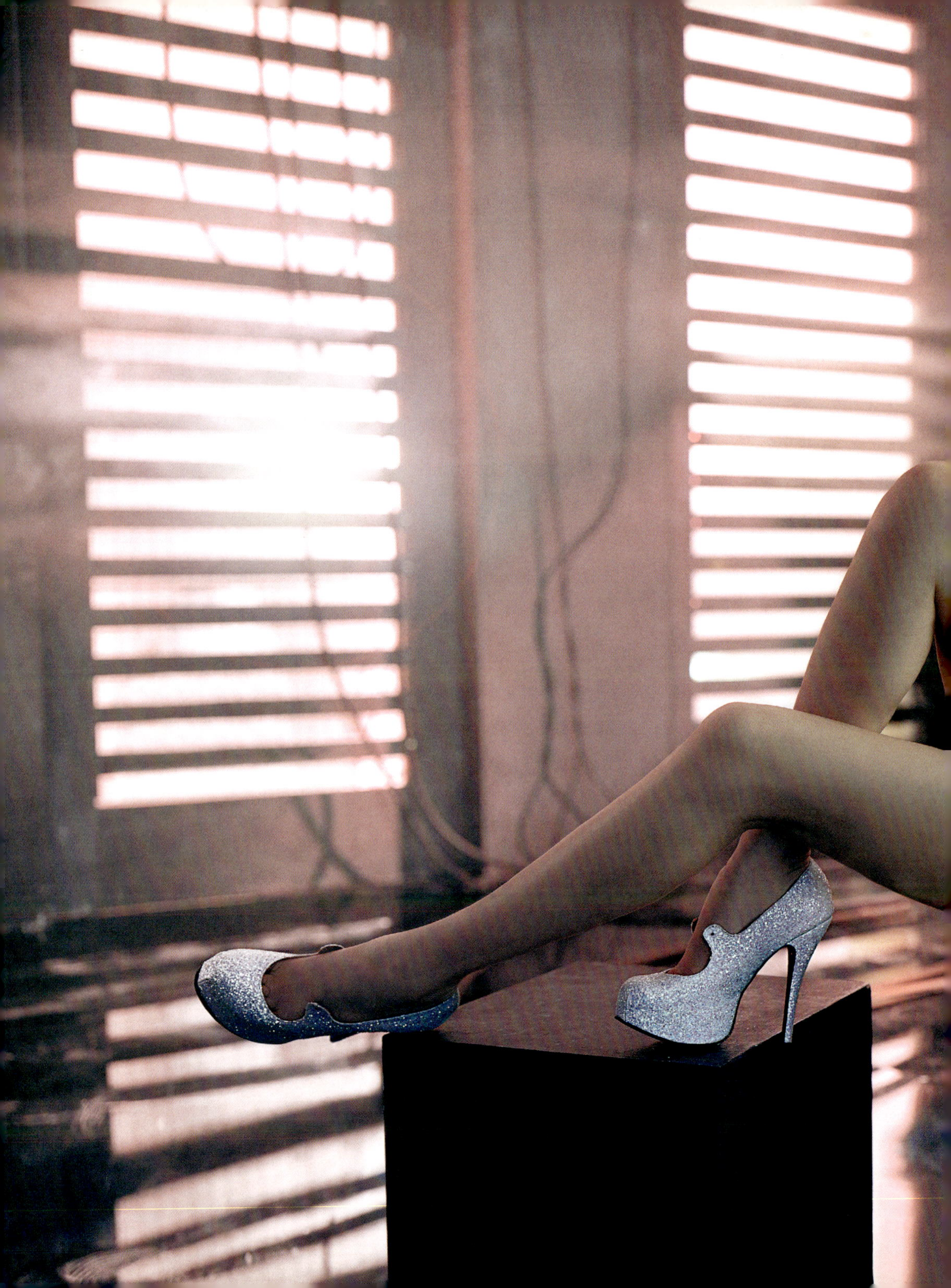

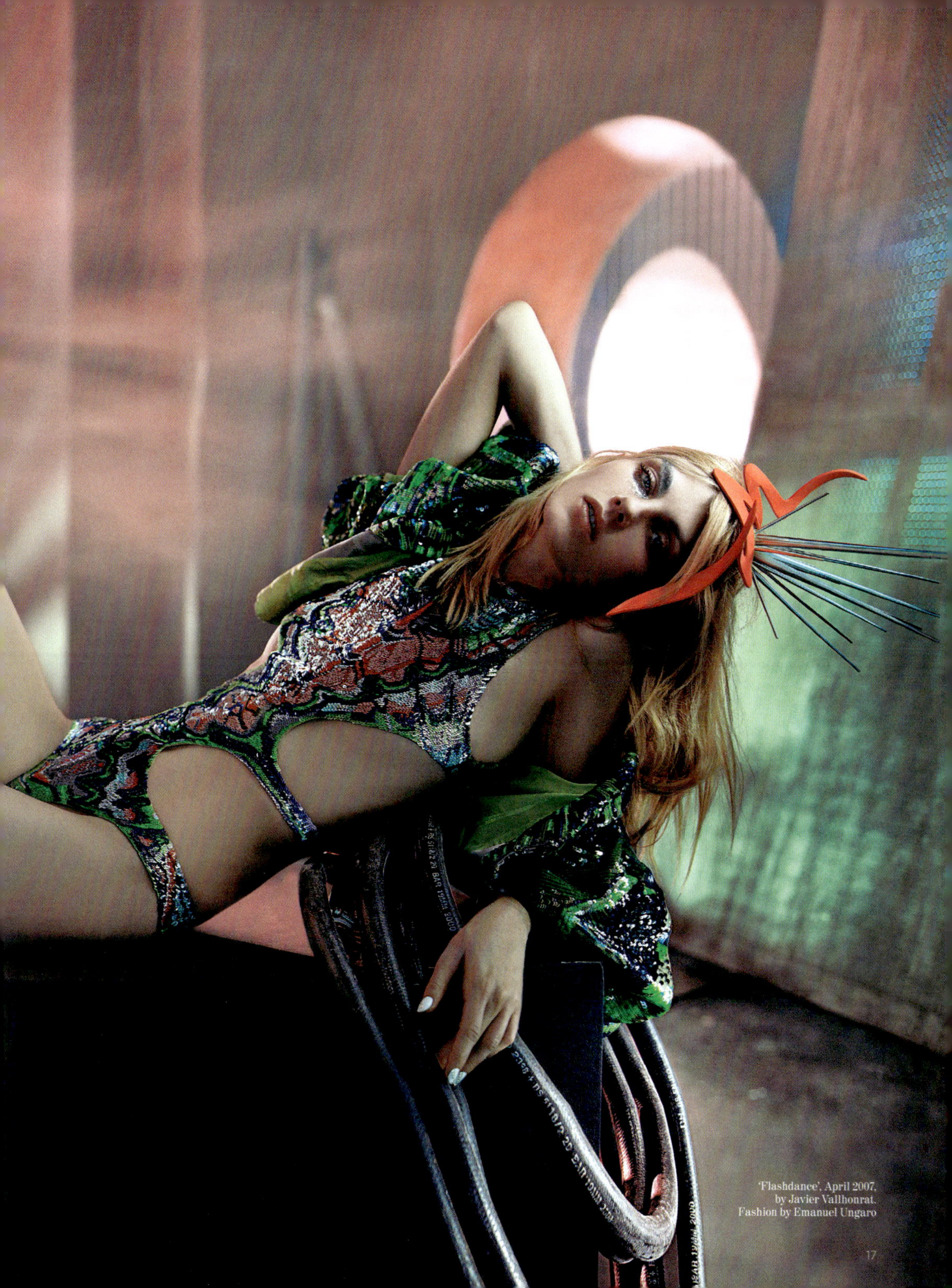

'Flashdance', April 2007,
by Javier Vallhonrat.
Fashion by Emanuel Ungaro

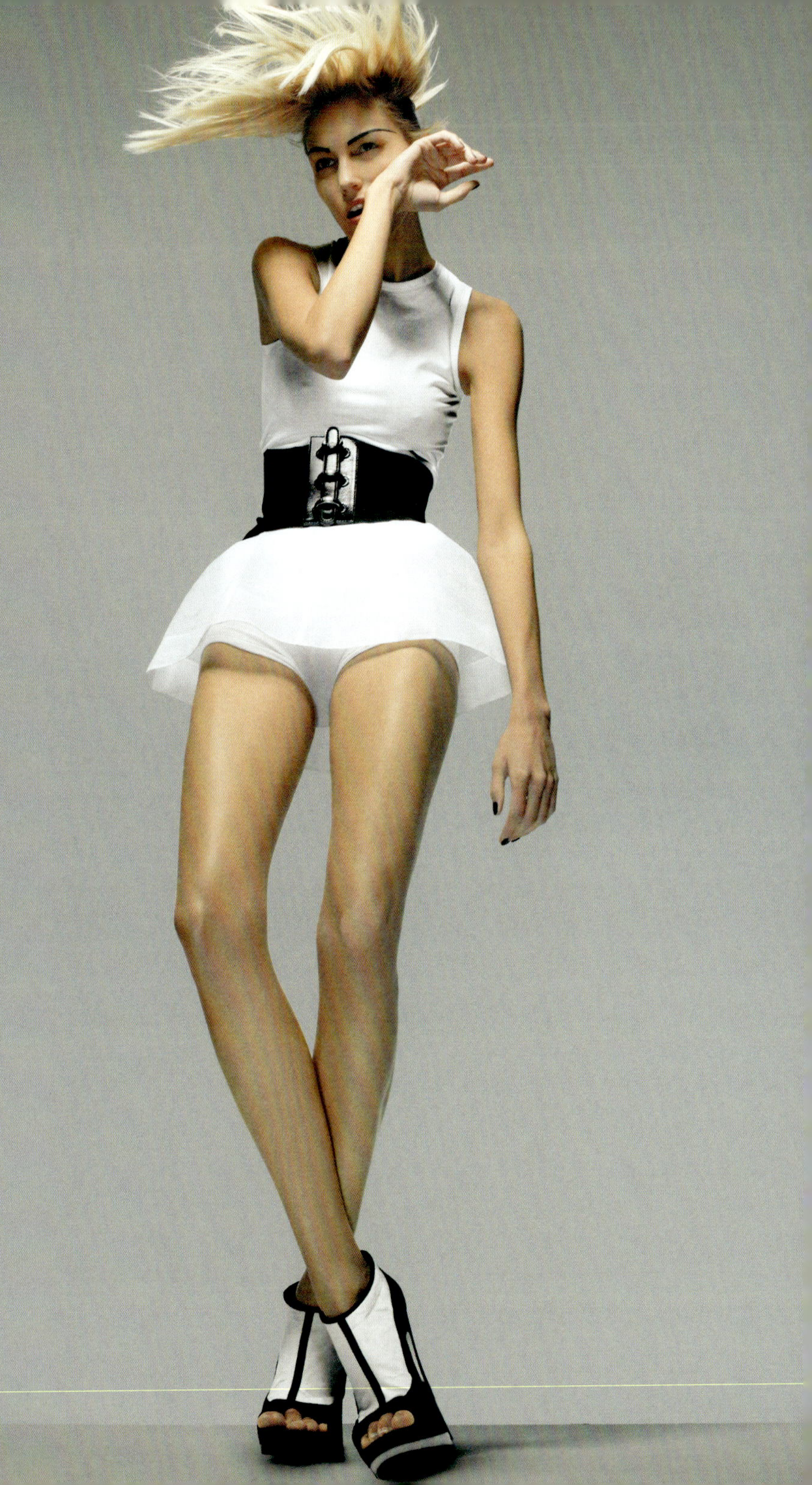

Anja Rubik

Lithe and, it would appear, endlessly flexible, 'the' model bombshell' was no stranger to the energetic shoot, most often in British *Vogue* for Nick Knight. 'Black and White' from March 2009 – all 24 pages of it – was perhaps the most demanding of her. Here she contorted for the lens in a variety of monochromatic, avant-garde creations. She bent herself double in a Martin Margiela silk-mix dress (more properly, according to *Vogue*, 'a bourgeois ruched chiffon cocktail dress blown out of all proportion, bursting like an over-inflated balloon'). She knelt with one leg tucked under the other in a plastic appliqué mini-dress with two-tone jersey leggings and found herself trussed up in a rope necklace by Florian and 'industrial chrome wedges' by Giuseppe Zanotti.

And in the further cause of experimental fashion, intricate and breakable garments made entirely out of paper and its derivatives, expensive or disposable, were created around her form. This demanded much of her patience. Only one confection defeated Anja and the *Vogue* team: a paper hoodie, made out of thousands of silver-sprayed balls of tissue fixed on to a zipped top, proved unwearable. Up until the last moments, the team were stitching and repairing. 'The moment when Anja was helped into a papier-mâché bustle before being tied into a circular skirt made from 27 sheets of paper was an especially surreal sight...'

Born in Poland in 1985, Anja's early life was peripatetic, taking in sojourns in Greece, Canada and South Africa. A conscientious student, she finished her academic studies before embarking on a career in fashion. An editorial and catwalk favourite, she remains by all accounts a joy to work with and endearingly easy-going, as per this account of a small transformation documented in *Vogue*'s pages: 'My hair has always been long and I really needed a change, so I just chopped it off. I love it! The best thing is it only takes me two seconds to style – at the shows I am ready in no time!'

Anja Rubik (b. 1985, Poland)

Opposite:
'Black and White',
March 2009,
by Nick Knight.
Fashion by Fendi

Anjelica Huston

In 1969, Anjelica Huston's career as a model got off to an inauspicious start. Sent to meet American *Vogue* editor Diana Vreeland by Richard Avedon, a friend of her parents, the would-be model fainted. '[Vreeland] was in the middle of a conversation about whether some gloves were beige or grey and there was a tremendous amount of clothes,' she remembered, years later. 'When I came to, she was patting my cheeks and sending editors off for ice – it was extremely embarrassing.' This did not deter either party. Vreeland proposed a trip with Richard Avedon to Ireland, where young Anjelica had grown up: 'We were in the bogs of Connemara, and on the Burren, actually, which is known for being like the moon. While we were there, an astronaut landed on the moon for the first time,' she recalled. 'It seemed so incongruous, so out of place, and I've resented it ever since – I've never liked the idea of men trampling on the moon.'

As the 1960s turned into the 1970s, American models tended to be sparkling and sportive, blonde (preferably) with a healthy disdain for life indoors and a penchant for the one-piece swimsuit and running shoes. Huston was the opposite: willowy with ironed-down curtains of black hair – 'I was concave and morose,' she put it. *Vogue* phrased it with more tact: 'Dark and mysterious as a raven, remote and graceful as a medieval heroine – a beauty. Her large black eyes are lustrous and she laughs with an inner warmth.' And perfect for the more adventurous European market. Huston had had a brief liaison with photographer Bob Richardson, who cast her in his opaque, faintly sinister and erotic photographs, but she left him to study acting and spend time in London.

Her modelling continued, mostly at British *Vogue* for David Bailey, with whom she had an instant and productive rapport. His pictures of Anjelica filled a book, *Is That So Kid* (2008) – the title taken from a habitual reply by her father, the film director John Huston, to almost any observation made by anyone else. *Vogue* admired Anjelica greatly and warmed to Bailey's pictures – 'She's a girl who dances divinely and perfectly suits this new look of Goya.'

As the years progressed, Bailey cast his model in more sensual and decadent roles, the pictures often somnolent and languorous boudoir shots where little daylight appeared to intrude. If *en plein air*, they tended to be in crepuscular gardens with Huston clad in slightly out-of-place fashion. An exception was a sun-suffused 20-page shoot in the south of France with Bailey, Helmut Newton and Manolo Blahnik. It resulted in a cover for Huston and Blahnik, Anjelica's first for British *Vogue* and only the third time a man had featured (actors Helmut Berger and Alan Bates had been there first).

Anjelica Huston's film career is now long and distinguished – she represents the third generation of her family to win an Oscar – but like her modelling, the start was low-key: her hands stood in for Deborah Kerr's in the portmanteau James Bond spy caper *Casino Royale* (1967). Her first starring role was in her father's Middle Ages curiosity *A Walk with Love and Death* (1970), an allegory of Vietnam. 'Yes. It's favouritism,' her father told *Vogue*.

After she met Jack Nicholson, with whom she had an on-off relationship, Huston put her career as a model and actress on hold for a while. She reinvigorated the latter with vivid roles in films starring her then boyfriend, notably *The Last Tycoon* (1976), *The Postman Always Rings Twice* (1981) and *Prizzi's Honour* (1985), for which she won that Oscar.

Huston's memories of her fashion days still perturb and amuse her: 'To be at a sitting with Polly [Mellen, fashion editor] and Dick [Avedon] was to be at something extraordinary. A *roomful* of shoes; a *roomful* of hats – it was accessorised beyond the beyond. Polly would go into tears over whether a hat looked good or not.' She added: 'Fashion at its best is a wonderful, adventurous medium and at its worst superficial and false. I was caught somewhere in the middle of that.'

Anjelica Huston (b. 1951, USA)

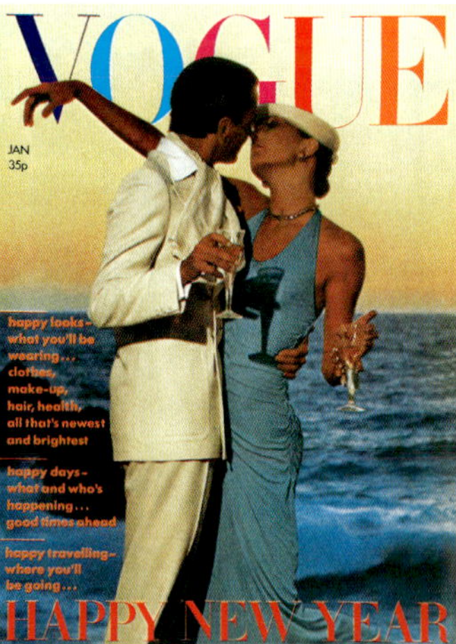

Above: 'Happy New Year', January 1974, by David Bailey. Fashion by Bruce Oldfield

Opposite: 'There's Nothing Like the Best', September 1973, by David Bailey. Fashion by Chloé

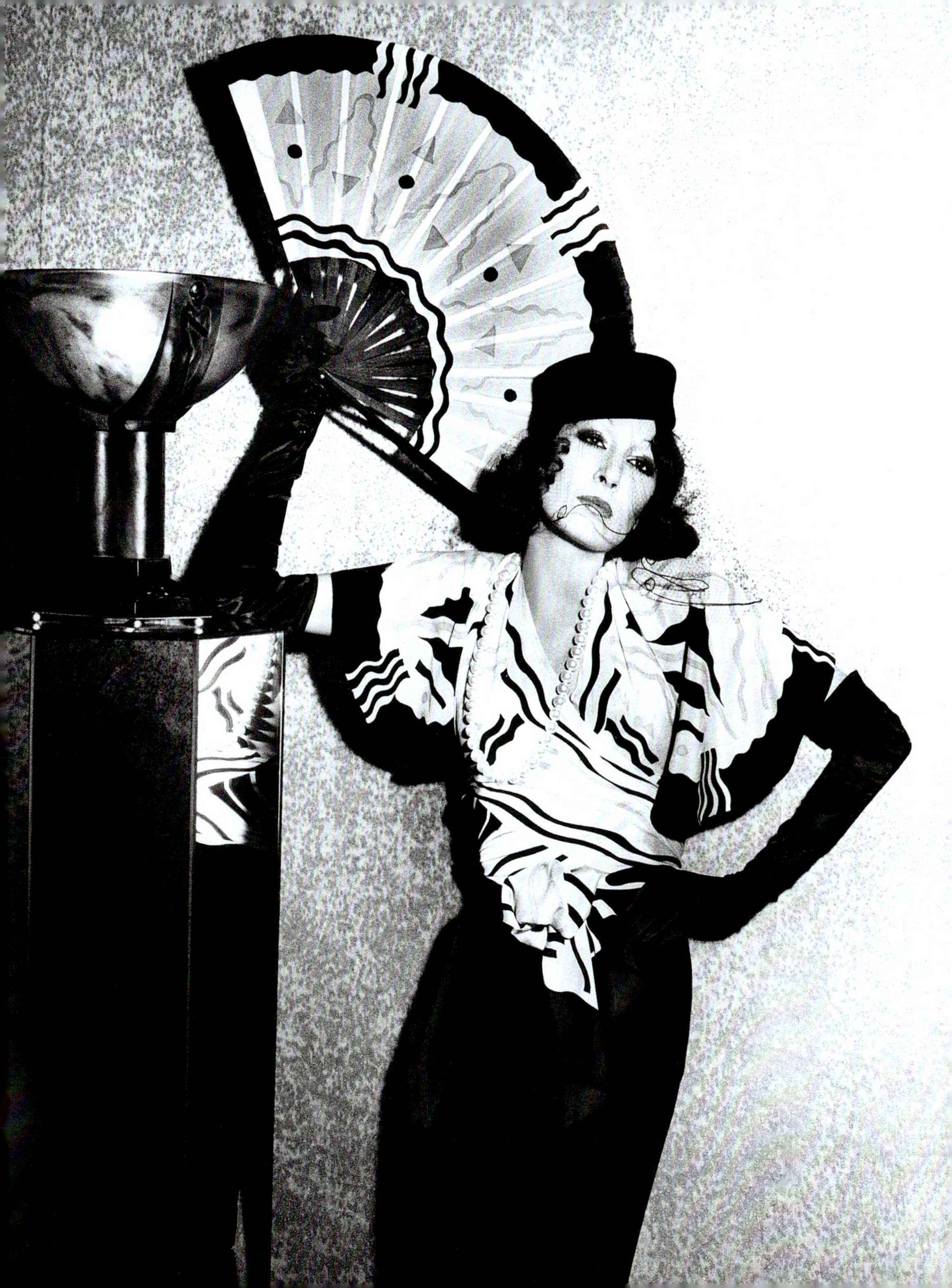

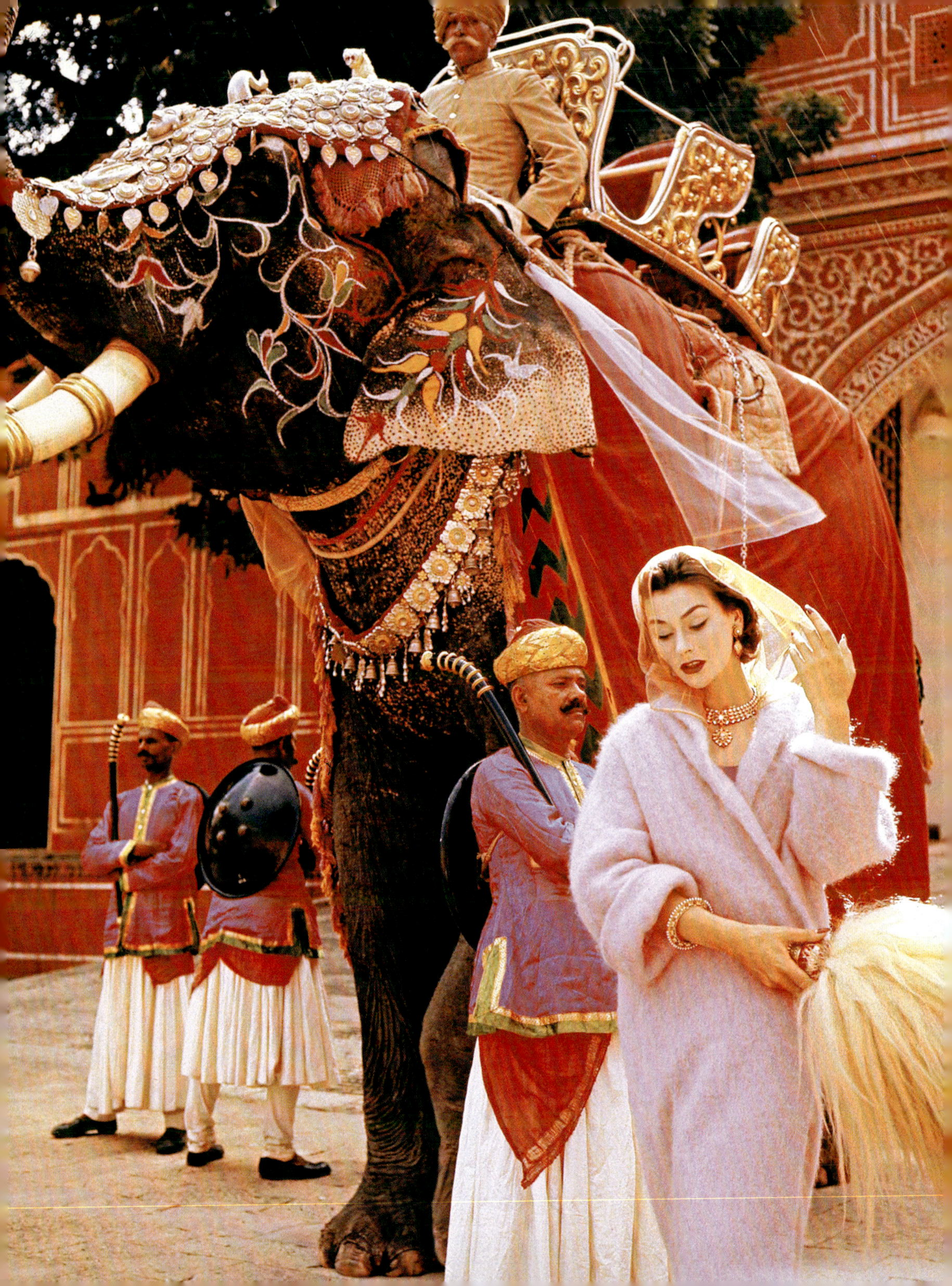

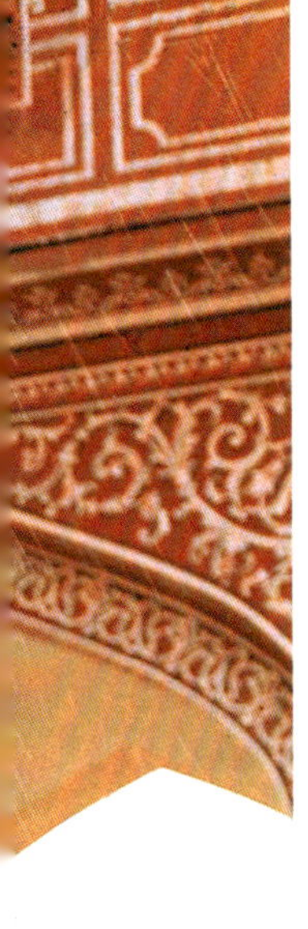

Anne Gunning

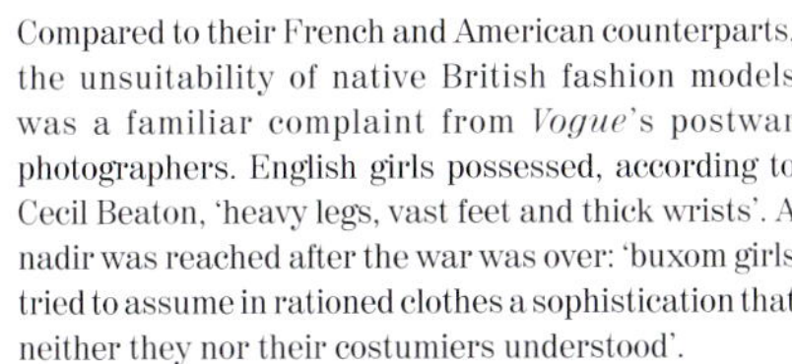

Compared to their French and American counterparts, the unsuitability of native British fashion models was a familiar complaint from *Vogue*'s postwar photographers. English girls possessed, according to Cecil Beaton, 'heavy legs, vast feet and thick wrists'. A nadir was reached after the war was over: 'buxom girls tried to assume in rationed clothes a sophistication that neither they nor their costumiers understood'.

Along with Barbara Goalen, former Rank starlet Anne Gunning was a notable exception. Though far more approachable than her rival, her career really took off after Goalen had retired in 1954. 'I smoked and drank a bit, and occasionally got podgy, but I was awfully sly, unlike Barbara – she was always out at social gatherings and nightclubs, but she *talked* about it.' *Vogue* was interested in the minutiae of Gunning's daily life, as well as her high cheekbones and perfectly chiselled face: 'She rides, she swims and dances but follows no slimming or maintenance diet, for as we so often find happens with slim people, she unconsciously chooses dishes which are high in protein and low in their calorie content. She likes to have an inexpensive boneless roll-on, but wears a made-to-order brassière and waspies from Rigby & Peller…'

Gunning made an impression. The doyenne of model agents, Eileen Ford, declared her one of the finest girls she ever had on her books, praising her 'withdrawn, Garbo-like quality'. It may have been in the blood: she was descended from the legendary Irish beauties known as the Gunning Girls, painted by Joshua Reynolds, one of whom died of poisoning from the lead in her *maquillage*. Gunning was proud of this ancestry – though not of her large hands and feet, which she took trouble to conceal cunningly.

'I started bang off,' she told one interviewer. 'No training, no model schools. And this was really due to meeting Henry [Clarke] and Dick [Dormer], being taken up by these very, very good photographers. I didn't have to do that awful thing of taking my photographs around and knocking on doors for work. I could never have done that.'

In 1961, Gunning all but retired from modelling after marrying the politician Anthony Nutting, the youngest member of Churchill's second government. She later became Lady Nutting, when her husband succeeded his father as third baronet. She was one of many *Vogue* models to make what the magazine described as 'good marriages'. Jean Dawnay became the Princess Galitzine; Fiona Campbell-Walter, the Baroness Thyssen; and Bronwen Pugh, Lady Astor. Anne Cumming-Bell reversed the trend, reaching the top in modelling only after her divorce from the Duke of Rutland.

Anne Gunning (b. Anne Gunning Parker, 1929, UK; d. 1990)

Left:
'India', November 1956, by Norman Parkinson. Fashion by Jaeger

Annie Morton

Annie Morton, an all-American blonde with a passion for vintage all-American cars, had a reputation for being reliable and hardworking with a natural easy charm and affability: 'a real trouper', according to British *Vogue*. 'She arrived for our sitting in New York after a long and arduous flight from Monte Carlo where she'd been working with Helmut Newton' – which, it was safe to assume, 'was no day at the beach either.' Nothing got in the way of her rigid beauty and yoga routine. Indeed, as *Vogue* observed: 'She's been known to advise whoever's around – at length – on how to look after their skin and to endlessly compare and contrast cosmetics with whatever make-up artist is on set.' 'She really works on a shoot,' said *Vogue*'s Kate Phelan, 'She always give that little extra bit to get the picture.'

Glamour magazine called her 'the modern-day Marilyn Monroe' – a compliment without any downside. She betrayed Monroesque kindness and quirkiness, arriving at a shoot with a puppy she found abandoned on the way in from the airport. 'I couldn't just leave him there,' she explained, christening him Paco and introducing him to the team.

Annie's big break came in 1995 when, at a fitting for Anna Molinari, she encountered the stylist Venetia Scott. Scott was impressed enough to suggest Morton to her then partner, photographer Juergen Teller, and together all three worked on a campaign for Blumarine. It was an era for girls with an 'interesting' look – which, as you might guess, meant a less conventional beauty. Photographers really wanted faces that were fresh to the market. As Juergen Teller said at the time: 'We were photographing urban, minimalist, spontaneous clothes, and it made sense to shoot them on a new kind of girl, one whose personality came across in pictures strongly enough to cancel out any so-called imperfections.'

Teller's colleague Glen Luchford summed it up: 'modelling is not about filling a sexy dress right now. It's much more important to project attitude and individuality.' Annie Morton had that, and an ability to be the sexiest model around without needing to expend the slightest effort (although she did). She also possessed, according to one fashion editor, 'the best smile in the world'. (Paco, by the way, ended up the companion to photographer Enrique Badulescu.)

Annie Morton (b. 1974, USA)

Opposite:
'Night Shifts', November 1996,
by Robert Erdmann.
Fashion by Giorgio Armani

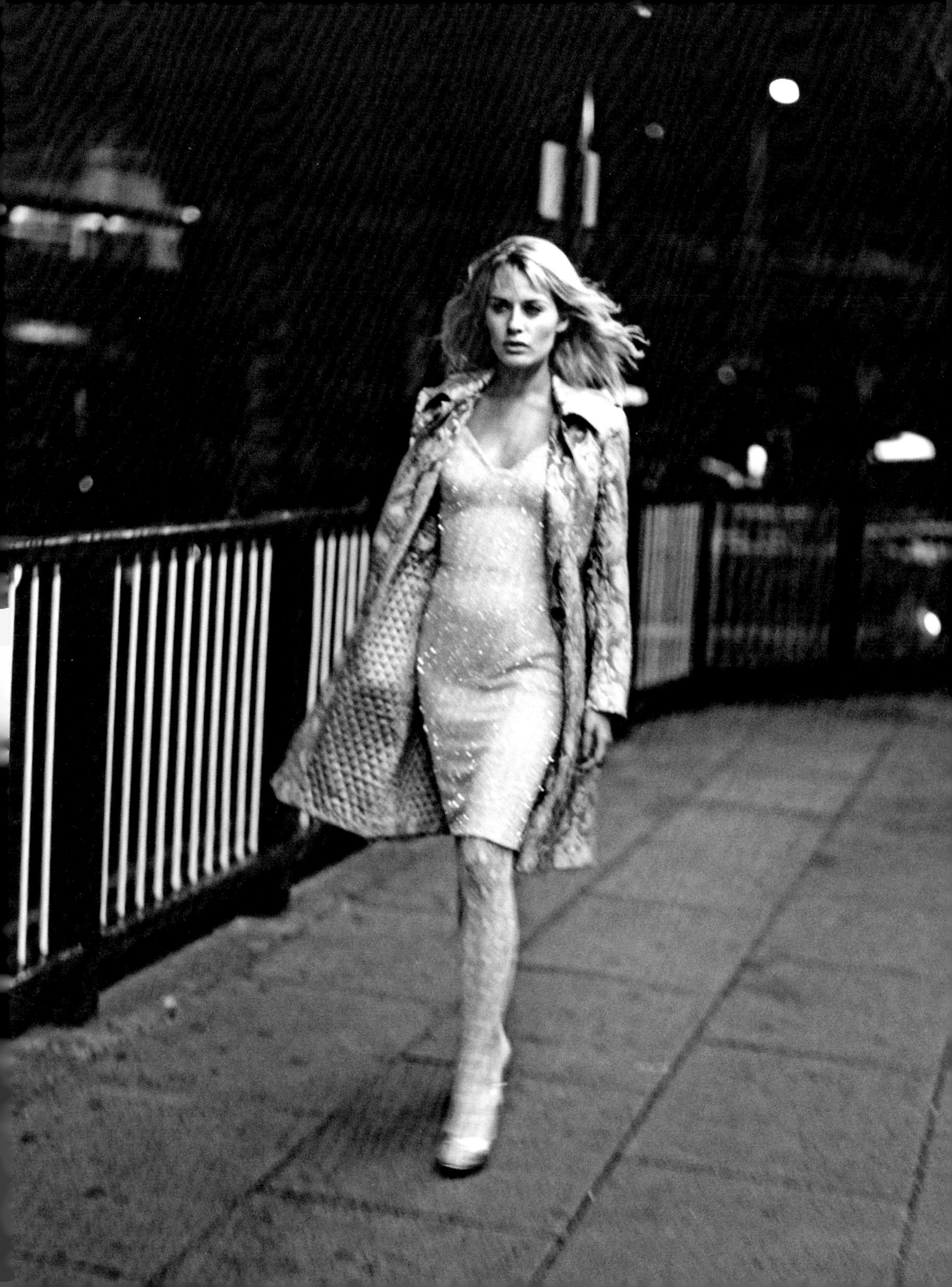

Apollonia van Ravenstein

She may have said, with deadpan accuracy, 'I was the model of the minute or the year or whatever,' but for Norman Parkinson she was the 'maddest, funniest, hardest-working model who ever earned a fortune'. Fashion, money and hedonism, none of it in sparing quantities, collided around 1973 in the impossibly long limbs, panther gait and bare grasp of English of Dutch-born Apollonia van Ravenstein, known to everyone simply as Plonja.

'It's all still to me dizzy,' she remarked as her career – which began on the catwalk – took in magazines across the globe, product endorsement (for which she was unnamed but vital), and more than 15 minutes with Andy Warhol. He sketched her with dark tumbling raven hair, but put her on his magazine *Interview* with an austere, Soviet-era bob and wearing a Dutch submariner's cap. 'I loved America. I never really looked at the culture too much; I just lived within it.' Her look – an ambivalent and anaesthetised disco-era brittleness – reached an apogee in hairdresser-turned-fashion-photographer Ara Gallant's shiny photographs of drug-fuelled fantasy; literally so in one slice of 1977 indulgence, as two male models snort lines of cocaine through silvered straws while Plonja challenges the viewer to match her desensitised gaze. More than one commentator alluded to her noble indifference.

It wasn't all glitter balls, rollerskates and bare-chested busboys in dickie-bows – Plonja had an energetic outdoors life too. A fraught trip to the Seychelles with Norman Parkinson and fashion editor Grace Coddington turned into a fashion-world *Heart of Darkness*. 'We wanted to re-create Rousseau's pictures of animals in the rainforest,' Coddington told *Vogue*, 'so we set off with two stuffed leopards in a boat… We were so miserably seasick the whole thing changed to a "shipwreck diary"' – complete with *objets trouvés* as footwear and a Man Friday in the form of a stray black mongrel. Plonja's personal bravery earned mention in dispatches from Parkinson. On Bird Island: 'birds by the million are most menacing and terns scream when they are disturbed; and with their half-fledged young puddling about your feet in centuries of guano the mother birds dive-bomb you in dozens. Plonja put on her usual energetic performance – no other girl could have managed it.'

Nearer to home, she turned a pedestrian shoot in Richmond Park into a memorable *jour de fête* for Arthur Elgort, on his first assignment for British *Vogue*: 'Apollonia had an individual, pixiesque look. She gave the clothes zest and life. In the pictures, she is moving and singing and dancing… she certainly kept us entertained.'

As her star waned, Plonja took to the screen, big and small, and then retired to a life on the high seas as wife to a cruise-ship captain. Her moment in fashion's brittle glare was brief but unforgettable. As Parkinson put it, 'I give a private round of applause to this intrepid and fearless girl, who has given me two or three of the ten best pictures I will ever take.'

Apollonia van Ravenstein (b. 1952, Netherlands)

Right:
'Barbados', July 1973, by Norman Parkinson. Fashion by Yves Saint Laurent Rive Gauche

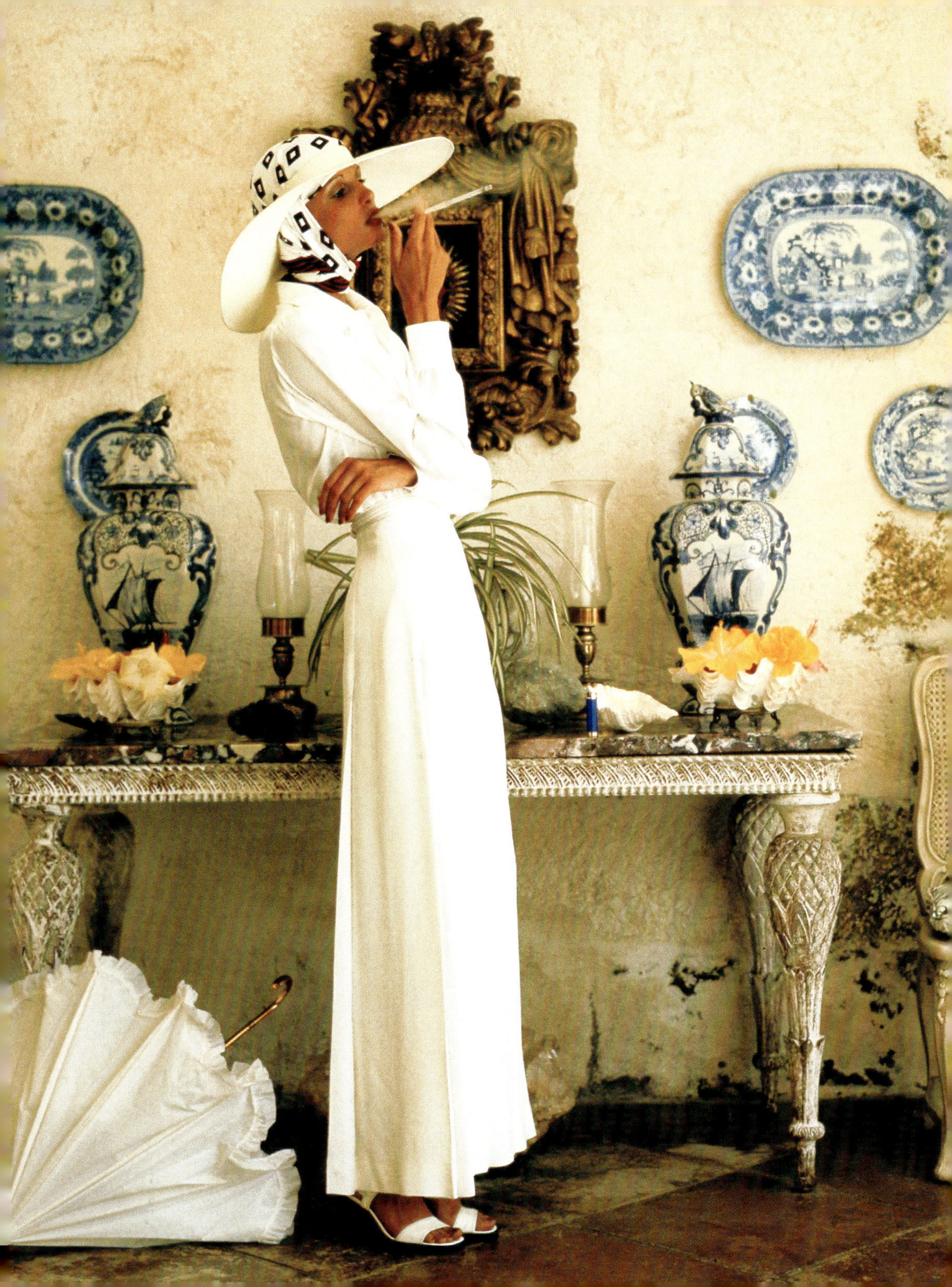

Audrey Marnay

'Hail the New Beauties!' *Vogue* proclaimed in 1998, ushering in a new generation of fashion models who had nothing to do with manufactured perfection and everything to do with personality, individuality and self-possession. The breakup of the Eastern Bloc had produced a horde of new girls, the beaches of Rio were emptying themselves of statuesque lithe-limbed Cariocas, and there was something of a *nouvelle vague* of French models popping up in British magazines. It was *trop petite* to be a full-on invasion, but it was a strike back from across the Channel nonetheless, something not seen in the pages of *Vogue* since the days of Estelle Hallyday (née Lefébure) in the 1980s. Storming the barricades were Aurelie Claudel and Katy Braitman, but *le grand fromage* was Audrey Marnay, petite enough herself to be labelled 'elfin' at every turn. 'What I like about Audrey is not so much her beauty,' Miuccia Prada told *Vogue*, 'but her personality and style. It's those strengths that make her the perfect face of Miu Miu.'

At 16, Audrey was then at *Vogue*'s bottom line for models portrayed in the magazine. A knock-on effect of a relentless search for novelty, as writer Mark Holgate has pointed out, 'is that girls are often hitting stardom at an age when the most pressing matter in their lives has, until then, been contemplating their GCSEs'. This was not likely to over-detain Audrey from Chartres, but the point was made and *Vogue* noted that her pre-shoot badinage made her seem 'just like any teenager': her latest buy was a scooter; her favourite band was the Chemical Brothers and she missed her friends back home. In fact, it had been her desire to earn enough money to buy a previous scooter that had led her into the industry – she left France at 15 for the Japanese modelling circuit. She presumably made enough, for she was back in Europe and under the aegis of Steven Meisel barely a year later (a 32-page cover story for Italian *Vogue* in May 1997 propelled Audrey to instant superstardom).

Audrey's youthful, pretty, freckled and almost perfectly symmetrical face made her a favourite for close-up beauty pictures. She was known as the Chameleon for her ability to change her look to whatever designers wanted and, never shrinking from a challenge, she was their favourite guinea pig. Here is *Vogue*'s description of a change of look: 'Audrey Marnay's slash of purple hair was tackled in much the same way. Here Laurent Philippon combed, detangled, conditioned and prepared the hair before adding his statement – a shock of colour. A hairpiece was dyed then cut sharp and blunt across the ends, at least four inches shorter than Audrey's own hair. It was attached to the parting with eyelash glue, combed over and ready in minutes… Audrey was so delighted that she pranced off with her purple hair intact for the rest of the day!' Ah, *la folie de la jeunesse!*

Audrey Marnay (b. 1980, France)

Right:
'About Faces',
December 1997,
by Regan Cameron

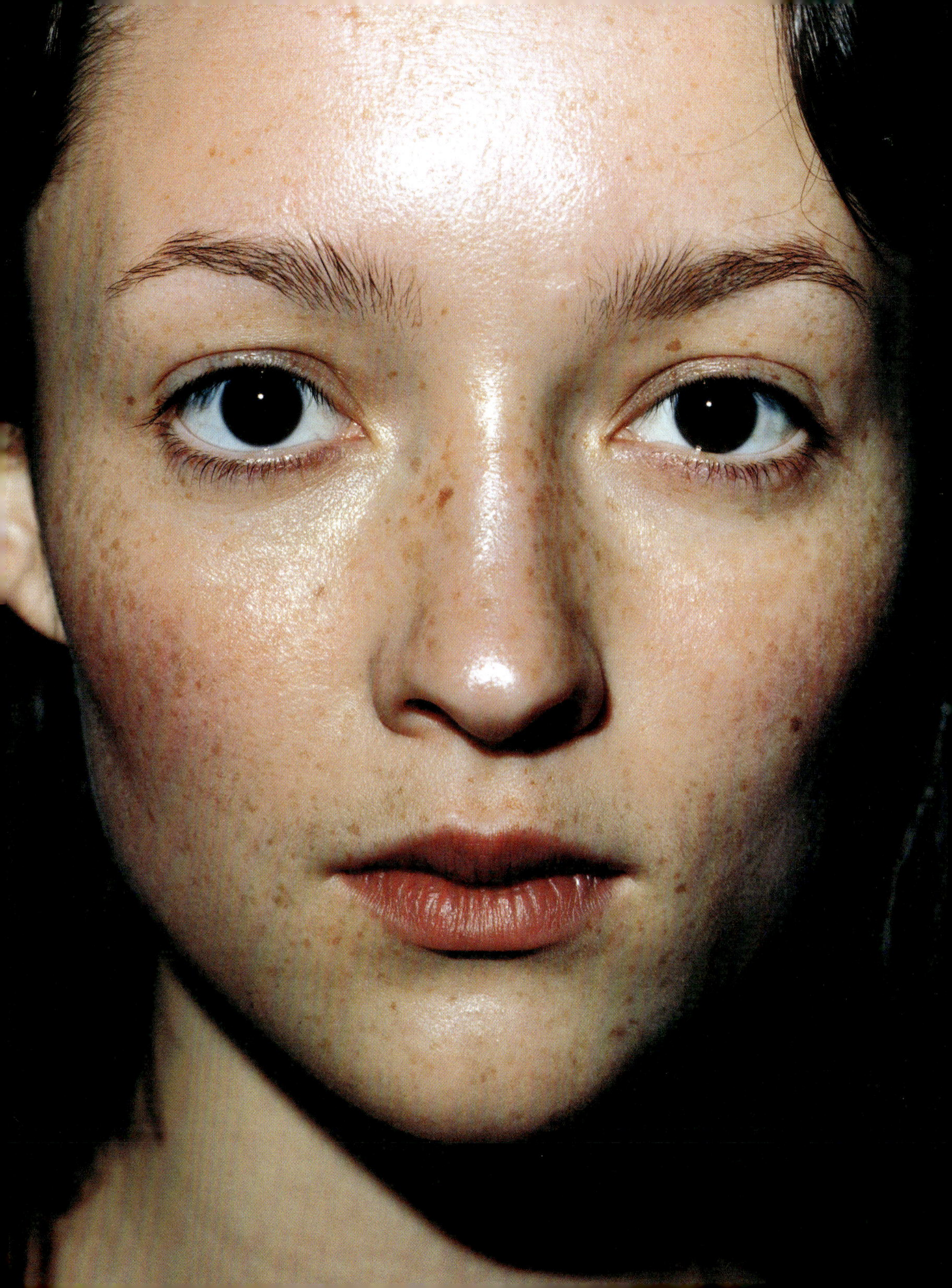

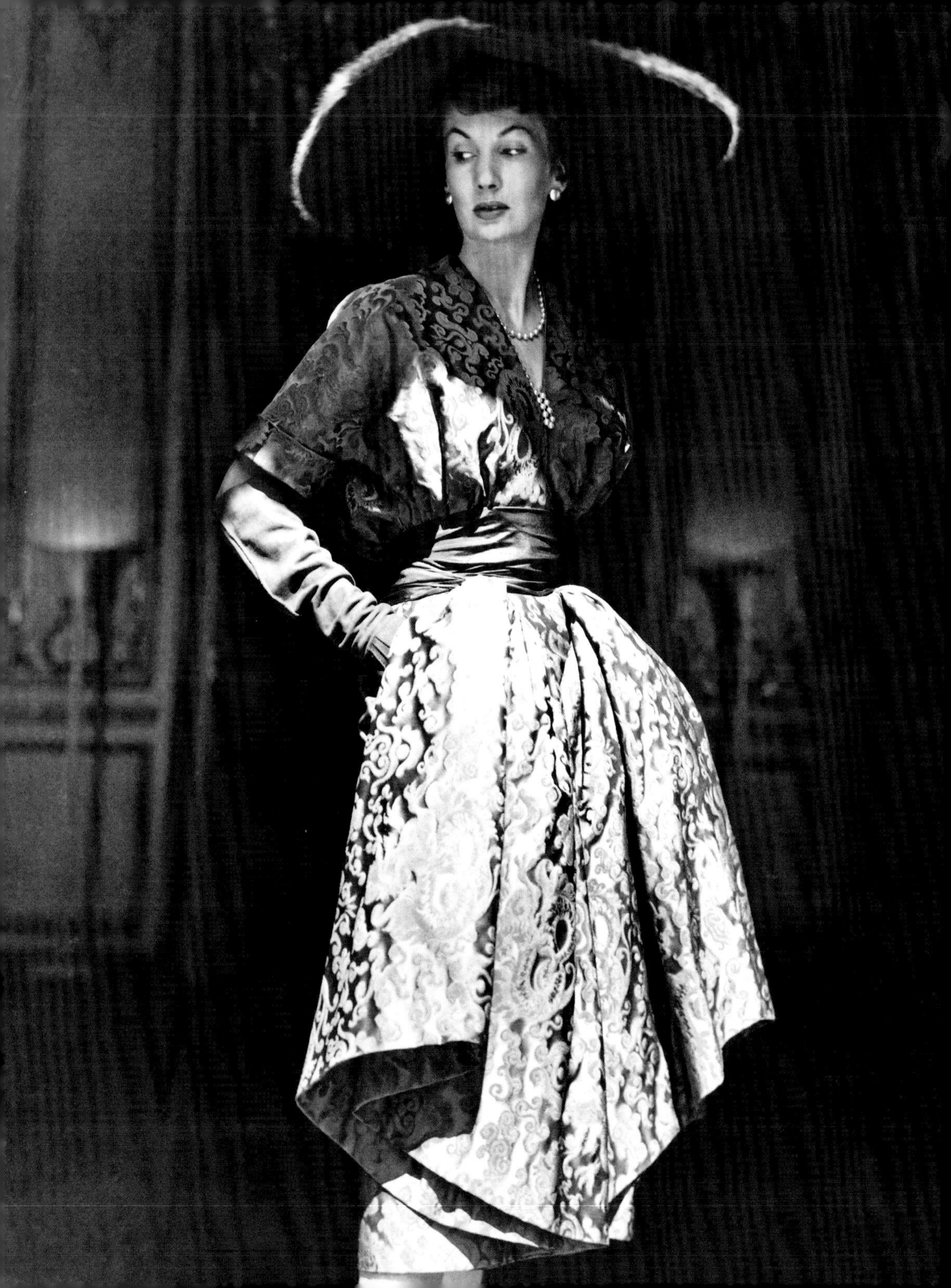

Barbara Goalen

In the days when fashion models were still known as 'mannequins' and when *Vogue* kept a regular spot for 'that mink and diamonds look', Barbara Goalen was pre-eminent. Her unsmiling hauteur – put on for the lens, as she was kindly and very funny – epitomised the spirit of the times for Norman Parkinson, Clifford Coffin, Horst P Horst and John French, whose photographs gaily decorated the drab pages of the *Daily Express*. Understandably, the dark days of the war and its immediate aftermath were not conducive to encouraging home-grown model girls, but the situation perked up (for Cecil Beaton, at least) 'when Miss Barbara Goalen appeared, as if from Cruft's'. This was intended as a tribute to her elegance and poise – like that of a champion greyhound, perhaps.

As Goalen herself observed: 'The English model? In my day there were half a dozen good models, but our style was totally different: more statuesque. I did all the best shows and all the high-fashion photography. I didn't do the bread-and-butter: I couldn't afford to – I'd lose the cake!' And modelling, for her, was born out of necessity. She turned to it when her first husband was killed in a plane crash, leaving her a widow with two young children.

She always carried herself imperiously erect, the better for displaying her 18in waist and 31in hips and – as she quaintly put it – her 33in 'charlies'. When she started out in 1947, aged 26, this was perfect for the designers of the New Look, who envisaged a clientèle of women, not girls. 'You put the dress on Barbara and she made it sing,' said the photographer Henry Clarke. Though well known across the Atlantic, she was much in demand for the Paris catwalks too. She drew the line, however, at modelling lingerie for the 300 wives of the king of Saudi Arabia. She demurred – 'It simply isn't done, you know' – adding, wistfully, 'but the underwear really is divine.' She had a rigid self-discipline, and was chic in well-cut suits and eveningwear at work and after hours: 'I only wear trousers if I'm cold,' she told one interviewer. 'Or in the garden.'

Though her career only lasted six years, Goalen remained a fashion authority and her advice and aperçus were much valued. On school uniform: 'It teaches girls chic, and they learn to wear plain, simple clothes.' On grooming for teenagers: 'Have a lesson in make-up at one of the top beauty houses. I have always found that it is a false economy to go to mediocre people.' She organised the Berkeley Débutante Ball for a number of years, remarking (with prescience for 1960), 'the Season has completely lost its point'.

She married the Lloyd's underwriter Nigel Campbell and advanced into middle age immaculately turned out. She made no concessions to the brevity of the hemline. Seven inches off the ground for an evening dress was bold enough. 'I'm not mad about getting older,' she told one interviewer, 'but I feel there is fun to be had in all ages. Don't ask me how old I am. I shan't tell you, and don't look it up in your files. It is so provincial to mention age.'

Barbara Goalen (b. Barbara Bach, 1921, Malaysia; d. 2002)

Opposite:
'Cocktails and Champagne', December 1949, by Horst. Fashion by Dior

Bettina Graziani

At the height of her career, Bettina was one of the most recognisable Frenchwomen in the world, not least because of her ill-starred love affair with Prince Aly Khan. Before they were able to marry (he was by then divorced from Rita Hayworth, his second wife), he died in a head-on car crash. But it had all started a decade or so before, more modestly.

'After the Liberation, I came to Paris from Normandy to make my living,' Bettina, formerly Simone, told *Vogue*. 'I had no idea what fashion was, but I knew how to draw.' She was hired as a *cabine mannequin* by the small couture house Costet. From there, after a brief marriage to Benno Graziani (she kept her first husband's name because, she said, it suited her), she moved to the more established Lelong. There she met a small round man, who insisted that if Monsieur Lelong would not take her then he would, as he was about to open his own *maison*. Lelong engaged her, however, so she never did get to work with Christian Dior.

Leaving Lelong – 'he had nothing to do with me and my age, he seemed faraway, boring, sad, from another world, the past' – she went on to Jacques Fath. And she stayed till 1950. In their first collaboration, Fath created 30 dresses for his new mannequin-cum-muse. He gave her the name Bettina because, he opined, 'you have the look of a Bettina; besides, we already have a Simone.' At 5ft 4in, she was *trop petite* for a house model, but what she lacked in stature she made up for in naturalism. Fath saw her – admiringly – as the ordinary woman in the street, natural and fresh.

When she left his atelier for a career as a photographic model, she was an instant success. At 25, Bettina was the most famous model in Paris, 'popular not only with the editors and photographers,' according to *Vogue*, 'but with every man who ever dreamed of meeting a French mannequin.' She did not cease inspiring fashion designers either. Helping Hubert de Givenchy (formerly an assistant to Fath) to establish his house, Bettina took full control of the ancillary tasks, from *directrice* and chief *vendeuse* to public-relations adviser, muse and house model. He created for her the famous and much-copied Bettina blouse.

By the mid-1950s she was commanding 7,000 francs for a sitting, according to *Paris Match*. This caused her trouble with the tax authorities. But it wasn't just in her native country that she was well known. In Britain, she starred on the cover of the mass-circulation *Picture Post*, while the oil company Shell revealed years later that the password to its first computer had been 'Bettina'. So unpretentious was she that Henri Cartier-Bresson asked her to pose in what turned out to be the nearest he would get to fashion photography. And she gave it all up for her love of Aly Khan (heartbreakingly short-lived, as it turned out), which she wrote about in *Bettina by Bettina*.

Bettina's connection to the fashion world continued long after she had given up modelling: for a time she was couture director for Ungaro and after that a muse to Azzedine Alaïa. 'In my time it was much more about fashion,' she told *Vogue*. 'If you were a model, fashion was part of your life. Now the girls are more beautiful than ever, but I don't know where the fashion is…'

Bettina Graziani (b. Simone Bodin, 1925, France)

Opposite:
'The Paris Collections',
September 1950,
by Irving Penn.
Fashion by Jacques Fath

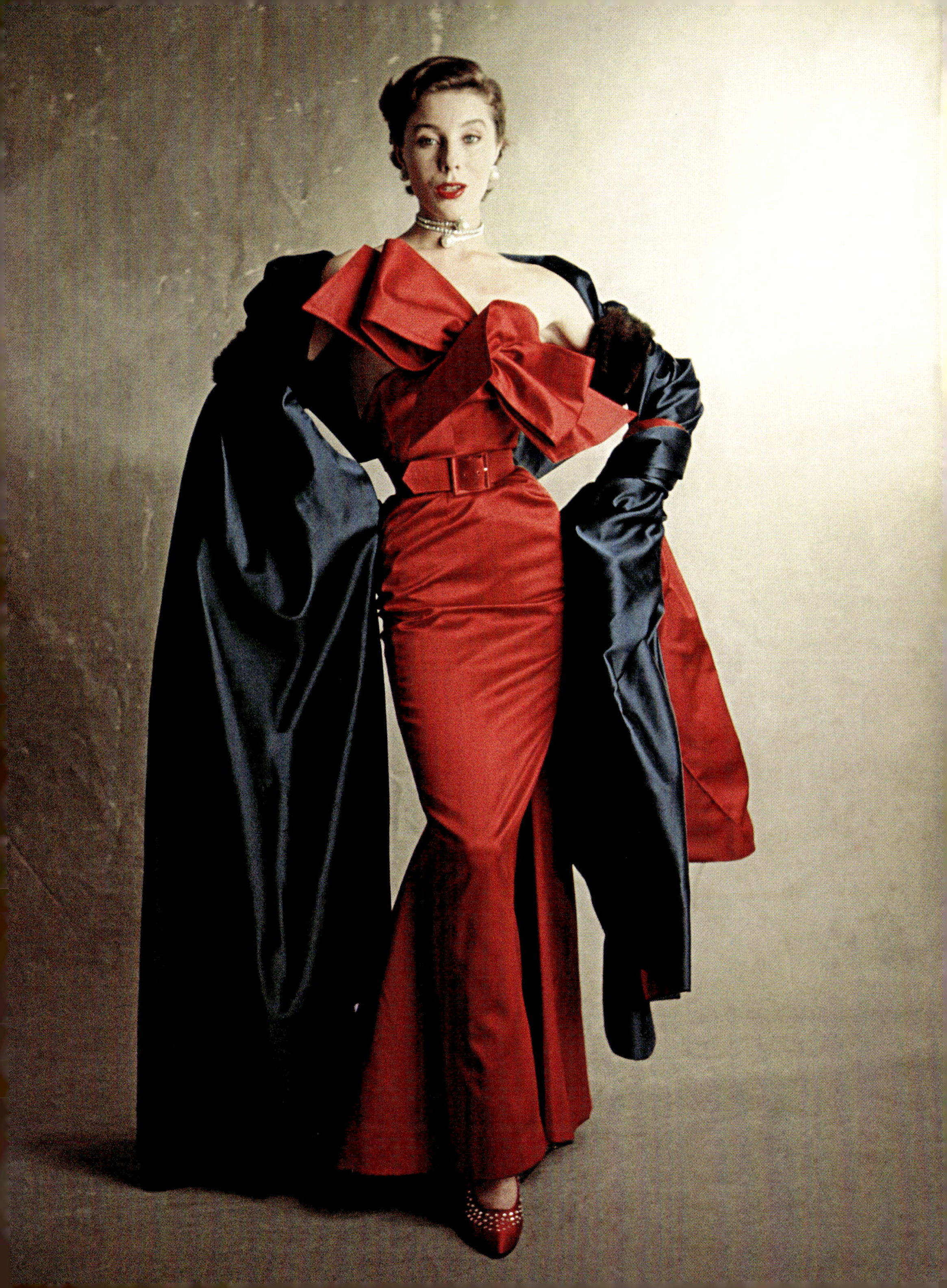

Bridget Hall

Bridget Hall, sporty and sun-kissed, happened to blow in from Dallas County at just the right time. Within a couple of years she was inescapable. She was in *Forbes*'s list of the top 10 supermodels by earning power, right up there with Cindy Crawford and Christy Turlington… How, you might wonder, did a ninth-grade dropout – that is to say, one who left school at 14, probably not academically notable – land up earning $10,000 a day and rising, with million-dollar contracts for Ralph Lauren, a four-litre Jaguar and a giant pick-up in the drive, a string of palominos, 22 acres of prime Dallas real estate and a trail of broken-hearted suitors, usually medium-grade to high-calibre film stars?

It's because America didn't want starved androgyne or emaciated waif, it just happened to want 1994's incarnation of wholesome teenage beauty – 5ft 9in; full, unenhanced breasts; full, unenhanced lips; chiselled cheekbones, but not Slavically so; a freckly, fresh-faced complexion; even a few front teeth that might benefit, as American *Vogue* suggested, 'from the attentions of an orthodontist'. And all that was wrapped up in Bridget Hall. Several fine minds tried to put their finger on just why it happened to this particular 16-year-old from hard-scrabble Farmers Branch, Texas.

The photographer Francesco Scavullo put it this way: 'She's just one of those miracles that happen. Forget that fabulous body. Just look at that face! There are girls I can make beautiful, there are girls Steven Meisel can make beautiful, or Richard Avedon, or Irving Penn. But if someone doesn't make this girl sensational, they should put away their camera'.

She started young. Very young. Bridget's mother Donna, a hardworking, impoverished single mum, drove her to a Dallas modelling agency and within two working days she was doing a catalogue for JC Penney at $75 an hour. It gradually escalated, with a few false starts and blind alleys, until Eileen Ford of the Ford agency rang. 'I'll never forget it,' Donna told *Vogue*. 'It was like having the Queen of England call…' Off went Donna and Bridget to New York City. Then, it was off to Milan. Within a day or two she was at Italian *Vogue* and the clamour could be heard back on the outskirts of Dallas. Bridget, in Donna's words, was 'going nowhere in high school', so instead she went to Paris and her first catwalk shows. She loathed them nearly as much as she loathed high heels, in which she had never walked before: 'I felt stupid.' She met Steven Meisel – always a fateful encounter, for the good, in a model girl's career: 'She is a very rare thing. The face,' he said, 'is almost perfect.'

Bridget did, however, lack a little worldly sophistication. (And who doesn't, aged 16 and newly away from home?) And the bright lights, big city… 'We tried a curfew,' Donna said, 'but it didn't work.'

There was talk of going back to school, but then contracts loomed with Ralph Lauren, Maybelline and Pepsi; tabloid romances with Leonardo DiCaprio and Norman Reedus; a huge party in her honour (fire engines had to disperse the crowds). 'What would you rather be doing?' Meisel asked *Vogue* rhetorically. 'Flying all around the world, making a million dollars, on the cover of every magazine, dating cute guys? Or hanging out at McDonald's, smoking pot or whatever they do, worrying about studying for some test?' Bridget Hall knew what route to take, and today Bridget Hall Inc (president, Donna Hall) flourishes.

Bridget Hall (b. 1977, USA)

Opposite:
'Native American',
June 1997,
by Robert Erdmann.
Fashion by Nike

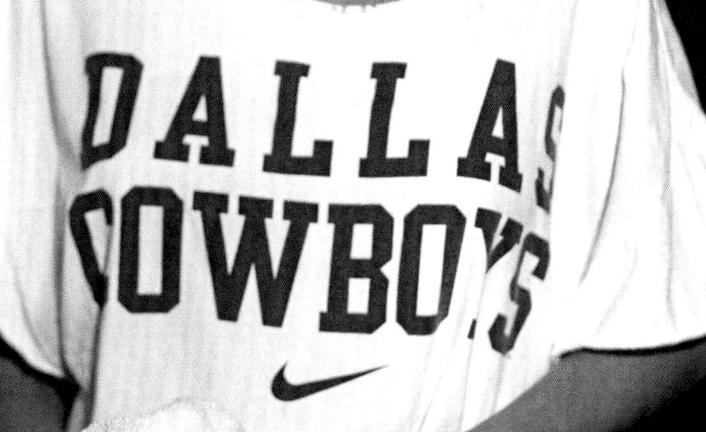
DALLAS
COWBOYS

Carla Bruni

Of course, it is Carla Gilberta Bruni Tedeschi's life after modelling that resonates nowadays. In February 2008, Nicolas Sarkozy married Carla Bruni in the Elysée Palace. As Carla Bruni-Sarkozy she became France's first lady, consort of its 23rd president, the eighth incumbent of the Fifth Republic – an unbroken line starting with Charles de Gaulle in 1959. She has, by most accounts, proved to be a great success, not least for her finely tuned fashion sense – ranging from headline-grabbing to demure as the occasion demanded – and a sparkling vitality upon which the spotlight rarely fails to land (often to the exclusion of her slightly diminutive husband).

This never detained Yvonne de Gaulle, who blended somewhat into the background, only coming to international notice when she and her husband escaped assassination in 1962. 'The presidency is temporary, the family is permanent,' she explained, as she retreated again into the shadows. But *autres temps, autres moeurs*: the modern republic requires its first ladies to do more than fling a protective arm around their husbands. 'It must be an embarrassment to other wives of heads of state to see this beautiful creature,' Karl Lagerfeld gasped in admiration to *Vanity Fair*, 'who can wear anything and speak like that' (she is fluent in several languages).

Not that Bruni, the Turin-born scion of the tyre conglomerate CEAT, is any stranger to the forces that once prevailed upon Madame de Gaulle. It has been suggested that the Tedeschi family relocated to France, where Carla was raised, in order to escape the threat of terrorist kidnappings, a wave of which swept through Italy's industrial families in the mid-1970s.

The notion of modelling was born out of a desire for an independent income, though her mother would later step in to be her manager. Bruni took to it with dedication, skill and, most importantly, with charm, which she possessed in superabundance. No-one, it seemed, had a bad word to say about her. *Au contraire*. Lagerfeld again: 'She was full of life and wit. She was beyond polite. She was always perfect.' Jean Paul Gaultier likened her presence to the 'heroine of a book or movie'. Her sheer likeability was unexpected in a model who had grown up knowing she could afford the entire collection. Hers was no good-luck story out of bad; she was not spotted eating a Big Mac in an impoverished backwater or selling fruit from a barrow.

She was an immediate star at *Vogue* – her beauty and breeding and her increasingly busy private life did not allow her to remain anonymous. The face of Prada's spring/summer '94 campaign and the catwalk star of Versace shows possessed, *Vogue* considered, 'a stare that is cool and mocking' and a body that poured itself down the catwalk 'like honey off a spoon'. Her actress sister, Valeria, photographed with her early on for *Vogue*, confided that 'Carla loves the seduction – showing her face, her body. She likes to be loved that way.'

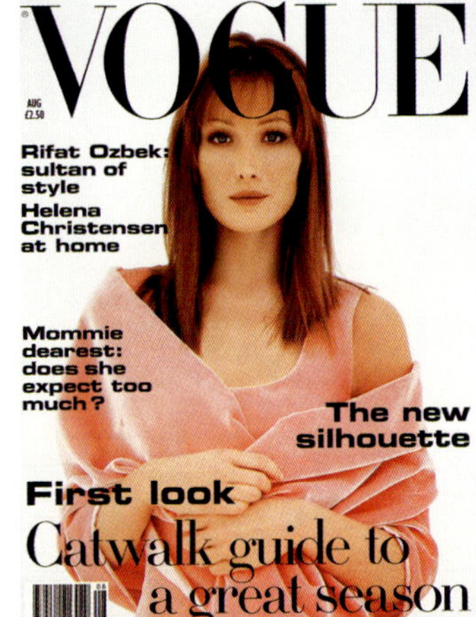

And she did like to be loved, at least as far as popular perception had it. She also liked music and musicians – she is an accomplished recording star. The public and private Carla Bruni, both self-assured, had trouble running in parallel lines. Romances with Mick Jagger and Eric Clapton made headlines. A propensity for the witty aperçu – 'Love lasts a long time, but burning desire, well, two to three weeks' – led to other liaisons. As Valeria Bruni Tedeschi put it in 1994: 'She knows her weapons.'

Carla Bruni (b. Carla Bruni Tedeschi, 1967, Italy)

Above:
'The New Silhouette', August 1993, by Neil Kirk. Fashion by Bella Freud

Opposite:
'Who's Afraid of the Little White Dress?', March 1994, by Max Vadukul. Fashion by Chanel

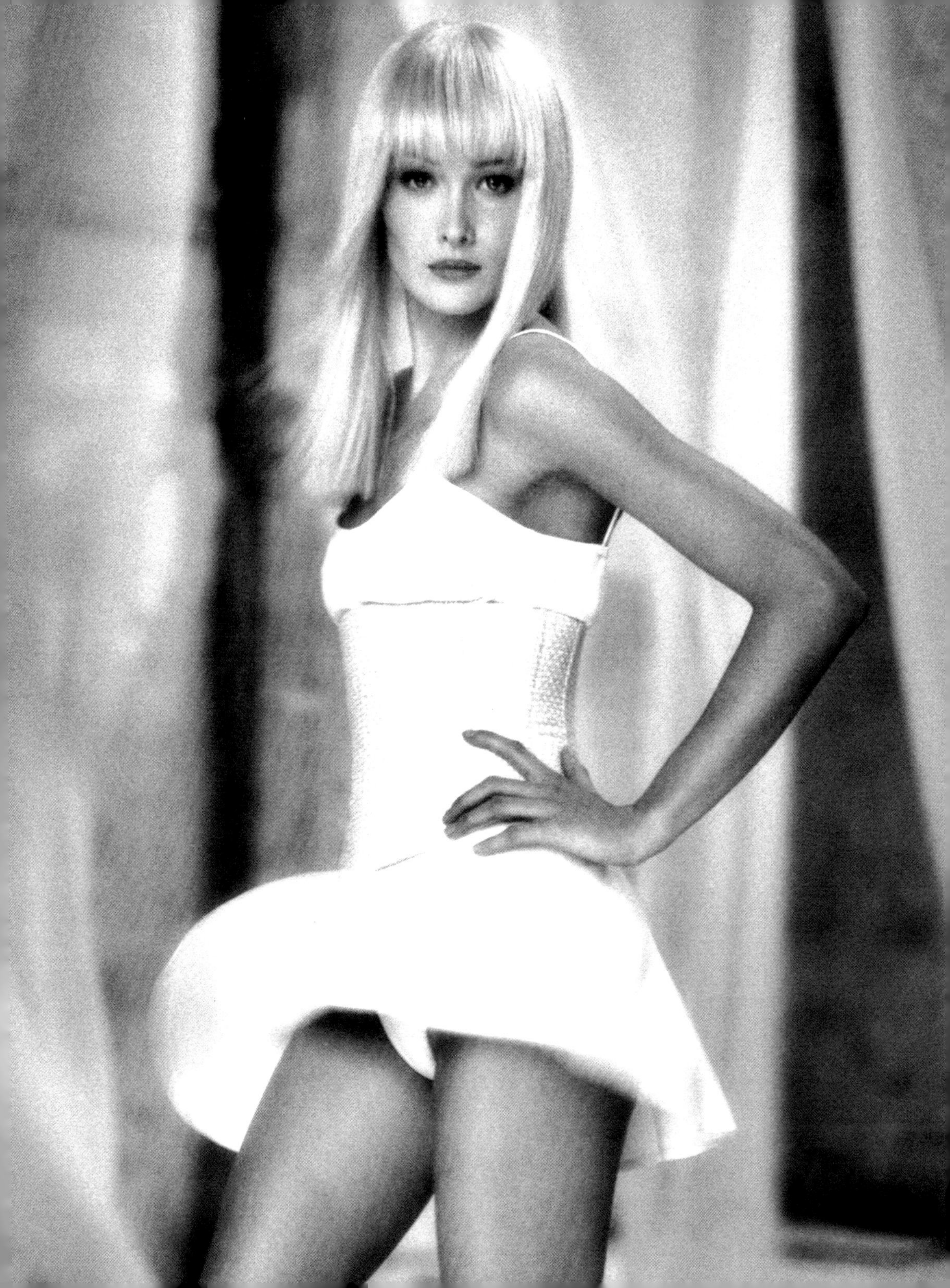

Carmen dell'Orefice

Carmen dell'Orefice has been a model for more than 60 years. Grown men squabble over her provenance: she was allegedly discovered on her way to ballet class by German photographer Herman Landshoff's wife, though Clifford Coffin claimed the honour too. Cecil Beaton maintained that he glimpsed her on a New York bus, alighting as he joined it; but fashion experts think this unlikely on the grounds that Beaton and public transport were an implausible combination. Besides, she was born into straitened circumstances, and legend has it she roller-skated to modelling jobs to save on bus fares anyway. Further, Carmen's family possessing no telephone, *Vogue* was obliged to send messengers to inform her mother where she should be.

Beaton called her 'a Renaissance child with a heart-shaped face, enormous aquamarine eggs for eyes and bad teeth. Soon, wearing a brace but never smiling, Carmen blossomed into a highly paid clothes peg.' But perhaps it was with Horst and Norman Parkinson that she did her most famous work. She moved the latter to hyperbole when both had late-flowering success: 'She is the Empress answer to all those dressed-up teenager nymphets who find themselves zipped into Yves Saint Laurent ballgowns by fashion editors who are in mourning for their own brief youths.' She charmed Horst, too. 'Although only a 16-year-old schoolgirl, she possesses an inherent gracefulness rarely found except among primitive races. Her almond-shaped eyes are a soft revelation when looking up…' She moved 'softly, like an animal' and possessed for him 'the two primary requisites of true elegance: the physical attributes of youth and the languor of the past. She is an American beauty of an antique other age.' She returned the compliment: 'He made me feel just so important and relevant and beautiful.'

Photography apart, she was also briefly a muse to Salvador Dalí. Aged 15, she posed naked for him at the St Regis hotel in New York, where he then lived. The finished painting, with Carmen on a clamshell as Botticelli's *Venus*, was acquired by Lord Mountbatten, who gave it as a gift to Princess Elizabeth. It currently resides in the Royal Collection, unseen for many years.

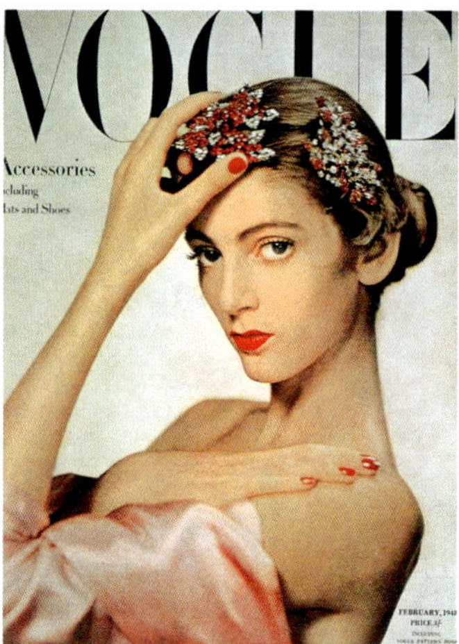

Whatever the magic that enthralled Dalí and *Vogue*'s photographers, she still possesses it, continuing to model occasionally to this day. 'I was very spoiled,' she said of Horst, Beaton, Penn and all the others. 'They showed me what manhood was about, really. I was madly in love… It felt like the world had given me all these wonderful lovers, and they were all photographers. It was all the gratification of that relationship though the lens, that moment of he's there and I am there and you have to feel and see what they want.'

Carmen dell'Orefice (b. 1931, USA)

Above:
'Accessories', February 1948, by Erwin Blumenfeld. Jewellery by Van Cleef & Arpels

Opposite:
"Summer Beauties', July 1946, by Cecil Beaton. Fashion by Salon Moderne

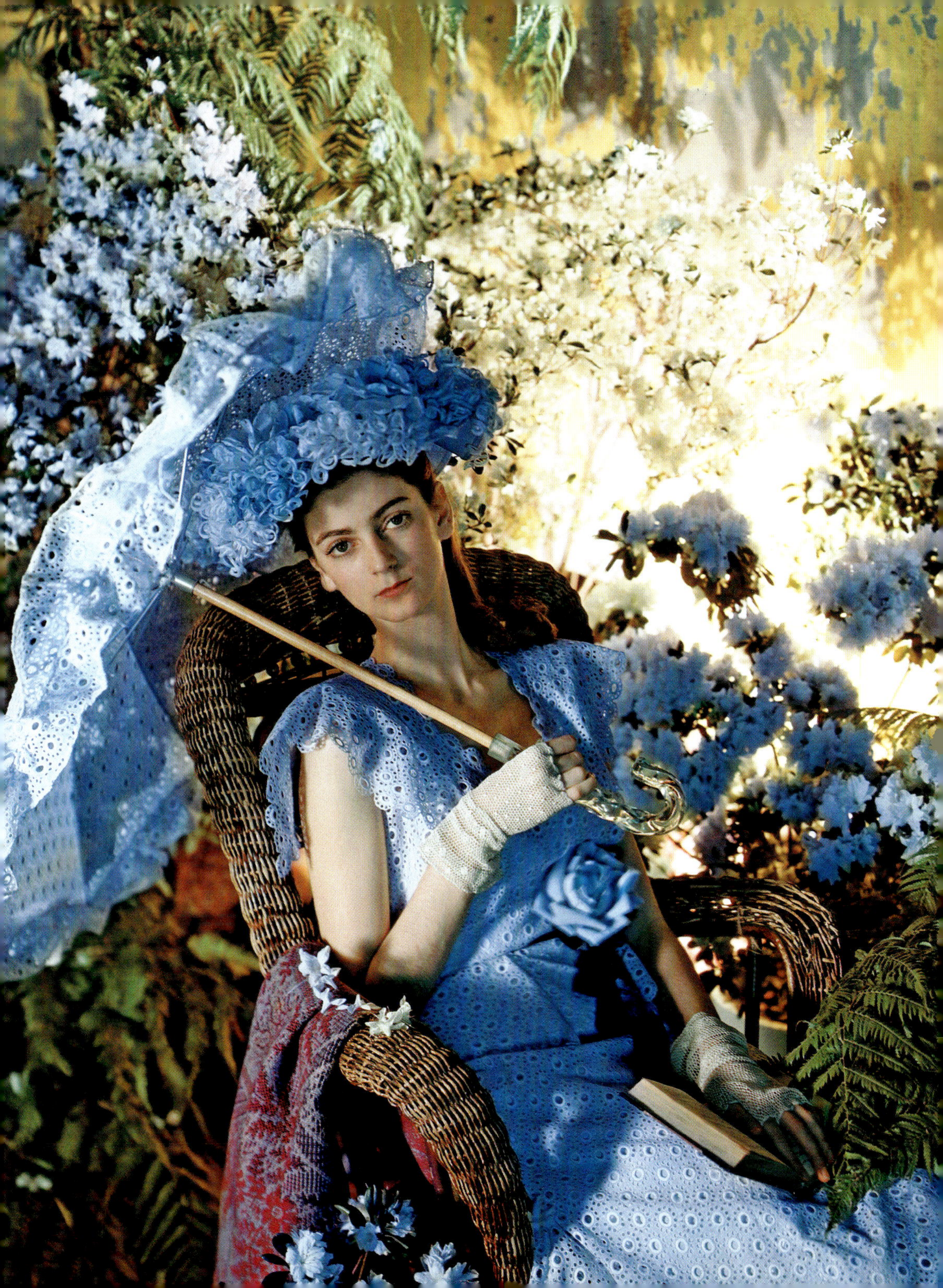

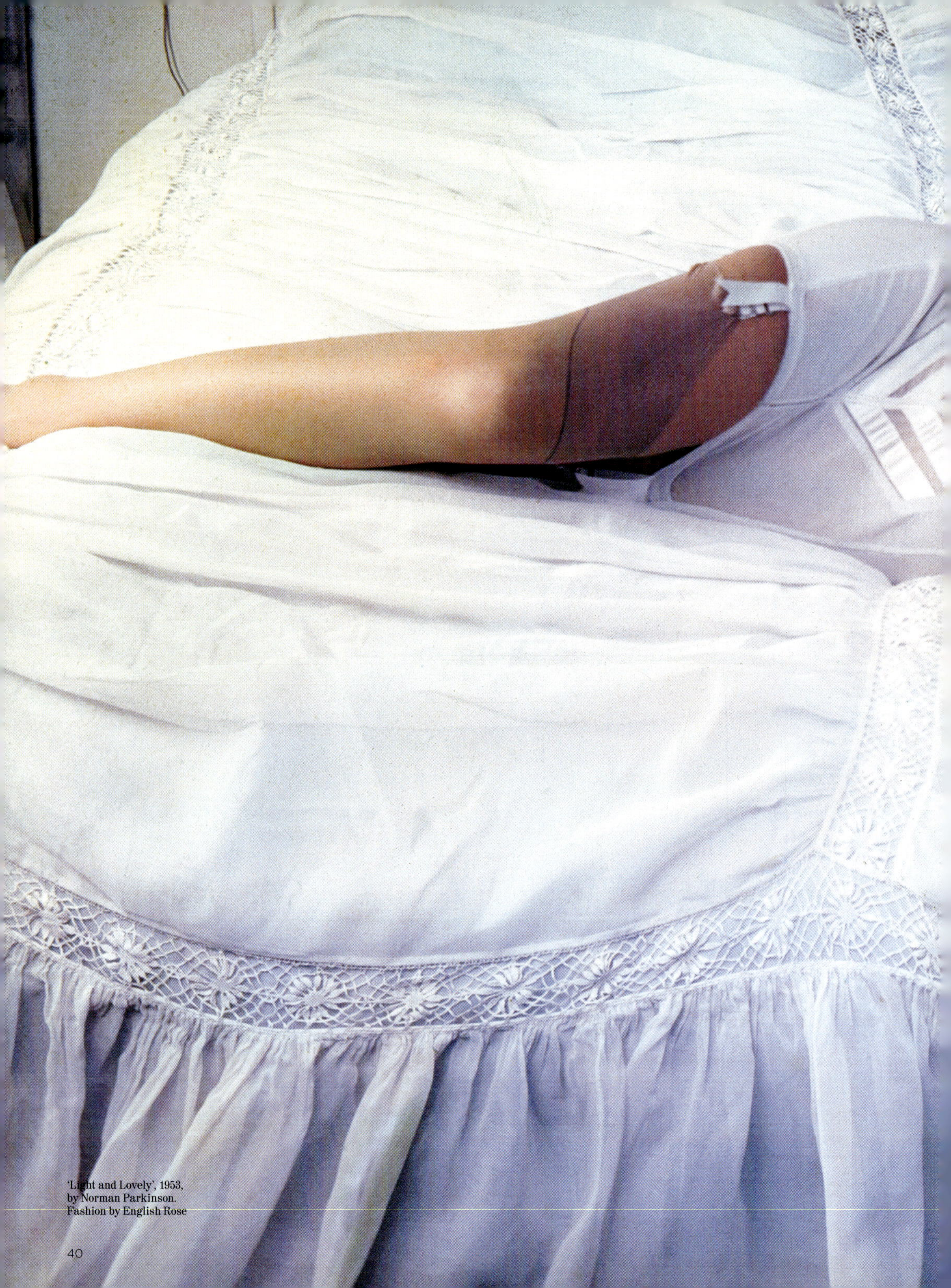

'Light and Lovely', 1953, by Norman Parkinson. Fashion by English Rose

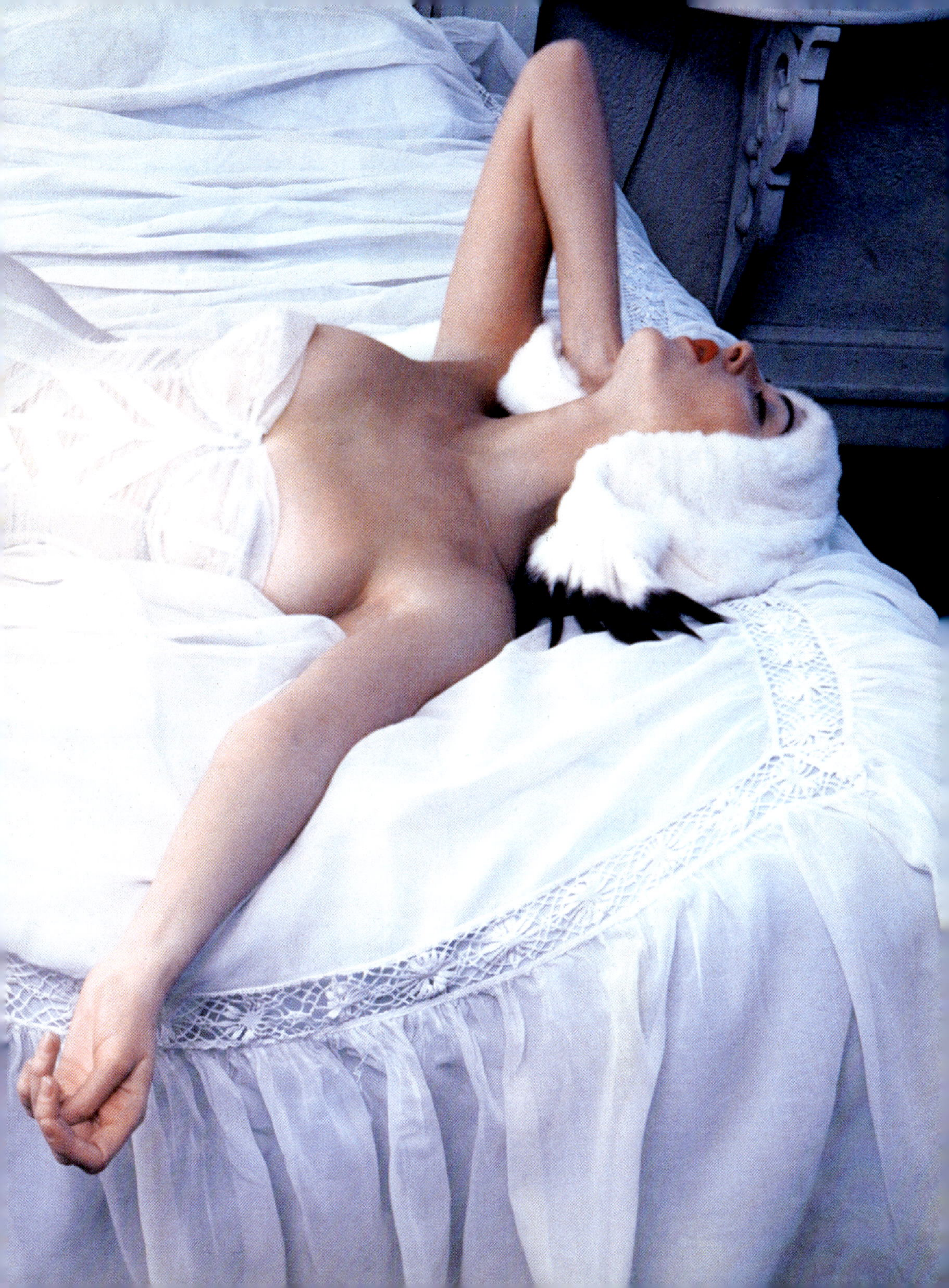

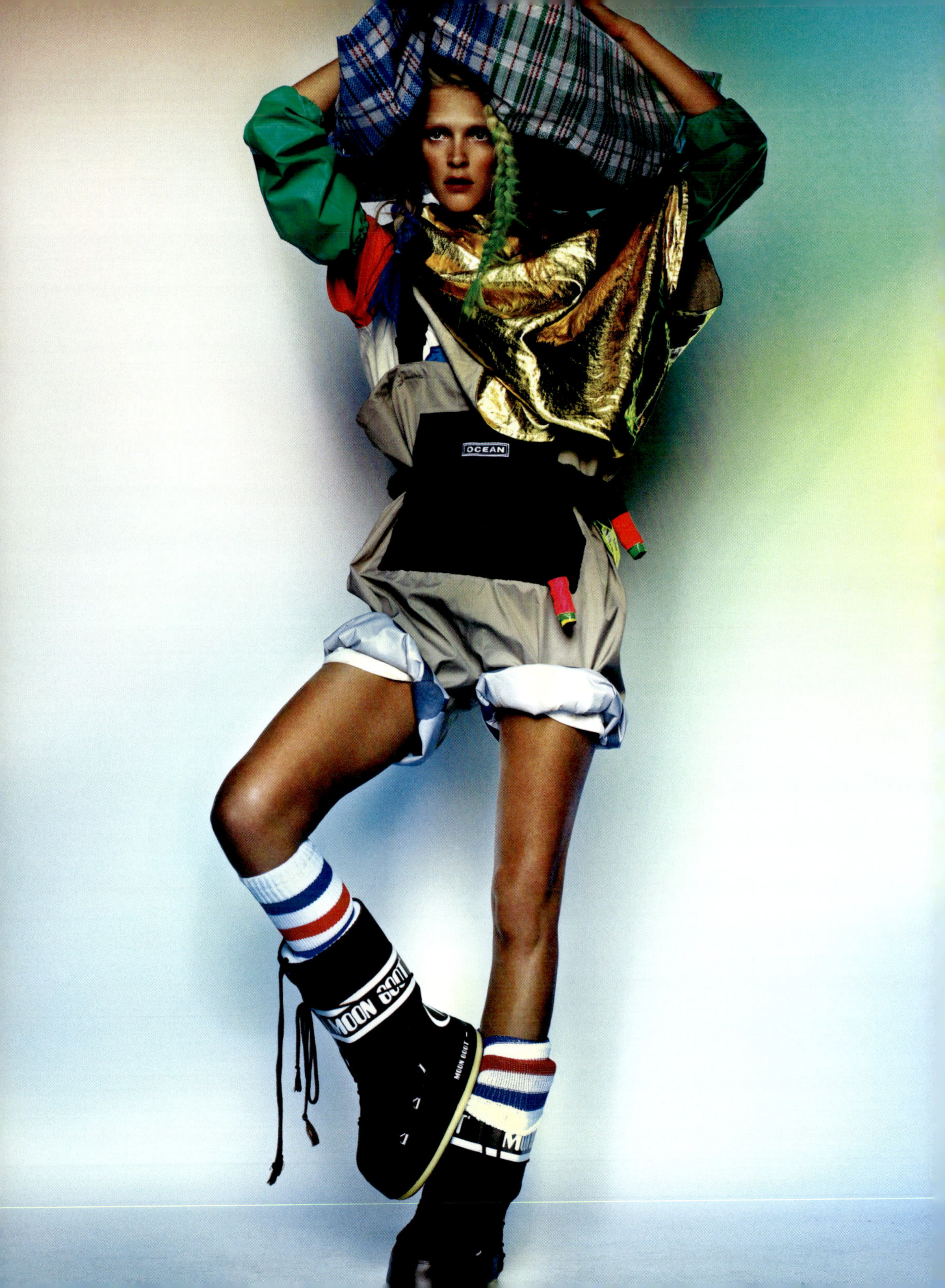
OCEAN
MOON BOOT

Carmen Kass

Where Carmen Kass comes from – Paide (pop. 9,600), in the Estonian county of Järva – nothing fashionable is ever worn, she says. In truth, the sleepy town does appear to have shied somewhat from the world stage. Apart from Carmen Kass, it is best known as the birthplace of Nobel Prize-winning novelist Herman Hesse's father.

It also has an annual Miss Paide pageant, which Carmen won. She went on to represent her hometown in the county championship and was duly crowned Miss Järva-maa. Apparently the title Miss Estonia only eluded her (she was surely a shoo-in) because she had been talent-spotted and was en route to Milan. She had been discovered in a supermarket in Tallinn. (Her first reaction: 'Who the hell are you?' Second: 'What is modelling?') She might have made it to Milan and back in time – however, her mother, a waitress, dithered over signing the documents that would allow her daughter to go. This proved a trifling hurdle for the ambitious and determined Carmen: 'I faked her signature,' she said. Ignoring any moral ambiguity, *Vogue* considered this a clever move: 'an impressive insight into the ways of the world she is well on her way to conquering.'

As it turned out, Carmen won a contest that was admittedly less likely to rouse her to patriotic fervour than Miss Estonia, but as a window to the world it was unrivalled: Model of the Year at the *Vogue*/VH1 Fashion Awards 2000. *Vogue* applauded her bare-minimum make-up look – 'the better,' it believed, 'to highlight the ethereal genetic features that can show up in people who hail from the shores of the Gulf of Finland.'

Besides being a face of Max Factor and Dior's golden-sheened J'adore woman, Carmen Kass is known in chess circles. Chess, to the Estonians, is like football to anyone else. *Chessbase News* considers her a 'kick-ass' player, and she was elected president of the Estonian National Chess League in 2004. As such, she was a roving ambassador for the game and lobbied hard for the 2008 Chess Olympiad to be held in Tallinn. (Unluckily for Estonia, it went to Dresden.)

While her modelling career seems unlikely to stall any time soon, the far-thinking Carmen has prepared an exit strategy on two fronts. She took acting lessons in New York and was cast as an Estonian professor and translator in *Welcome to America* (2000). She followed this with the 2004 thriller *Täna Öösel Me Ei Maga*, mistranslated from the Estonian as *Set-Point*. She also expressed an interest in standing for the European Parliament in 2004 and, to that end, joined the then ruling Res Publica party: 'I'm entering politics because, for the past ten years, I've gotten a lot from the world,' she told the Associated Press. 'And everything I've gotten, I've gotten from Estonia. I want to give something back.' Sadly, this was one Estonian contest she didn't win.

Carmen Kass (b.1978, USSR)

Opposite:
'Style Hunter',
November 2009,
by Mario Testino.
Fashion by Ocean Rainwear

Carolyn Murphy

Vogue liked Florida-born Carolyn Murphy for many things: dirty-brown hair (it went honey-blonde later), piercing ice-blue eyes, and her breath-of-fresh-air attitude. 'To me, modelling is all about opportunities – it's money, travel, a creative outlet. This business can seem like high school – at times it makes no sense the way some people behave. I just turn up, do my job, mind my own business and be nice.' This is not the weariness of modelling's battle-hardened praetorian guard, but a volunteer in the first flush of the big time. In truth, she had been a footsoldier for several years, having enrolled at modelling school at 16 and worked subsequently, with great success, in and around her home state.

The next step was further education at the University of Virginia. For a while she was able to mix her studies with modelling part-time. And then it all took off. She swept across Mario Testino's well-honed antennae; they twitched and crackled, and Carolyn was suddenly in French *Vogue*, *Harper's Bazaar* and American *Vogue*. The inevitable campaigns followed, chiefly Prada and then, much later and more remuneratively still, Estée Lauder. She succeeded Elizabeth Hurley as the face of the cosmetics giant. This was a big deal. American *Vogue* pointed out that her face would be blinding us from department store to duty-free shop the world over: more than 85,000 cosmetics counters. 'We picked her,' explained Aerin Lauder, 'because of who she is: one minute she's posing for a shoot, the next she's running to feed her baby. She's got the right values [*Vogue* already knew this, of course]. She's solid, secure, not spoiled.' In short, if you were to tick the various boxes on the demographic spreadsheet, she'd be 'someone I'd like to be' and 'someone I'd like to know'. This is borne out by her own characteristic reaction: 'I'm not the kind of person who looks in the mirror every day and says "My God, I'm gorgeous." I'm still in the stages of "Why me?"'

It turned out not to be false modesty. After years in the spotlight and a fleeting (so far) liaison with Hollywood – specifically her debut in 1999's *Liberty Heights* – Murphy slipped a little from view. She relocated to Costa Rica, embraced beach life with surfer dude Jake, bought a restaurant (he was a chef) and that was that. 'There was such a sense of freedom and I totally immersed myself in the lifestyle' – and she did it all, as *Vogue* reminded her, 'without so much as leaving a forwarding address'. She had put her Manolos in storage, she said, and ran around barefoot in bikinis and sarongs. It was the antithesis of her pressure-cooker life so far. She got pregnant too (a daughter, Dylan Bleu, born in 2000). It ended unhappily ever after with the dude, but the hiatus led to a resurgence in her modelling career. Carolyn modified her wardrobe again: 'I haven't been in high heels in so long…' she marvelled to *Vogue*.

Everyone fell in love with her again. Ever rigorous and forthright, this time round, Carolyn maintained, 'my priorities will be completely different. My job won't run my life like it used to, and there won't be any last-minute flights.'

Carolyn Murphy (b. 1973, USA)

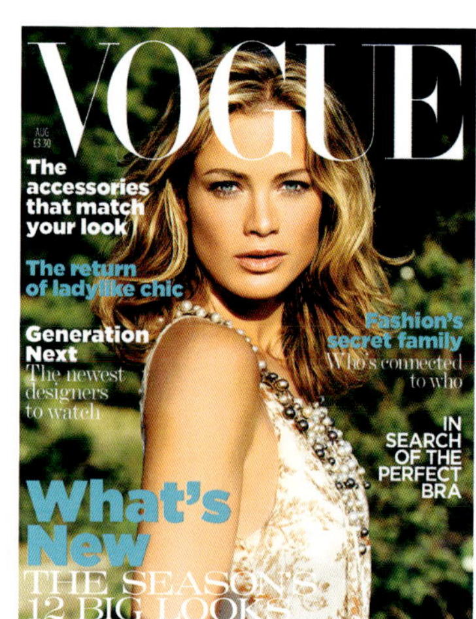

Above:
'What's New', August 2004,
by Mario Testino.
Fashion by Chanel

Right:
'Siren Call', November 2002,
by Regan Cameron.
Fashion by Alexander McQueen

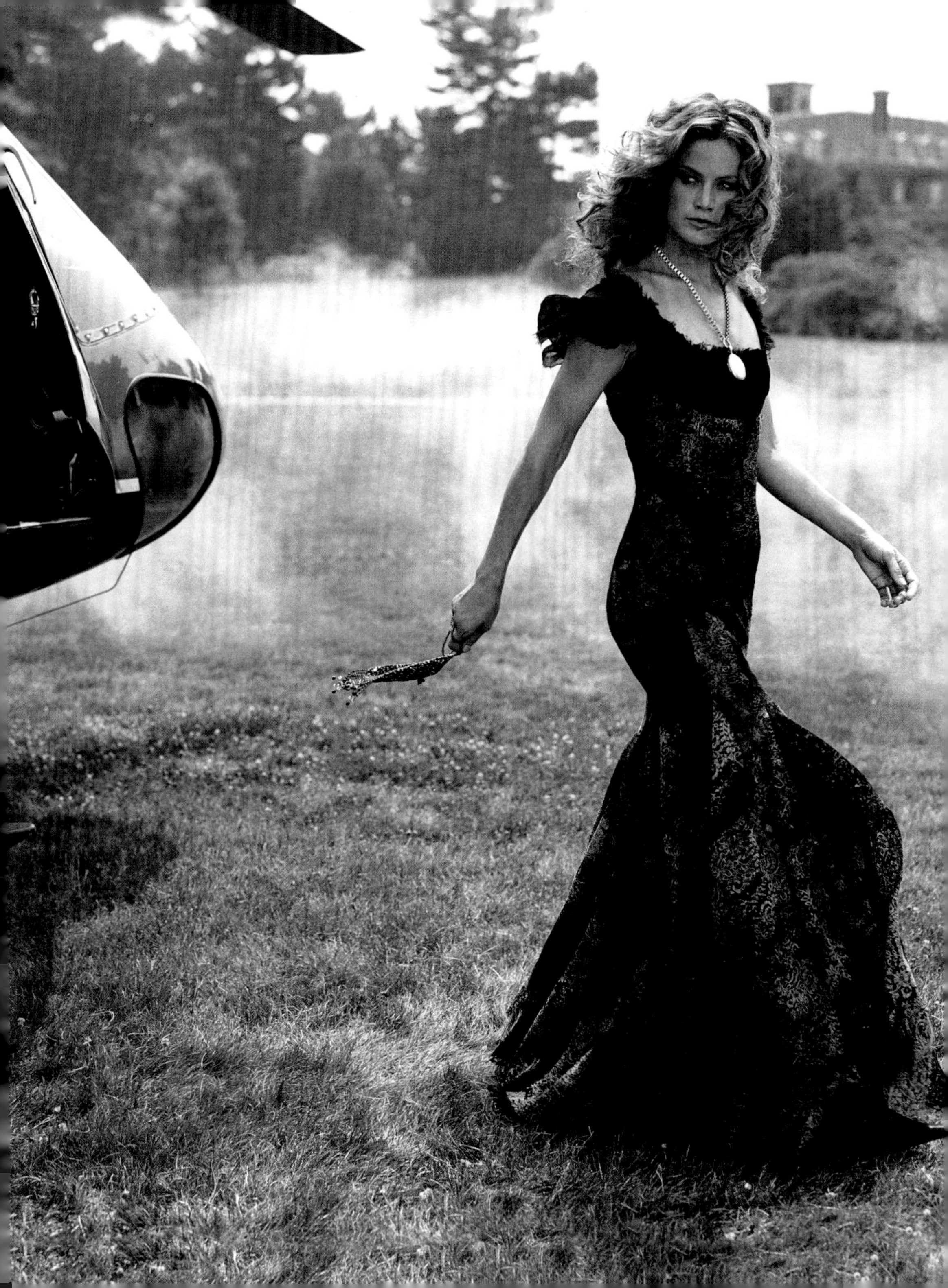

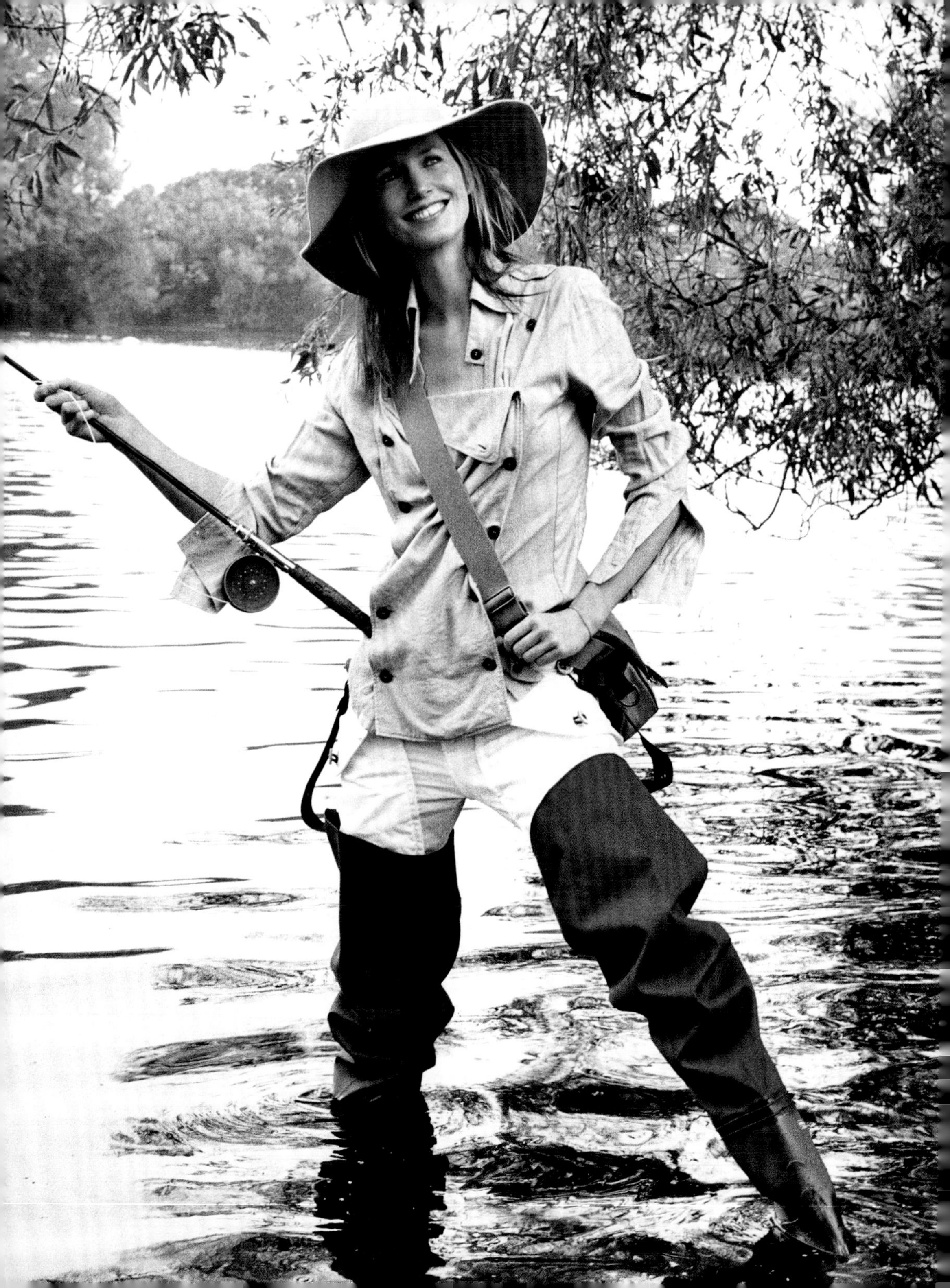

Cecilia Chancellor

By the early 1990s, *Vogue* was delighted to report that the 'London Girl' had come into her own. The high-maintenance, carefully manicured standards of beauty set by 'glowing superwomen', as the magazine put it, had had its day in the sun (or not, depending on prevailing trends for skin tone). It was perfectly acceptable, considered *Vogue*, to bin the capsule wardrobe in favour of 'poor-boy sweaters and spandex trousers'. 'This means,' the magazine continued, 'that it's now OK to look a bit ragged round the edges. It's even fashionable to wear slightly fraying cardigans from the menswear department at Marks & Spencer.'

For *Vogue*, Cecilia Chancellor was the living embodiment of the London Girl, though she had started her career in the 1980s as something of a glowing superwoman herself and, to be fair, she clearly found it more difficult to look ragged round the edges than some of her newer colleagues. Which was unfortunate because, as she revealed later, the spirit of grunge (as it became popularly known) was much more her kind of off-duty look anyway.

She remained impossibly elegant, even when her hair had been carefully de-lustred and preternaturally re-greased by hairdresser James Brown. His 1993 take on 'Fashion's New Spirit', in collaboration with photographer Corinne Day and fashion editor Lucinda Chambers, remains one of the most influential sets of *Vogue* photographs of the modern era. It introduced Kate Moss to a wider audience and starred Cecilia doing her best to look elegantly dishevelled. The shoot, set on school playing fields in south London (said to belong to Kate Moss's alma mater), saw Cecilia gamely playing football in Jasper Conran's navy crepe jacket with white collar, a chiffon vest, a long devoré chiffon and velvet skirt and crocheted tights.

A pupil of St Paul's Girls' School in Hammersmith, Cecilia's first modelling assignment was helping out a classmate, Camilla Nickerson, later an influential fashion stylist. Working on some test shots with photographer Perry Ogden, Nickerson asked her to come along, and the resulting £75 seemed like easy money. Chancellor's modelling career occurred in two phases. After the highly polished 1980s, she stopped to attend art college but then, as fashion's new spirit kicked in, she found herself in demand again. She was on the catwalk for the moment at which fashion experts acknowledge that grunge – the style adjunct to a prevailing mood in rock music – was born: Marc Jacobs's spring/summer 1993 collection for Perry Ellis (cashmere beanie hats, silk trainers, accessorised with thrift-store *trouvés*). Jacobs later named a quilted leather handbag after her – the Cecilia (aficionados favour it in a shade of papaya).

Two decades after she started out, Mario Testino cast her in 'Another Country', a 20-page shoot celebrating 'splendid settings, beautiful people and traditional country pursuits'. Cecilia's chosen pursuit was angling, something she had never undertaken before. 'To weigh down the rod, we attached a silver spoon to the end of it,' she recalled, 'but every time I cast off, the dog goes for it!' The artifice of the scenario apart, Cecilia herself was uncontrived and natural and spontaneous. Suddenly, 20 years didn't seem so long an interval.

Cecilia Chancellor (b. 1967, UK)

Opposite:
'Another Country',
October 2004,
by Mario Testino.
Fashion by Ann
Demeulemeester

Celia Hammond

'Celia Hammond – always so serene, it was as if she was in some other place,' mused Twiggy of *Vogue*'s Facemaker of '66. If it were some other place, it would surely have been populated by happy cats and dogs; preferably the former, though the Celia Hammond Animal Trust makes no distinction among animals in distress. As a model, her advocacy of fur was born out of ignorance, as she is the first to admit. A trip for Beauty Without Cruelty to witness first-hand the horror of a seal cull convinced her that the promotion of fur was morally untenable. A natural extension was to set up her low-cost neutering and vaccination clinics, which have saved countless feline lives, and her re-location of stray animals to urban and rural homes has made her reputation far more than her life in fashion ever could. Her own rural home is set in 12 beautiful acres of East Sussex, near Hastings – shared, she reckons, with around 300 lucky cats. For this and many other animal causes, Hammond was accorded the RSPCA's highest accolade, the Richard Martin Award, in 2004.

Norman Parkinson, it is generally agreed, discovered her, having arranged a 'cattle market' (his words) at the Lucie Clayton modelling school. The principal thought it a thankless task, surmising that she had nothing to offer. 'On the contrary,' he replied, 'you have a star up there. Celia Hammond.' The principal demurred that she looked 'Burmese or something', but Parkinson booked her for *Queen* magazine and Hammond was launched. The shoot produced her first cover.

Norman Parkinson was smitten, *Queen*'s proprietor tried to place her under exclusive contract, and Diana Vreeland at American *Vogue* was similarly entranced. But most deeply affected of all was Terence Donovan; as David Bailey is inextricably linked to Jean Shrimpton, so Donovan is to Hammond. The pictures they made together were some of postwar British photography's finest, defining the era for those who followed. This creative partnership vexed Parkinson greatly: 'He liked working with a raw canvas,' Hammond told the writer Michael Gross. 'And your getting involved with someone else is not part of his picture…'

Also not part of his picture was her concern for all creatures. 'On one occasion, driving down the motorway to a location,' Parkinson recalled in his memoirs, 'inadvertently as can happen, I hit a small bird. Celia let out a scream that could be heard in the next county and, seizing my neck in her strong hands, she attempted to strangle me at 60mph; "Stop, you murderer, pull over, stop!"'

For a while Hammond's modelling career went comfortably hand-in-hand with her charity work but the late nights on building sites took their toll; something had to give (and it wasn't ever going to be the animals). Modelling, she had decided, was for the self-obsessed; she was not interested in 'standing on a piece of paper in a funny way' – or, peculiarly, in front of a plastic model of the DNA molecule while wearing a grey Wollands tweed skirt. She left at the height of her career, walking away as the 1960s dream began to turn sour. Abandoned strays had finally lured her – a better breed, as one commentator noted, than those she had been lately hanging around with.

Celia Hammond (b. 1941, UK)

Right:
'Your Next Great Looks',
October 1968,
by David Montgomery.
Fashion by Jean Allen

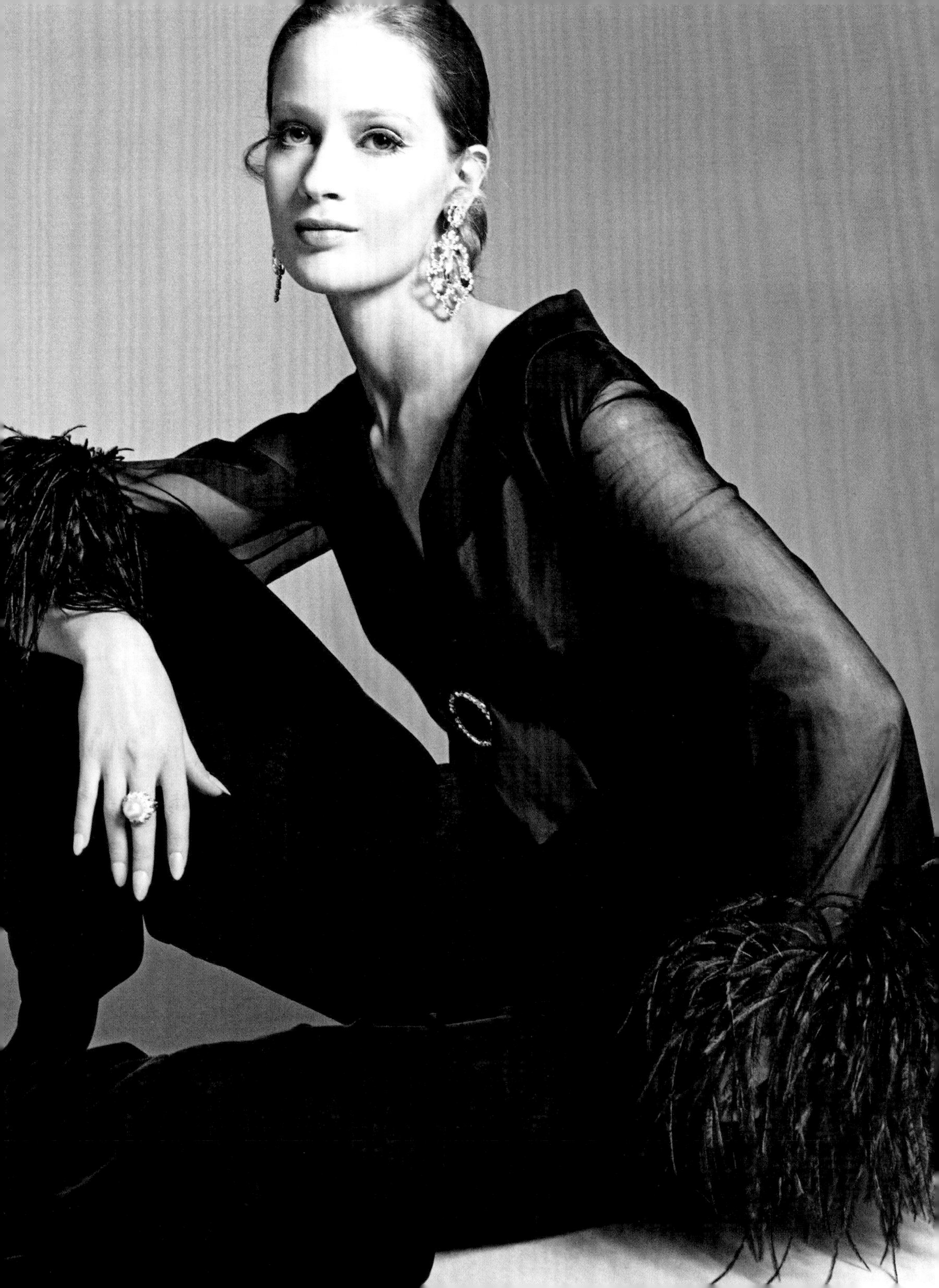

Christie Brinkley

'Up north, camping out in Alaska, you carry the minimum of gear and dress only for protection. You crawl out of your sleeping bag – as Christie Brinkley does – and dash on skin protectors and a very good moisturiser....' At the outset of the 1980s, *Vogue* looked a little inward to examine the great whatever-remained-out-there. With or without Chanel's Emulsion No 1 and a lip enhancer such as Mat de Chanel Lip Blush, which Christie's survival pack contained, there was something atavistic in this pull to reacquaint oneself with the raw nature and the elements. 'At one extreme end of potency,' wrote the travel writer Jan Morris, 'it spawns ecology movements and national parks; at the other it simmers somewhat morbidly within ourselves, intermittently surfacing to send us jogging in the park, planting herbaceous borders or sailing catamarans single-handed to Australia...'

Actually, we didn't. Instead we let Christie Brinkley do it for us. There she goes, kayaking into the white wild noise – and the icebergs – of Alaska. Where you and I might say cold, wet and very tired, 'if you had asked her at the end of the day how she was,' opined *Vogue*, 'she'd say soothed and cleansed.'

Rock climbing, jungle trekking, deep-sea diving – the smiley, sun-kissed surfer girl from Brentwood, California, did it all with a smile. (And that smile led to a 20-year contract with Cover Girl cosmetics, which, after a break, started again in 2005 – by which time its leading lady was 51.) Such escapades were the hallmark of Christie Brinkley's modelling career, and owed much to her appeal as the 'all-American' girl, chiming with a prevailing sportive aesthetic. *Vogue* could rarely get enough of her and, if she wasn't parachuted into the wilderness, she was in demand for swimwear shoots all year round. In fact even in the wilderness there was always time for a little R&R, in a Fendi thin-strap Lycra one-piece with a double twist of bandeaux making a belt and a deconstructed straw boater from Byblos. Like all the best fashion pictures, they were never quite as glamorous as they might finally appear: 'See my pink healthy glow? It was the remains of the worst allergic reaction [to sunblock] in my life! We were in St Barts photographing a story about sunburn when my cheeks started stinging and welled up, up, up...'

When the sun went down over another Bahamian beach club, another side of Christie emerged, to make the night come alive – 'a little touch of taboo,' ventured *Vogue*. She was a regular in Chris von Wangenheim's darkly glamorous pictures. His sense of the sinister scenario was politely tagged as 'heightened reality', but was really about the down, dirty and dark side of sexuality. It was, he suggested, all about 'flirtation and titillation: physical sex is not necessary, but the promise will do...'

Outside the fashion pages, Christie made an impact on the world at large with her on-off liaison with singer Billy Joel. (She starred memorably as the 'Uptown Girl' in his 1983 video.) Though she has modelled with increasing frequency in recent years, her third and fourth marriages have kept her name – unsought for – in the tabloid headlines. More positively, so did her campaigning on animal rights and environmental issues. Those Alaskan trips – 'the need for nature' – paid off.

Christie Brinkley (b. Christine Hudson, 1954, USA)

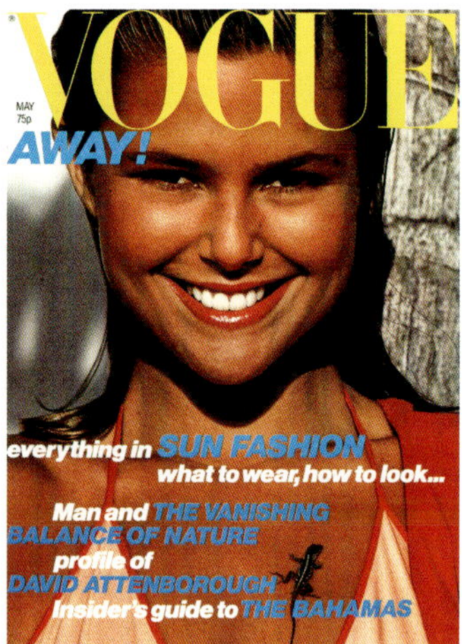

Above:
'Away!', May 1979,
by Alex Chatelain.
Fashion by Gianni Versace

Opposite:
'Snap Throats!',
February 1977,
by Chris von Wangenheim.
Fashion by Geoffrey Beene

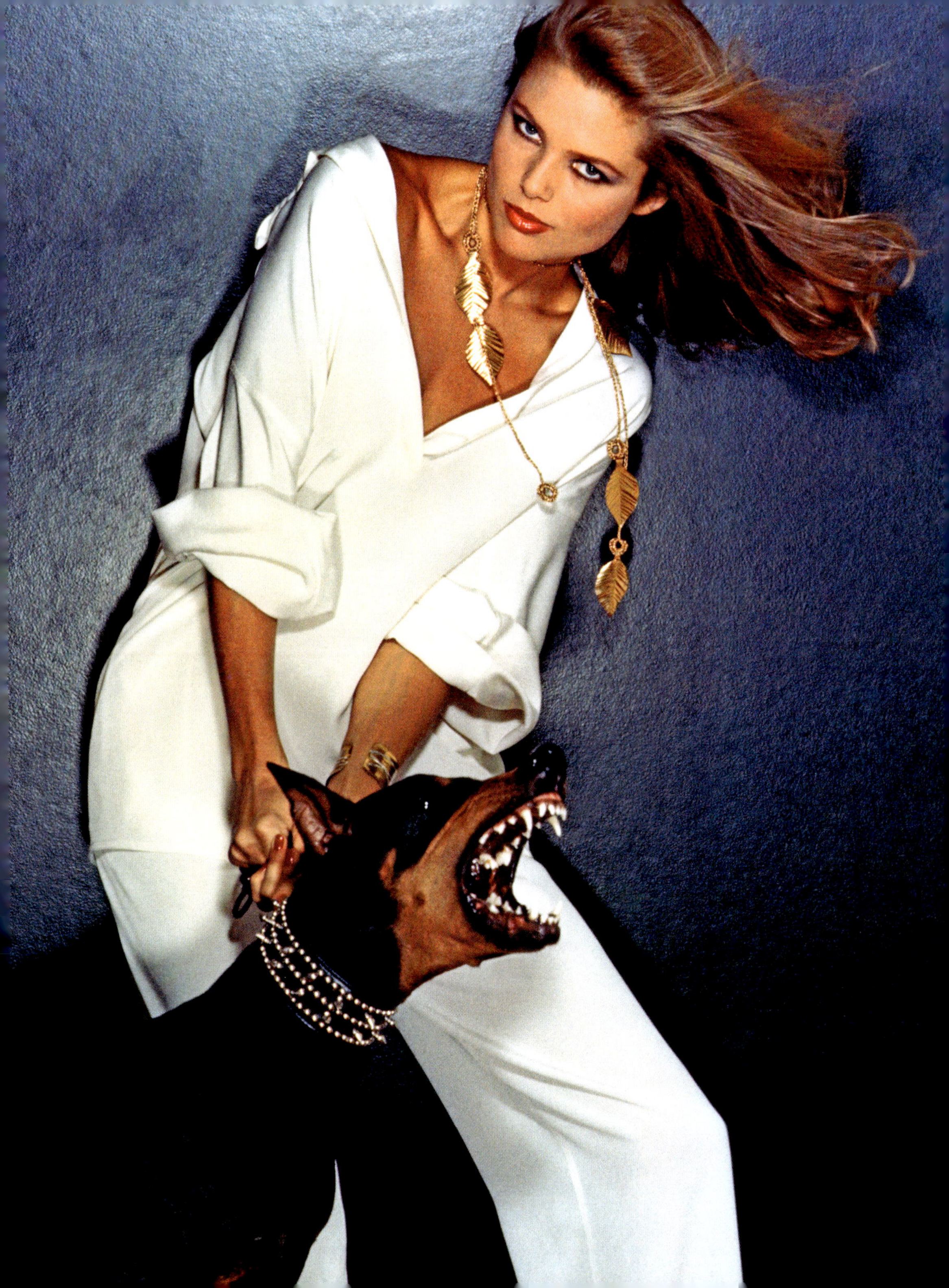

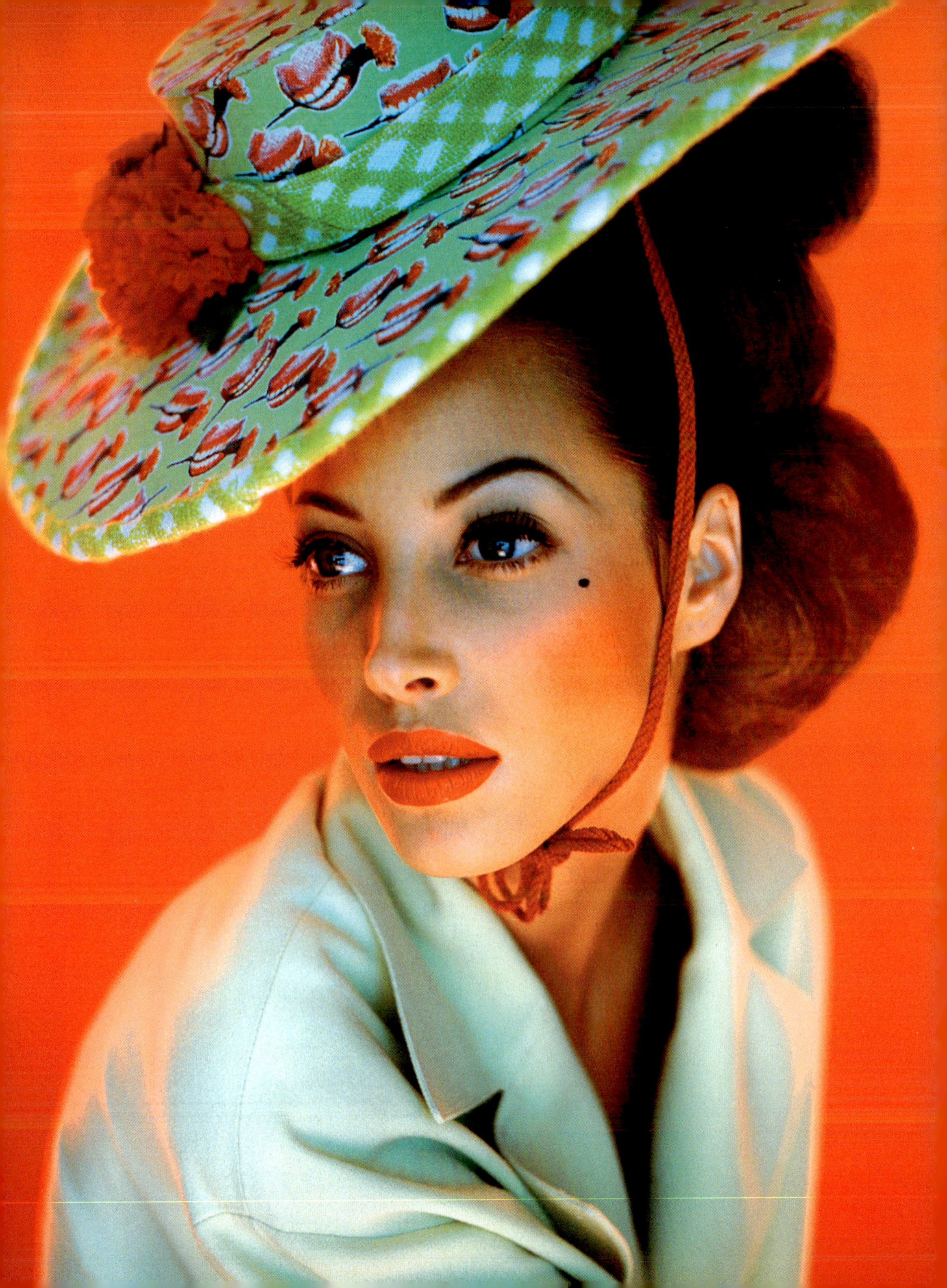

Christy Turlington

'Supermodels are the stars of my shows,' said the late Gianni Versace, and he, more than anyone else, planted them firmly in the spotlight. 'I respect them highly. I don't like to transform them or re-invent them, but use them just the way they are.' A vital component of the tripartite alliance – Christy, Linda and Naomi – Christy Turlington's rise to stardom was meteoric. Figuratively, of course. She has since found the term 'supermodel' a little absurd, as if 'we change into our capes in telephone booths'. The author Michael Gross has written that the supermodels were the result of a 'collaboration of smart agents, photographers and perceptive designers', of which Versace was the sharpest, paying the girls around $60,000 per show. By 1990, Christy was 21 and very rich in the 'lucrative purdah', as *Vogue* put it, of an exclusive two-year arrangement with Calvin Klein's perfume Eternity, rumoured to be worth around $6 million.

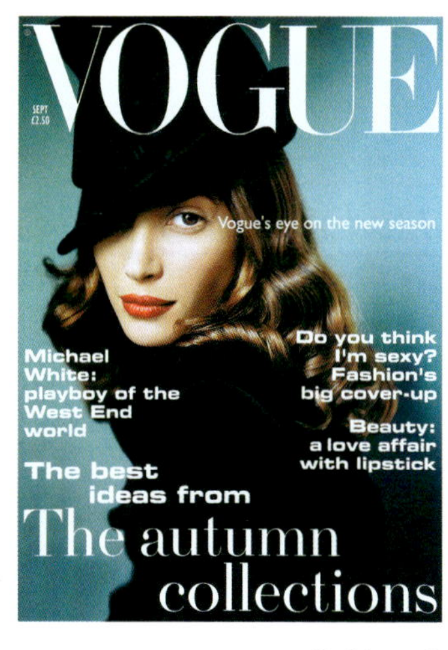

These were the days of conspicuous wealth worn with deliberate effect and usually without irony: power suits, puffballs, exaggerated jewellery. Of all the photographers that captured that time and place and its leading characters, the late Herb Ritts remains one of Turlington's favourites. His foremost ability was to marry two worlds hitherto kept separate – celebrity and fashion – and turn them into pictures that belonged to neither: still, relaxed, unhurried, sunlit. 'Most of the photographers of the 1980s were caught up in the clothes and the make-up, whereas Herb's work was very clean…' says Turlington. 'Everything [was] pared down but he still managed to capture a sense of heightened glamour. I don't think anyone has come close to Herb and certainly no-one will be able to match his style.'

Christy was discovered while horse-riding near Miami, though some sources are convinced by a more prosaic scenario – eating a cake in a café. In any event, a photographer stopped her and asked her to pose. 'Look bitchy,' he said, which nonplussed her. Her father's work as a training pilot for Pan Am had taken the family to Florida, though she was born in northern California. She modelled at weekends. By 16 she was working for *Vogue*, which helped her avoid much teenage introspection. 'I kind of figured that if *Vogue* thinks I look OK,' she told the magazine later, 'I probably look OK.'

Once compared – favourably – to a particularly pulchritudinous breed of mountain goat, as she grew older her face lost whatever fullness it ever possessed to become angular, her high razor-sharp cheekbones more pronounced. 'Fawn-like' and 'gazelle' were better appropriations from the animal kingdom. The writer Joan Juliet Buck admired the 'rare geometry' of her face, 'a diamond shape made up of clean facets'. (That bone structure was easily translatable into injection-moulded display mannequins for the Costume Institute at New York's Metropolitan Museum of Art.)

Like Cindy Crawford, her colleague in the pages of *Vogue*, Christy made the move from supermodel to entrepreneur. Her best-selling yoga-inspired fashion line, Nuala, and natural ayuverdic beauty line, Sunari, were assiduously promoted with personal appearances (though she and her Nuala collaborators, Puma, have since parted ways, and Sunari no longer boasts Christy's imprimatur). This had sprung from pilgrimages to India, meditation and an immersion in Eastern comparative religions, which led her to give up modelling full-time in the mid-1990s. It's all a far cry from her appearances in lingerie for Calvin Klein: 'There was all kinds of craziness – people asking me to sign their underwear, you name it.' What kept her sane amid the chaos of a life lived in the eye of the fashion storm? 'I've been practising yoga since the age of 18. I hope I have found a life/work balance. At least I know the tools that can help create a sense of space. It just doesn't happen – you have to put the effort in.'

An activist for causes close to her heart, having studied and gained an MA in public health at New York's Columbia University, Turlington is also a widely travelled envoy for the relief agency CARE. She is by every account, a gifted communicator. One director of CARE found Christy's resilience, intellectual gifts and capacity for humanitarian work astonishing: 'How can someone who's been modelling since she was 14,' she asked, 'be such a *mensch*?'

Christy Turlington (b. 1969, USA)

Opposite:
'Bewitching Beauty', March 1992, by Javier Vallhonrat. Fashion by Red or Dead

Above:
'*Vogue*'s Eye on the New Season', September 1993, by Mario Testino. Fashion by Philip Treacy

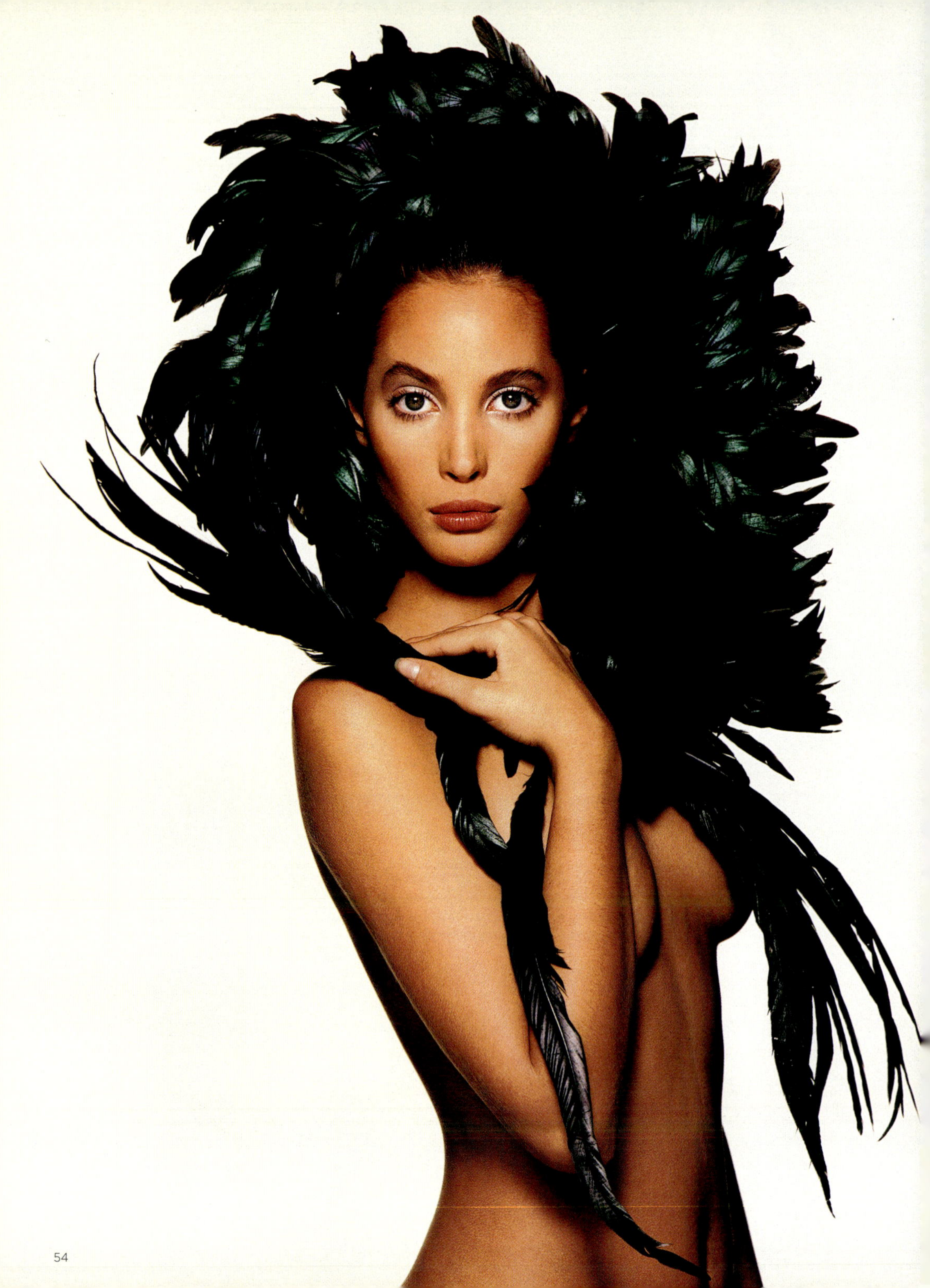

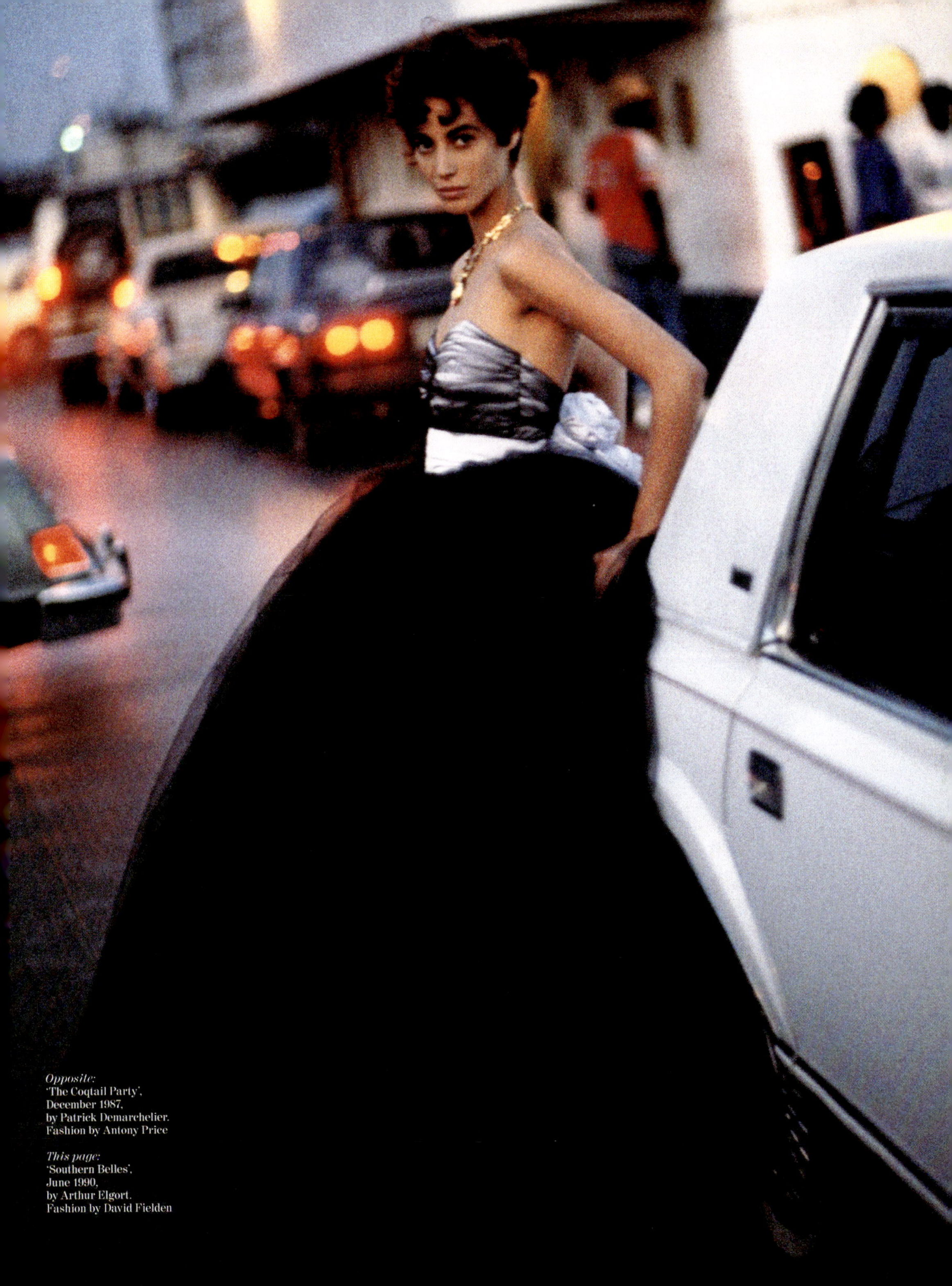

Opposite:
'The Coqtail Party',
December 1987,
by Patrick Demarchelier.
Fashion by Antony Price

This page:
'Southern Belles',
June 1990,
by Arthur Elgort.
Fashion by David Fielden

Cindy Crawford

For *Vogue* – all of 18 of them across the globe and, let's face it, probably every other magazine down the food chain – Cindy Crawford represents hit-between-the-eyes, full-on glamour. She is the American dream girl *ne plus ultra*. She's the one whose poster teenage boys put on the wall, the writer John Heilpern observed, though they are likely never to have opened a fashion magazine. 'Their mothers are happy their sons have posters of me and not Madonna,' Cindy replied. 'For some reason I come over as unthreatening and fun, even in a bikini.' And in *Vogue*, at least in her earliest incarnation, she was in a bikini rather a lot. That and power suits. It was the late 1980s and she was a vital part of the first wave of supermodels (with Linda, Tatjana, Naomi, Claudia, Christy). As *Vogue*'s Sarah Mower put it early on: 'These girls, none out of their twenties, are paid so very highly not so much to sell products as dreams. On them are projected the fantasies of fashion editors, designers, photographers and, ultimately, the public. Their appearance is a symbolic index of where women stand now, of what we approve of in each other, of how we want to be...' They wanted to be Cindy because she is everything America admires the most: successful, hardworking, charming yet modest, non-threatening, approachable, clean, unpromiscuous and, of course 'drop-dead good-looking'.

In the years that followed, she rode out the crest of that first wave, and those wholesome girl-next-door curves gradually gave way to a leaner silhouette. She ensured cannily that her trademark mane of glossy hair and a readily identifiable mole above her top lip remained as twin trademarks. That mole: 'It's going to have its own talk show soon,' she once told *Vanity Fair*. (Prescient, as it later starred in its own confectionery ad – Cindy pretended to lick it off, so delicious was the chocolate-coated product.) The girl from DeKalb, Illinois, moved to Chicago to start her career – 'And in Chicago modelling is a job not a lifestyle,' she told *Vogue*. 'I did hard-core commercial things... You had to do your own hair, your own make-up; bring your own shoes, your own pantyhose.'

But there would be far more to Cindy Crawford than Sears catalogues and K-Mart flyers. And more to her, too, than the mole, the hair and the extraordinary body. There would be a whole lot else: her first *Vogue* cover, by Richard Avedon (about as high an accolade for a first-timer as you can get), the first of 15 American *Vogue* covers alone; the marriage to Richard Gere and that full-page 'personal statement' *Times* ad; the shoot for *Playboy* with Herb Ritts ('I want to reach a different audience. Let's face it, most college guys don't buy *Vogue*'); the *House of Style* hostessing for MTV; George Michael's 'Freedom '90' promo video; even a foray into films, although her lead role in *Fair Game* (1995) was underwhelming ('I cringed through the whole thing,' she admitted).

Balanced against the latter, a rare high-profile disappointment, was a continuing fascination with, in her own words, her 'clean, approachable, fairytale image', which led to diversification and the mini-industry known popularly as Cindy Inc. Cindy knows that Cindy sells – the $7 million Revlon campaigns, the Pepsi ads, the exercise videos, the celebrity endorsements and, of course, the obligatory calendars (the proceeds of which go to leukaemia research).

'As a model, I see myself as a product,' she told *Vogue*, 'so I can decide how and when to sell the Cindy Crawford product. It helps me stay grounded. It sounds cold, but I don't think it is. It's a business...' Naturally, it wouldn't work for anyone if Cindy obliged with a cigarettes or beer ad, though it would certainly capture attention. 'It wouldn't make sense,' she says. 'I understand what the entity ["Cindy Crawford"] represents.' Neither, less obviously, would a Cindy doll: 'I kept seeing the promotional picture of me holding a doll dressed in exactly the same clothes as I was wearing. That picture would speak a thousand words – and they're not the thousand words I want spoken...'

Cindy Crawford (b. 1966, USA)

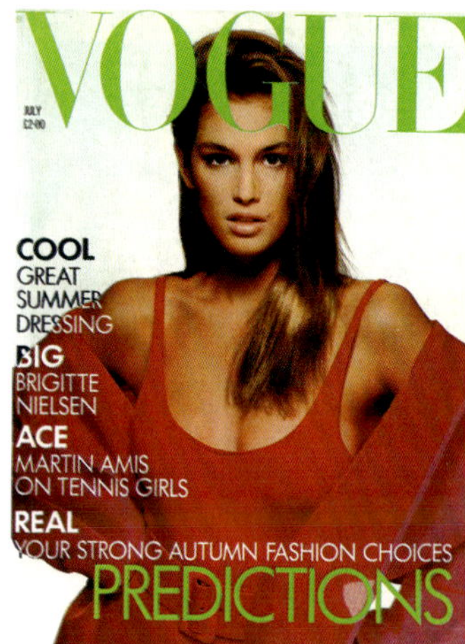

Above: 'Predictions', July 1988, by Patrick Demarchelier. Fashion by Giorgio di Sant'Angelo

Opposite: 'Double Agents', January 1990, by Patrick Demarchelier. Fashion by Norma Kamali

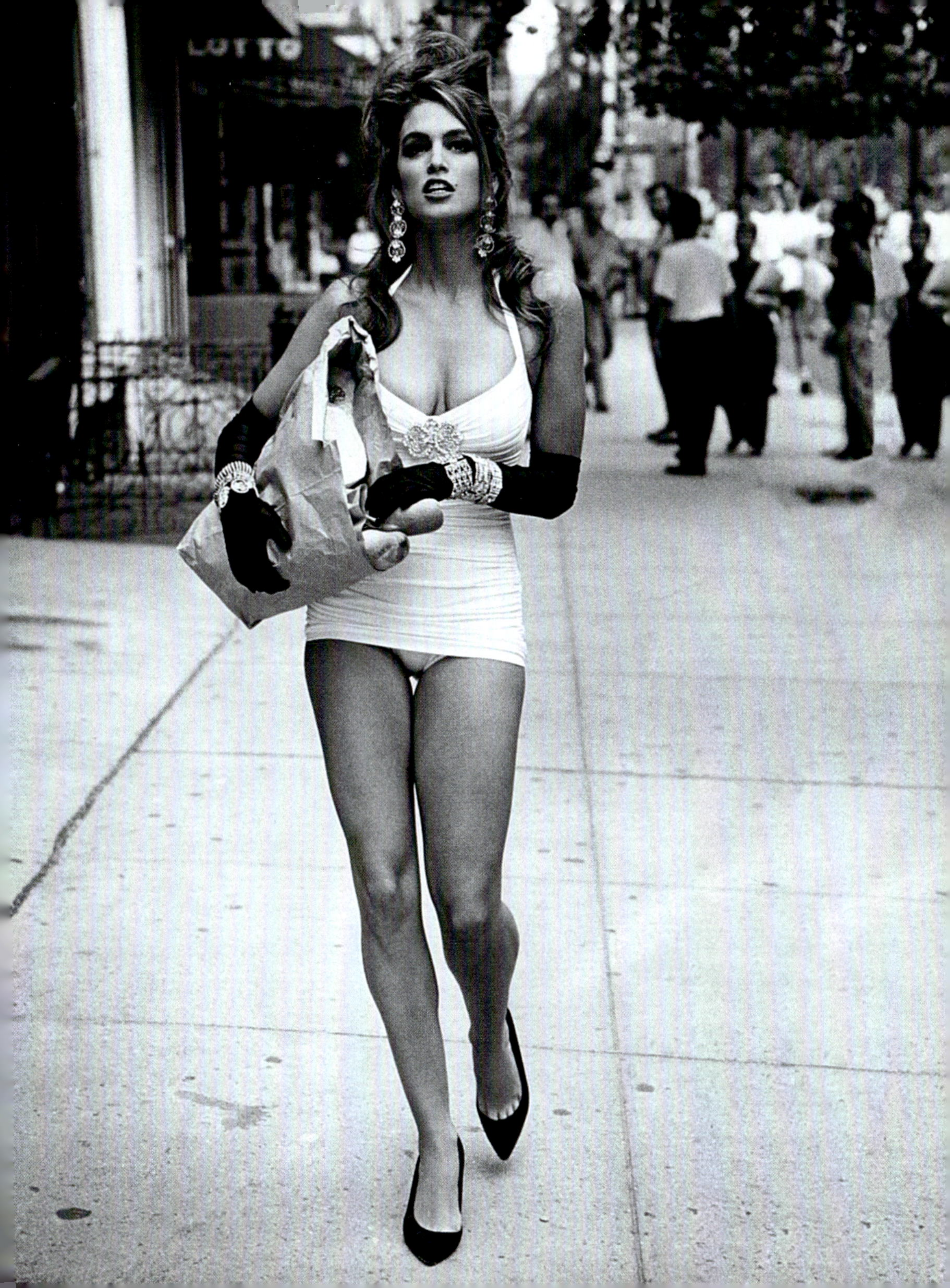

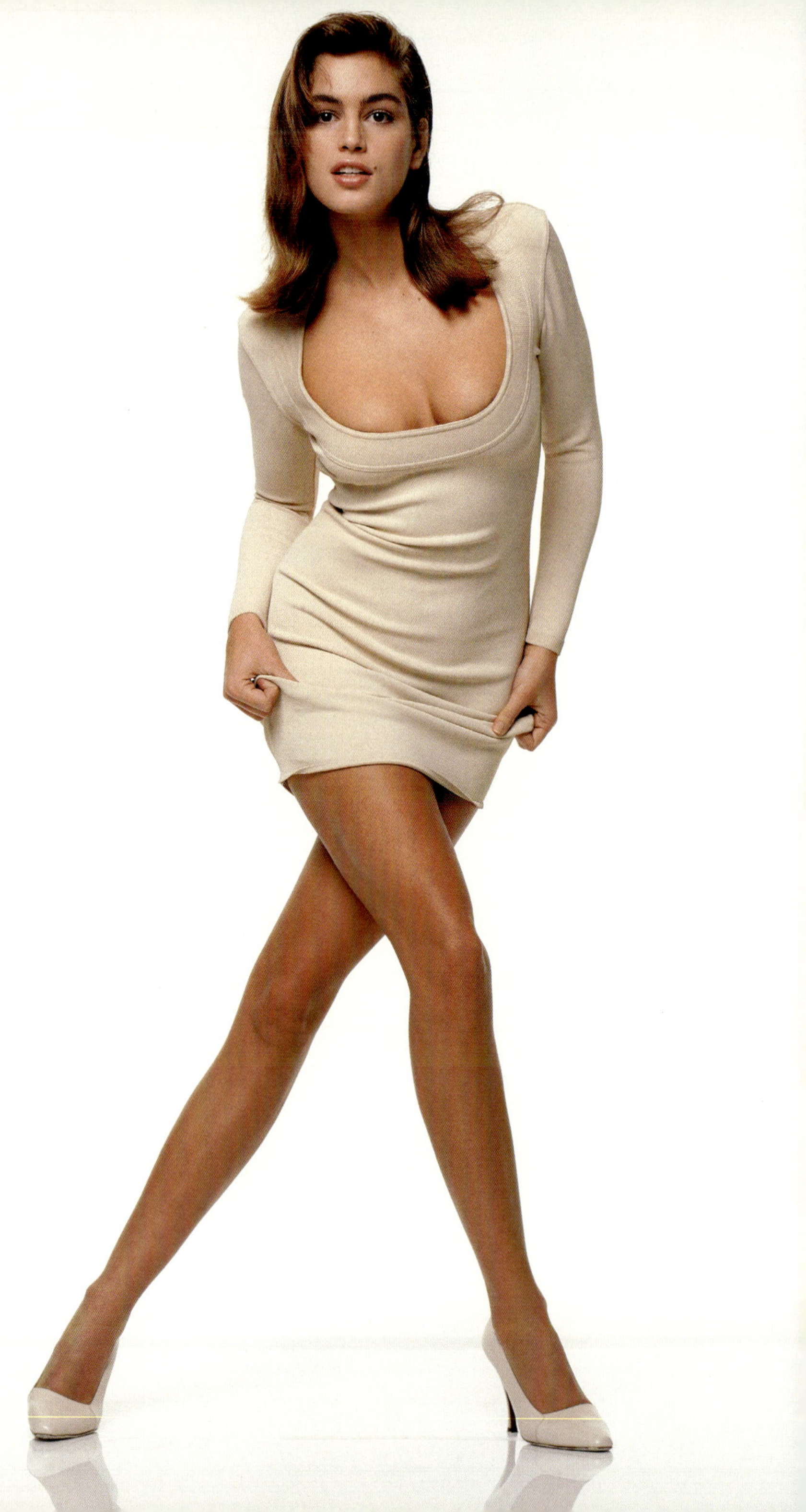

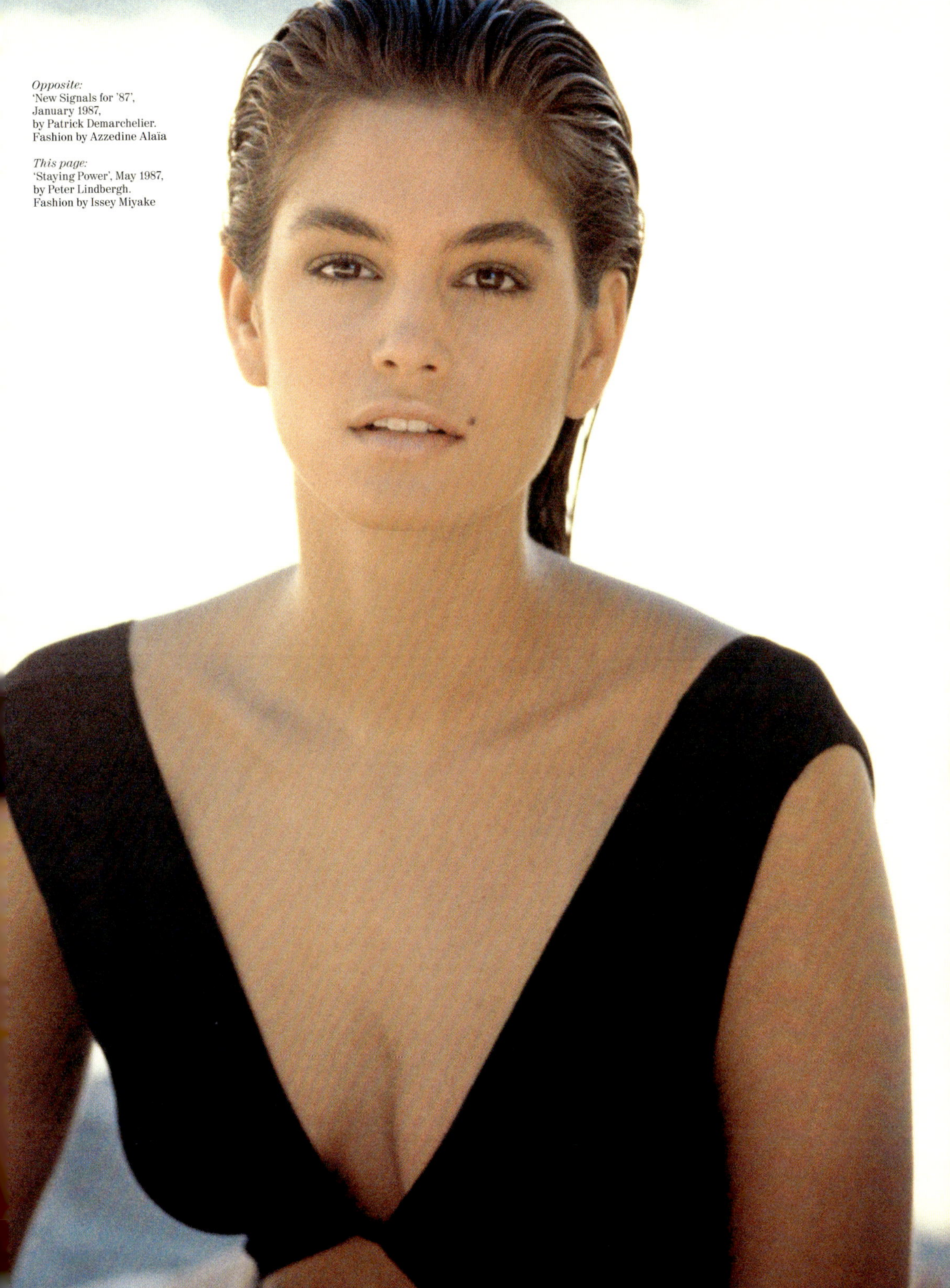

Opposite:
'New Signals for '87',
January 1987,
by Patrick Demarchelier.
Fashion by Azzedine Alaïa

This page:
'Staying Power', May 1987,
by Peter Lindbergh.
Fashion by Issey Miyake

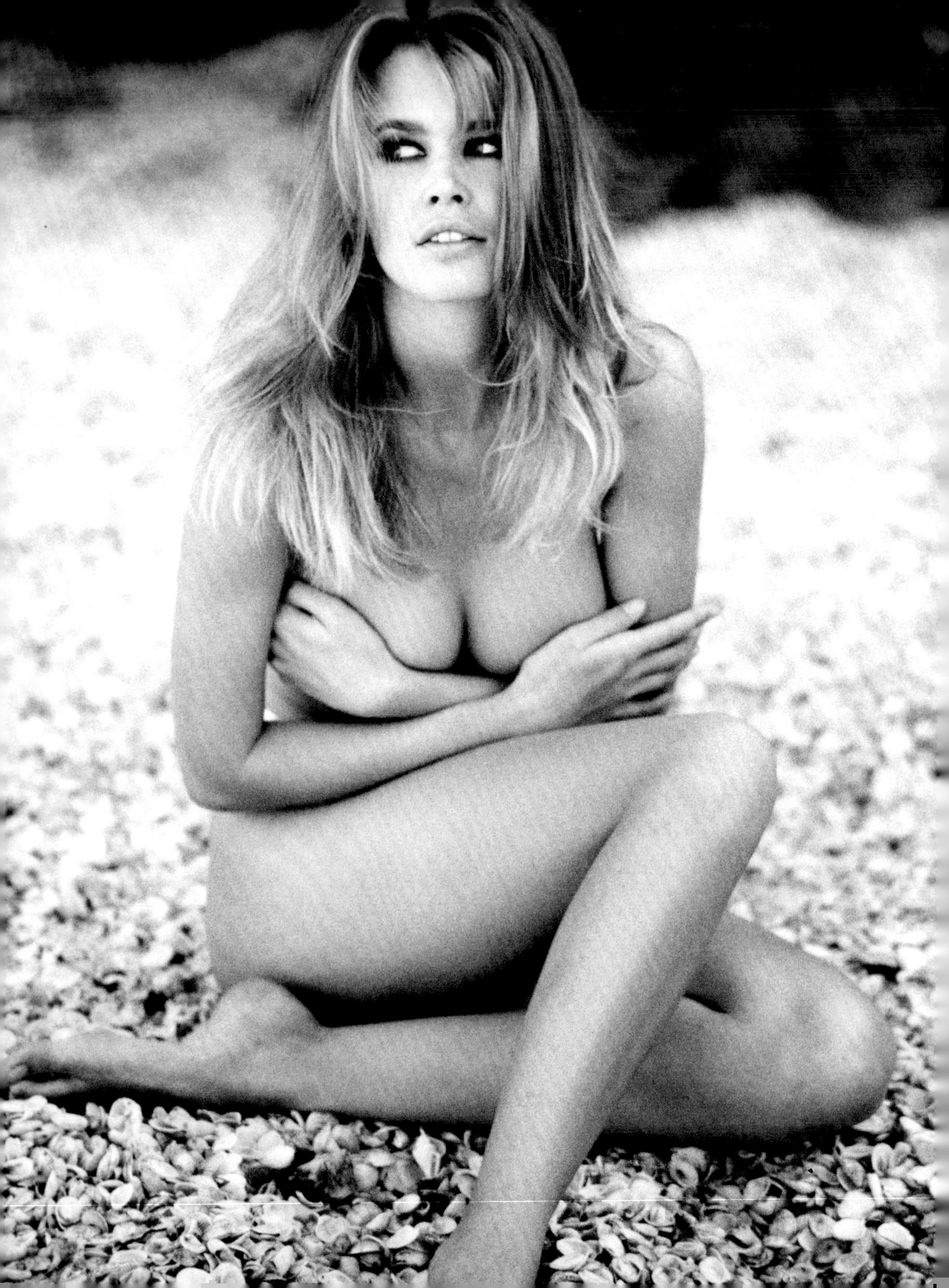

Claudia Schiffer

'She's more like a movie star than a model', said photographer Arthur Elgort of the statuesque (5ft 11in), Bardot-like (36-24-36) German model with the commanding presence. 'Strangers will approach Claudia on the street for autographs – once on location I couldn't believe the lines at our table while we were eating. She just smiles and signs.'

One of the most recognisable models of the 1990s, Schiffer epitomised just how much of a rival to movie stardom modelling might be. She was estimated by *Forbes* magazine to be the richest model as the new millennium loomed. Initially, this had much to do with campaigns for Guess jeans, which, when they propelled both model and product firmly into the popular consciousness, became increasingly lucrative; there was also a $10 million, three-year deal with Revlon and, most prestigious of all perhaps, she was the face of Chanel when times were exceptionally buoyant.

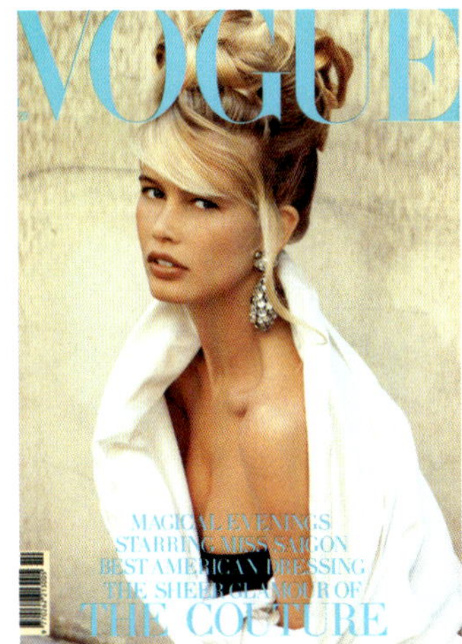

Dissenting a little from Arthur Elgort, Karl Lagerfeld refuted any comparisons: 'When she started, people thought she was a kind of new Bardot. In fact she was not. I have always thought she was very different from any other girl. She had, and still has, a unique *éclat*, as the French say…' Lagerfeld had persuaded her on to the catwalk in 1990: 'The press went wild because I was this new thing,' she told *Vogue*, 'and I had the craziest walk you had ever seen...' It was not so peculiar as to inhibit a fee of $30,000 per appearance.

The looks, the productivity rate, the 'hip-swaggering, seductive prowl' (in *Vogue*'s words) – all conspired to raise her to supermodel status. This accelerated considerably when she realised the power of abstinence and a stellar fee. 'A supermodel was a status symbol,' she explained. 'If designers couldn't afford all of us, or even one of us, it meant they didn't have a big enough budget.'

There is something of the Mittel-European romance about the beginning of the story. Schiffer was born in Westphalia into wealth and privilege. 'It all fell out of the sky,' she told American *Vogue*. 'I was in high school in Rheinberg, the typical sort of shy well-behaved child. My afternoons were busy with tennis, piano, ballet. My girlfriends and I did not even look at fashion magazines. I was the sort of girl who blushed when the teacher spoke to me.' An outing to a Düsseldorf discotheque led to her discovery by a talent scout, and some test shots were made: 'I was sure that they would realise they had made a mistake and send me back.' They hadn't, and she was on her way to Paris; in an embarrassingly short time she had been plucked by Karl Lagerfeld to be his latest muse.

A fearsome work ethic has kept Claudia in the spotlight for nearly 25 years (she has been the spokesperson of cosmetics giant L'Oréal for roughly half of them). She balances that with her charity commitments – she is a Unicef ambassador – and her domestic life. This threatens, at first glance, to spiral into unruliness: she has three children, homes in Notting Hill and Suffolk, three dogs, two sheep, four chickens, a pig and piglets, two more smaller pigs, two swans (black), four ducks, three tortoises and a parrot. Apart from prolonging the fairytale leitmotiv (it gets more romantic – one of the tortoises was an alternative to an engagement ring), the menagerie is the product of an ever-inquiring mind: 'I always dreamed that one day I would like a farm with lots of animals, so I thought I'd get little amounts of each and find out how it works…'

Her commendable Teutonic stoicism and self-control keep it in all in check. With a line of Schiffer products on the horizon, Claudia's earning power fails to diminish in the slightest. And when not pregnant, clearly, the capacity for hard work kicks in time and again. For Yves Saint Laurent's spring/summer '09 campaign, she was required to abseil down the Hollywood Hills and disport herself on a narrow plinth. About this she was creditably equanimous: 'It was about 100°F and I was balanced on a high box, with huge heels… It was pretty unnerving; if the whole thing had collapsed, I would have been thrown down the cliff, finished.'

Claudia Schiffer (b. 1970, West Germany)

Opposite:
'St Barts', May 1991 (unpublished), by Patrick Demarchelier

Above:
'The Couture', October 1989, by Herb Ritts. Fashion by Yves Saint Laurent

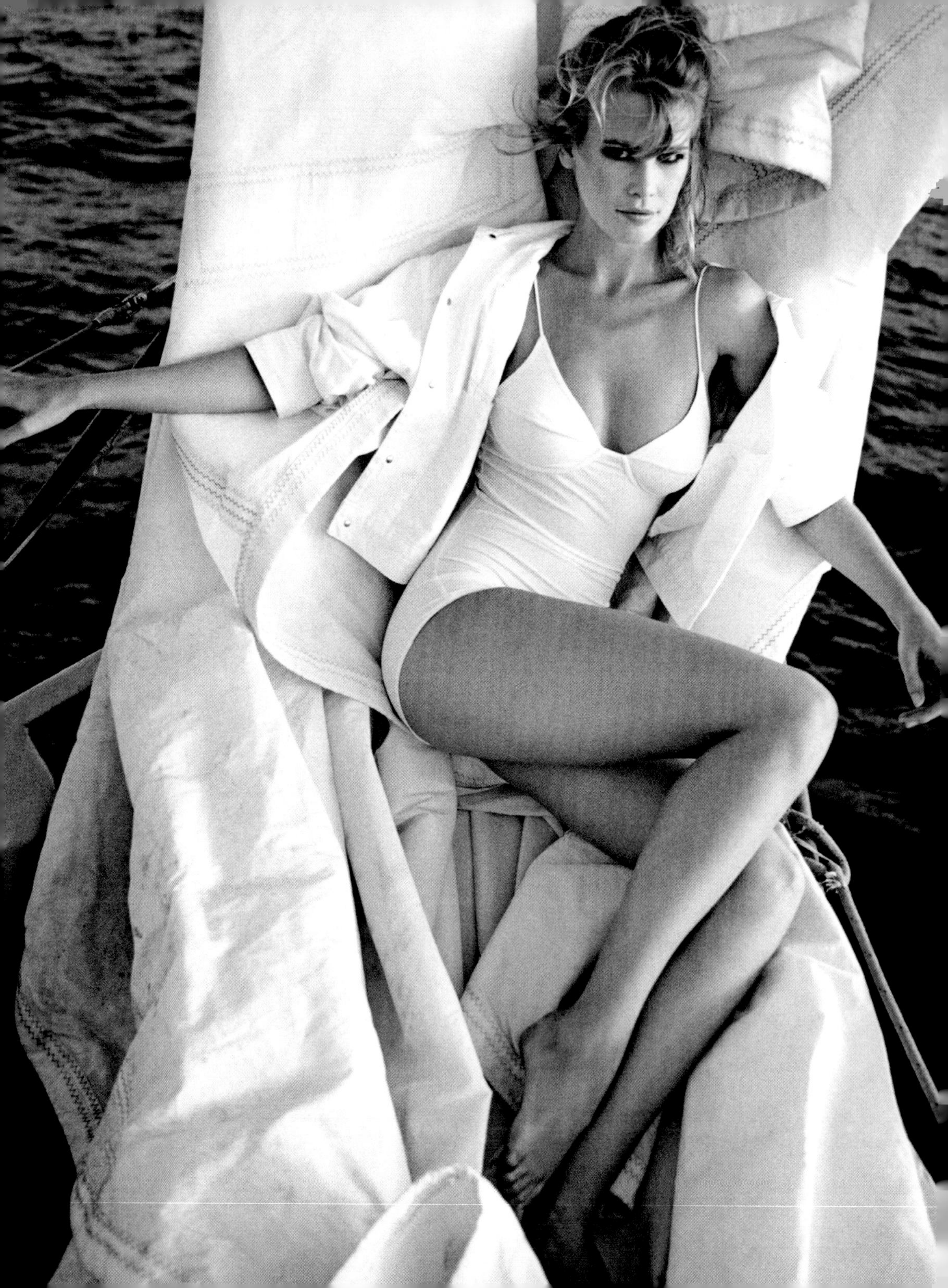

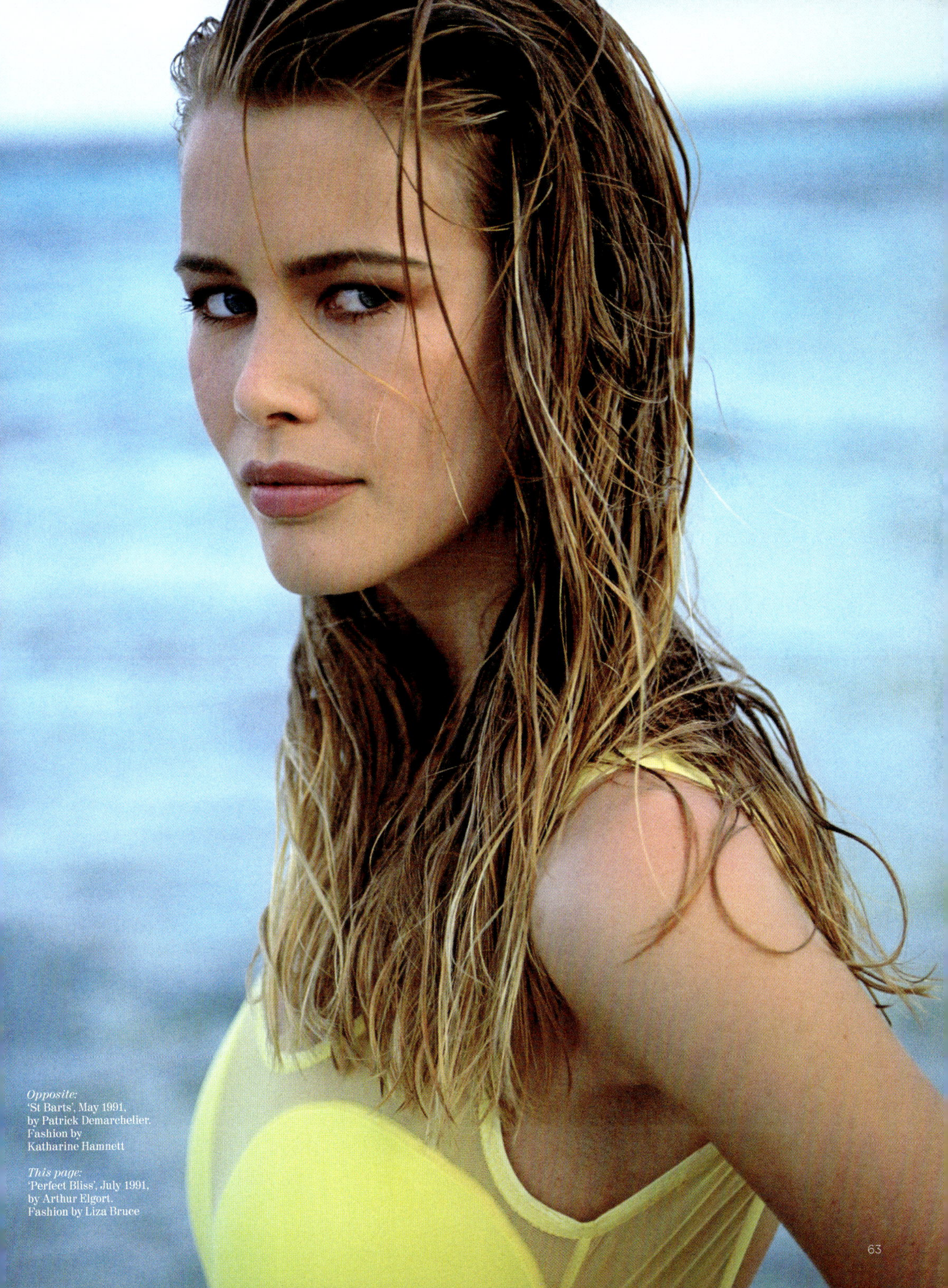

Opposite:
'St Barts', May 1991,
by Patrick Demarchelier.
Fashion by
Katharine Hamnett

This page:
'Perfect Bliss', July 1991,
by Arthur Elgort.
Fashion by Liza Bruce

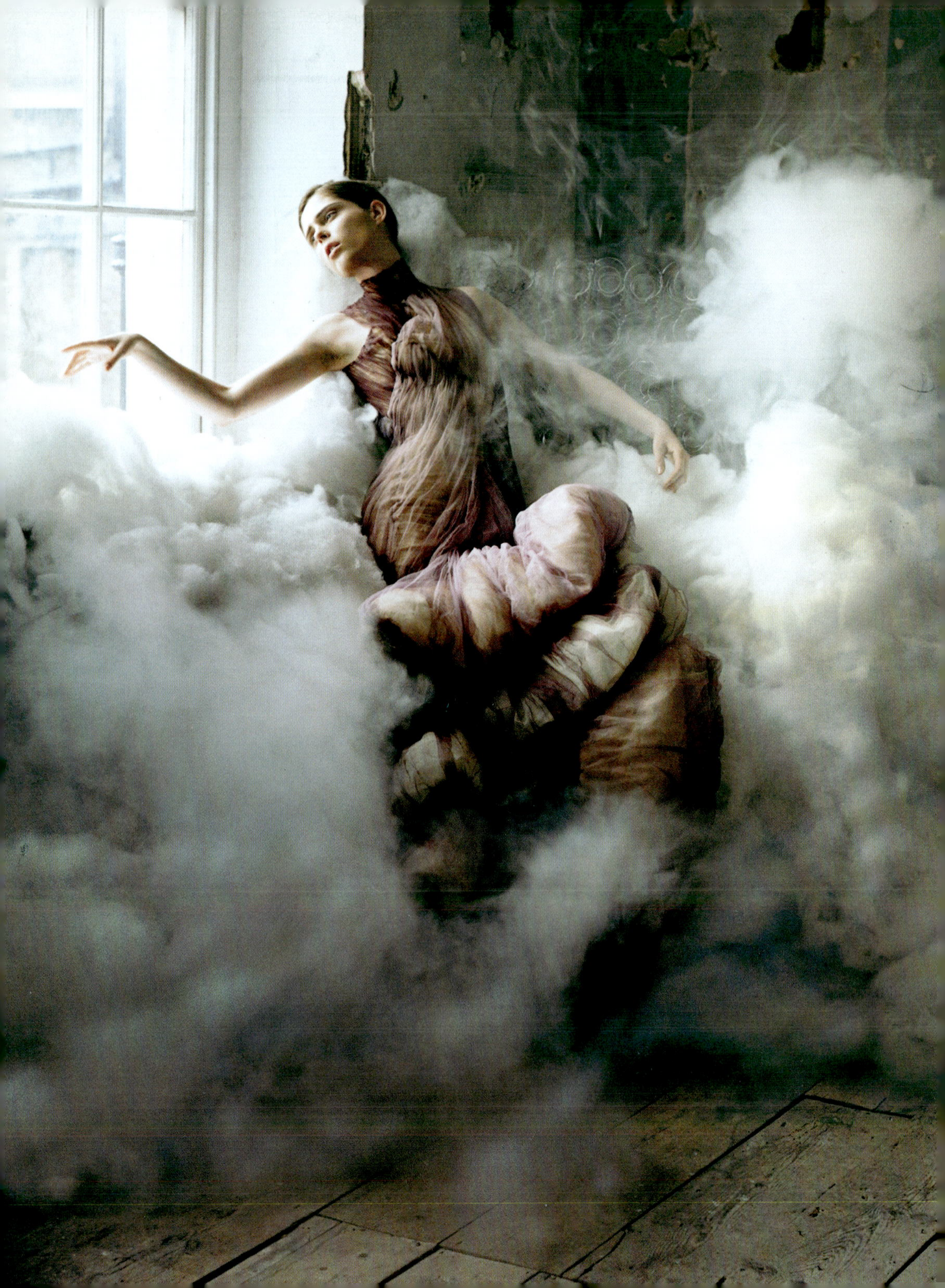

Coco Rocha

What has gone down in fashion history as 'the Coco moment' occurred at the autumn/winter shows in 2007. Clad in a red jacket, tartan skirt and a head decoration of plumed feathers – it was a Jean Paul Gaultier paean to Scotland and the Highland tradition – the model Coco Rocha high-stepped, jigged and Riverdanced her way down the catwalk. The applause was fervent, the reception ecstatic, the collection a hit. And the cult of a new personality formed. At that moment, wise fashion minds concurred, they might just be missing the era of the supermodel, the personalities, the big number.

Coco is of Irish, Russian and Welsh-Canadian descent (and the first portion must have been the most decent-sized, viz the Celtic toe-tapping). In fact, she was first noticed by a modelling agent at an Irish-dance competition in Vancouver. She was 14 and very good at it (she'd been jigging and stomping all over her native Canada and then on to Switzerland) and had not given modelling a second thought. She did, though, when the agent, shrewd and determined, dogged her every move. She gave in. 'They had to teach me from the ground up,' she told American *Vogue*. 'I was not raised thinking about Dolce & Gabbana, Gucci, Dior…' Similarly Steven Meisel and Anna Wintour: 'No clue who he was. Never heard of her. Now I know. Now it's my life…' Meisel in turn had not – understandably – heard of Coco Rocha from Toronto, but 'I just saw this little Polaroid and thought, this face is for me!'

If she wasn't one of the world's greatest models, she says she would 'probably be teaching kids how to do Irish dance'. The dancing betrays a physical edge to Coco's world. Off-duty and away from the seething hothouse of her everyday world, she loves to take trips that challenge her (such as to Botswana or Namibia). This is tempered by a streak of practicality: 'If I had to do something daring like sailing a boat or climbing Mount Everest, I would want to take along someone athletic, like David Beckham.'

Not, of course, that her day job is without its perils. Starring in one of Tim Walker's elaborate *mise-en-scènes*, a large-scale production based on Surrealism's first wave – Dalíesque melting watches, Magritte *trompe-l'oeil*, lobster telephones – she was required to put herself into a fictive world. Setting Coco's hair alight was vetoed at an earlier stage, though one got the impression it was for aesthetic reasons rather than a question mark over her fire-retardancy. As professional fire-raisers set to work, Tim shouted over his shoulder 'Nice knowing you', as a tuba ignited right beside the model of the moment.

Vogue divined early on that she had the fierceness of spirit for just such challenges and an innocence that made it all work beautifully: 'Porcelain skin and an "old soul" mien are the hallmarks of Coco.' The magazine was on standby when she dyed her hair red, having taken advice from style counsellor Steven Meisel. The fashion world's most illustrious redhead, Grace Coddington, approved: 'People don't book her [Coco] as a classic beauty, because that is not her strength. You book her because you love her, and she can do something strong and bold and it will always look good. She could go green and she'd look great.'

Until green day arrives, Rocha will continue to be confoundingly contrary, impossible to pin down, so *de nos jours*: spiky, innocent, kittenish, gothic, surreal, down to earth.

Coco Rocha (b. Mikhaila Rocha, 1988, Canada)

Left:
'Curiouser and Curiouser',
February 2007,
by Tim Walker.
Fashion by
Alexander McQueen

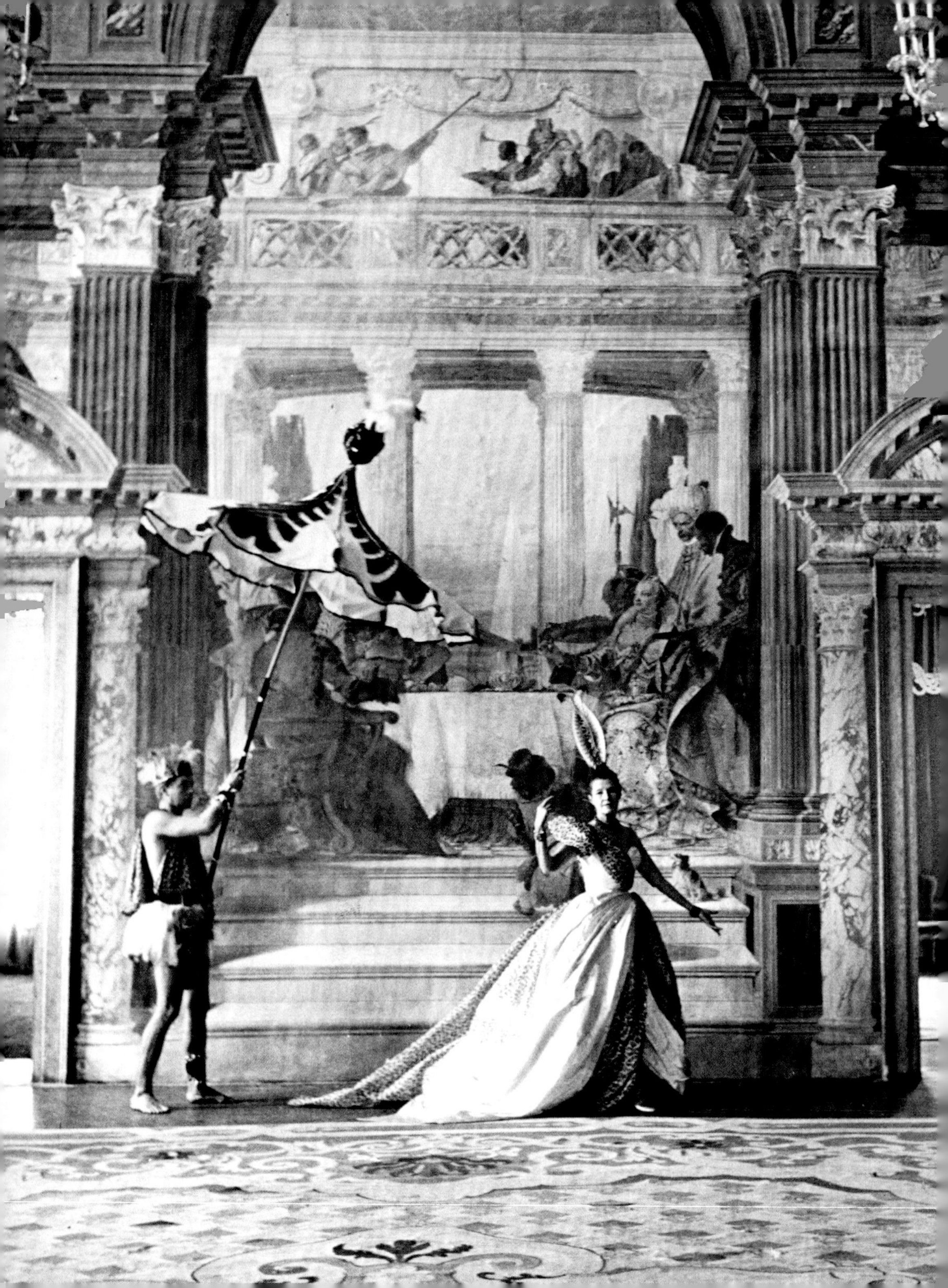

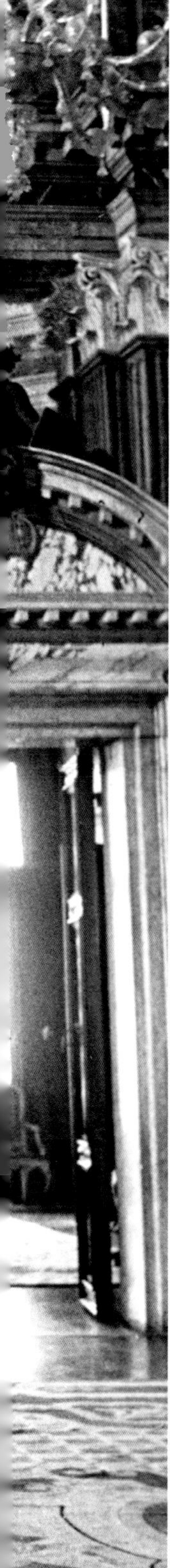

Daisy Fellowes

She had the air of having just disembarked from a yacht, one observer noted, adding 'which she very likely had'. Rich and soignée, half-French and half-American (either of which she played up if the occasion demanded), the Hon Mrs Reginald Fellowes was considered the best-dressed woman in the world. That might have implied frequent changes of wardrobe, but in fact the title was hers on account of a rigorous simplicity of style. This extended to her *après-bain* wear, a Cellophane cape, which she wore with outsize jewellery, and a sequined coat cut like a man's smoking jacket. The latter she wore, said Cecil Beaton in admiration, 'with audacity and a green carnation sprouting from the buttonhole, until indeed she wore it out.'

'Whatever she wore, she wore conspicuously. She created dramas wherever she went to stave off boredom and she cared not a whit what anyone thought of her, as long as they thought something,' observed *Vogue*'s Bettina Ballard. Daisy was herself a direct influence on the fashion scene as an unignorable, Paris-based editor-at-large for *Vogue*: 'Here Mrs Fellowes shows her approval of the feather-boa revival…' She was an early champion of Elsa Schiaparelli.

She went to great lengths to combat ennui, enjoying her friends' discomfort by wearing plain silk shifts when everyone else had overdone it. Her restraint made other women appear overdressed, garish and faintly ridiculous. No-one, thought Diana Vreeland, could be that beautiful without making a pact with the devil – she had, the doyenne of fashion continued, 'the elegance of the damned'.

Fellowes was a legendary hostess, although a low boredom threshold occasionally led to her hospitality taking on a macabre twist. For one dinner party, she invited all her worst enemies – together with the worst enemies of those worst enemies – and, as the photographer Horst recalled it, 'treated them to a dinner of sausages and sauerkraut'. Horst also recalled her wit, which was no less devastating for being delivered in a curiously thin and high-pitched voice. One admirer likened it to the tinkling of 'a little porcelain temple bell'.

She cultivated eccentricities, such as crossing herself each time she passed an advertisement for Singer sewing machines, the source of her earliest fortune. When there was someone else in her favourite cinema seat, she simply sat on top of him.

Daisy was born Marguerite Decazes de Glücksbierg, heiress to the Singer fortune, in 1890 (officially). As a young lady of striking beauty, she was sketched by John Singer Sargent, a likely kinsman. Thereafter, two generations of *Vogue* photographers took her likeness: Adolph de Meyer, Cecil Beaton, George Hoyningen-Huene and Edward Steichen, as well as Horst, Wladimir Rehbinder and Havrah of Paris. Her first and brief marriage to Jean, Prince de Broglie, propelled her into the society pages. Her second, in 1919 – to Reginald Fellowes, a financier and cousin of Winston Churchill – propelled her further. *Vogue* approved of his pedigree: 'The Hon Mrs Fellowes is the wife of the son of the Lord de Ramsey.' As the 1920s turned into the 1930s, the magazine's devotion to its latest ornament was unswerving. 'The Hon Mrs Reginald Fellowes is the embodiment of the 20th century in the variety of her interests. She is a noted hostess, sportswoman and author. Mrs Fellowes's first book, published recently, is called *Cats of the Isle of Man*.'

Thereafter she enjoyed a long life and a considerable fortune and many appearances in *Vogue*. 'Like most genuinely witty commentators on the human condition,' ran the magazine's 1962 obituary, 'she had a relentless eye for the silly, the pretentious or the incongruous in conduct.' It concluded, 'the world in which she habitually moved provided an ample range of specimens of these.'

Daisy Fellowes (b. Marguerite Decazes de Glücksbierg, 1890, France; d. 1962)

Left:
'Ball in Venice', November 1951, by Cecil Beaton

Daria Werbowy

Clearly at US *Vogue* no superlative is superlative enough when it comes to Ukrainian-Canadian Daria Werbowy (it means 'willow' in Ukrainian): she is 'a model of scorching sexiness and the supreme avatar of tawny-limbed fashion desires'. Nor for *Glamour*: 'Right now, supers don't get hotter than Daria…' In her, and *consoeurs* such as Lily Donaldson and Karlie Kloss, the magazine identified a prevailing trend, one which designer Alexander Wang called 'model off-duty'. That is to say that the personal style of models as they dress for themselves – individualistic, idiosyncratic, occasionally unique – is as momentous as the creations they disport on the catwalk.

After several false starts – not least the ill-fortune of her being booked for the first time as an adult for half a dozen New York fashion shows in the week of September 11, 2001 – her rise was irresistible; years, she told one interviewer, of 'non-stop travelling, waking up in places and not knowing where I was.'

Steven Meisel, for whom she worked on the Prada campaigns and Italian *Vogue* covers (a modelling rite of passage), propelled her into the stratosphere. 'Sometimes I might just stand in a certain way and Steven will refine the pose. Other times he'll want you to do nothing and he'll direct you on the tiniest thing: where you're looking, giving the hint of a smile…' She was also the subject of Helmut Newton's last fashion sitting for *Vogue*. She described the experience as 'an honour, as it is rare to get the chance to do stories with a deeper meaning'. While the meaning remains oblique – and the maestro is not here to fully explain it – Daria recalled 'he made me wear rubber nipples and had me lying on a bed of nails and eating grass with a fork. It was all really… *grrr*!'

By 2009, as *Forbes* magazine pointed out, she was the eighth richest model in the world, with annual earnings of $4.5 million and rising. She has been the face of Gucci, of Lancôme's Hypnose perfume, and occasionally of Prada fragrance (and the subject of its meditative, jazz-inflected, Ridley Scott-directed ad). For several years, she opened the most catwalk shows in one season. This is, in modelling terms, a mark of great achievement.

Known as something of a tomboy, a notion that her lithe 5ft 11in frame does little to deter, she was a disciplined rugby player at school, excelled on the basketball court and is an accomplished sailor and snowboarder. (She was thrilled to be photographed for *Vogue*, in a midnight Alexander McQueen ballgown, alongside Olympic gold medallist Shaun White.) She also affects a sportif and perceptibly masculine off-duty wardrobe: she likes boys' Levi's and leather jackets, and loves hoodies. 'Plain. Gap. Men's. Always with a double-layered hood,' she told *Vogue*. Why? ''Cause they stay on your head!'

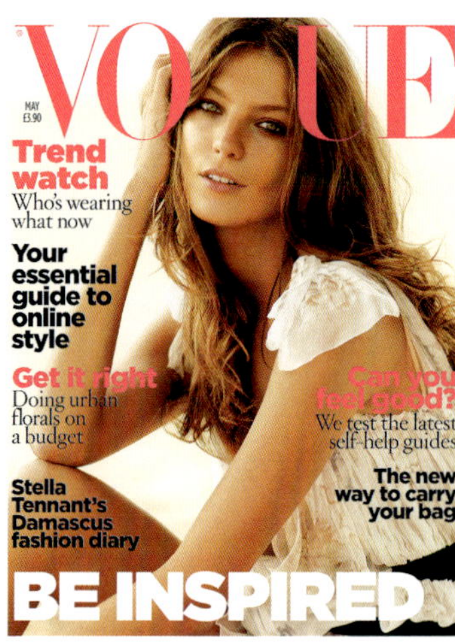

Her beauty is enhanced by an unaffected thoughtfulness and a down-to-earth practicality: 'A few years ago, my luggage got lost and I had no clothes for five days during Milan Fashion Week, so Burberry gave me a trench and a bag and I still wear both.' She is determinedly unstarry, unmoved by the absurdities, let alone the trappings, of supermodeldom (a Burberry trench and bag don't count) and cannot begin to analyse her allure. 'If I did,' she said, 'I'd be in a straitjacket.' Helping preserve her sanity, *Vogue* did it for her: 'Those eyes. That range.'

Daria Werbowy (b. 1983, Poland)

Above:
'Be Inspired', May 2009, by Mario Testino. Fashion by Christian Lacroix

Opposite:
'Spring Forward', February 2008, by Patrick Demarchelier. Fashion by Chanel

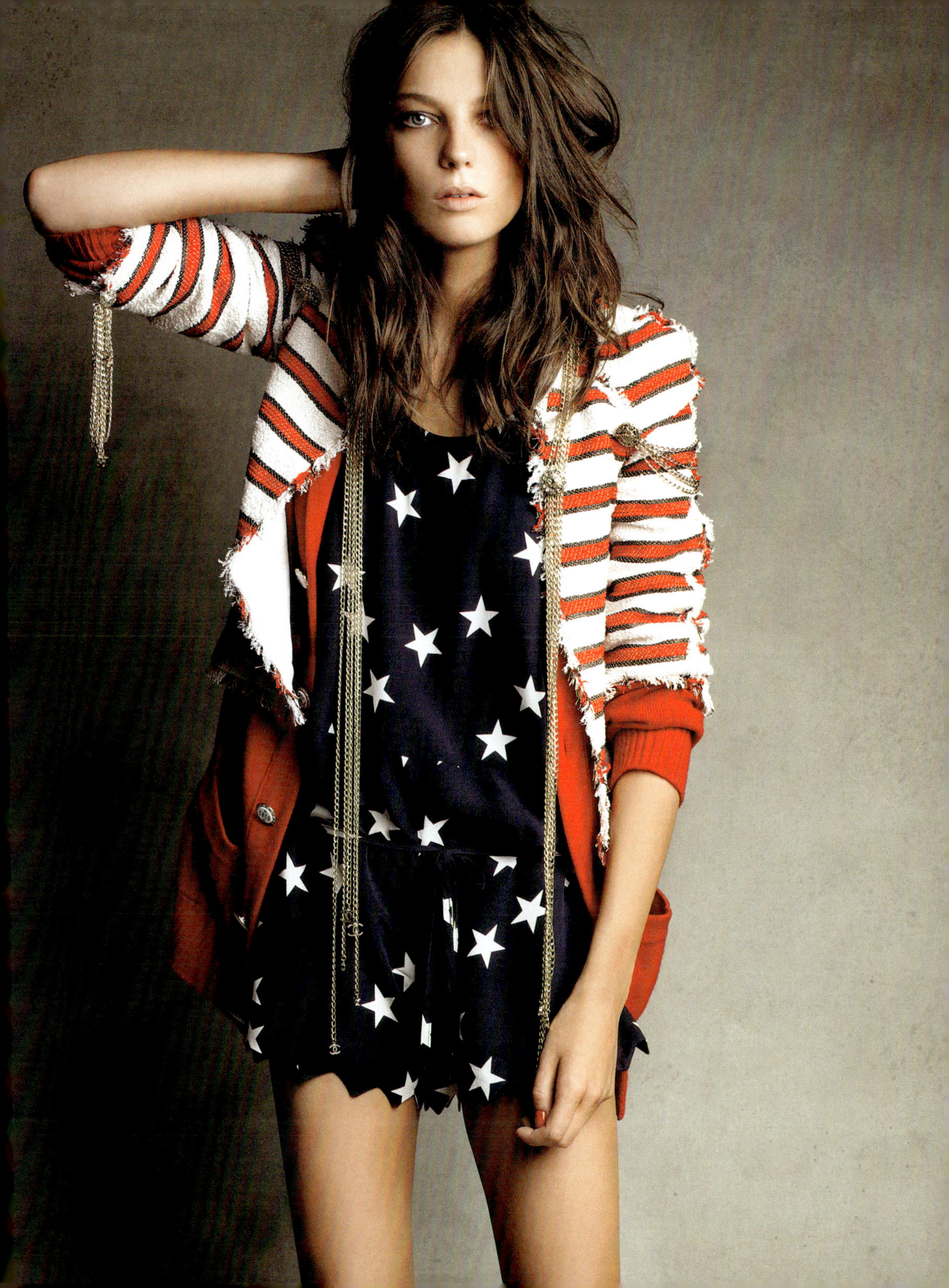

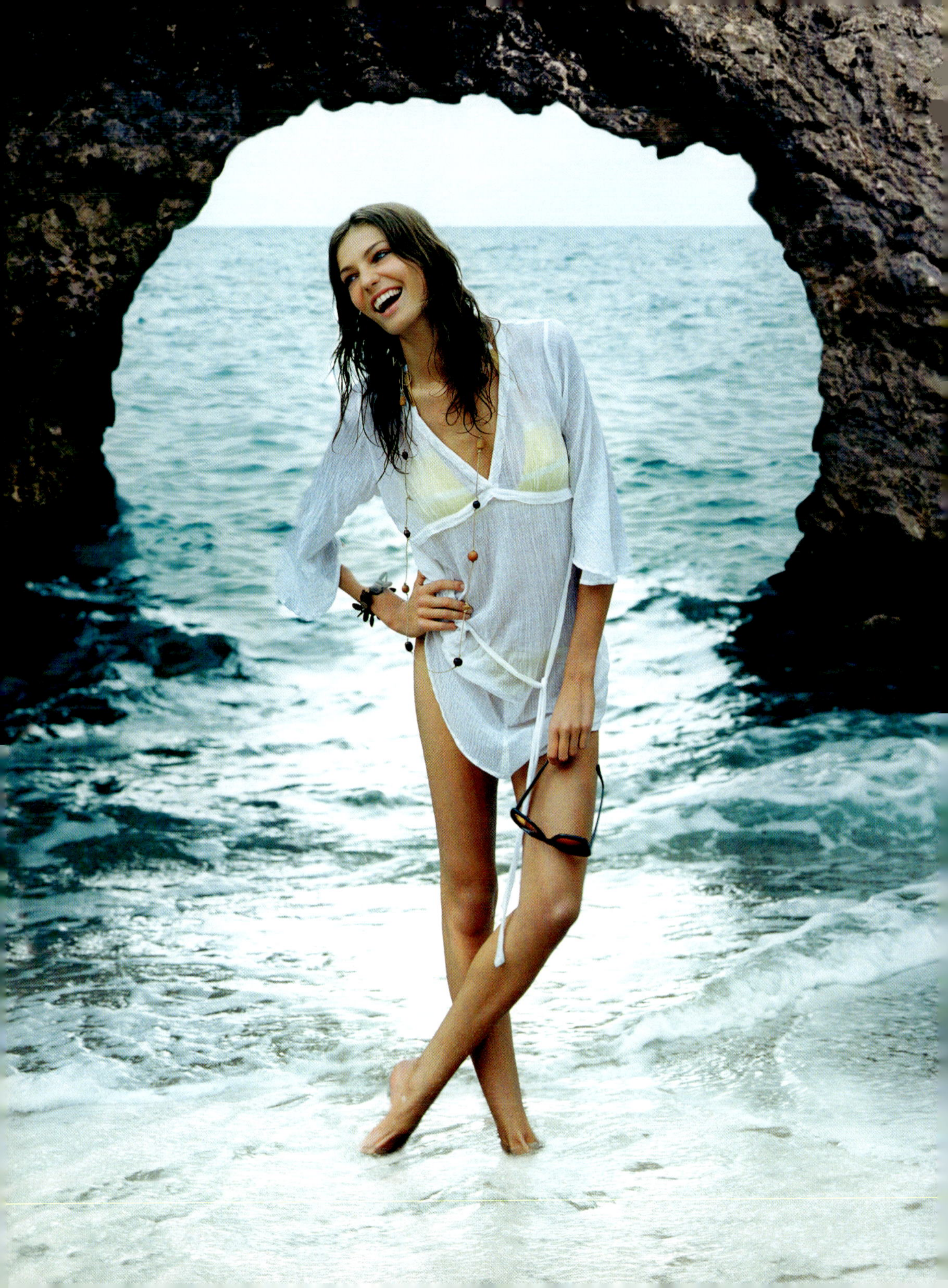

Opposite:
'Summer Days',
July 2004, by Corinne Day.
Fashion by Melissa Odabash

This page:
'True Romance', May 2007,
by Paolo Roversi.
Fashion by Gardem

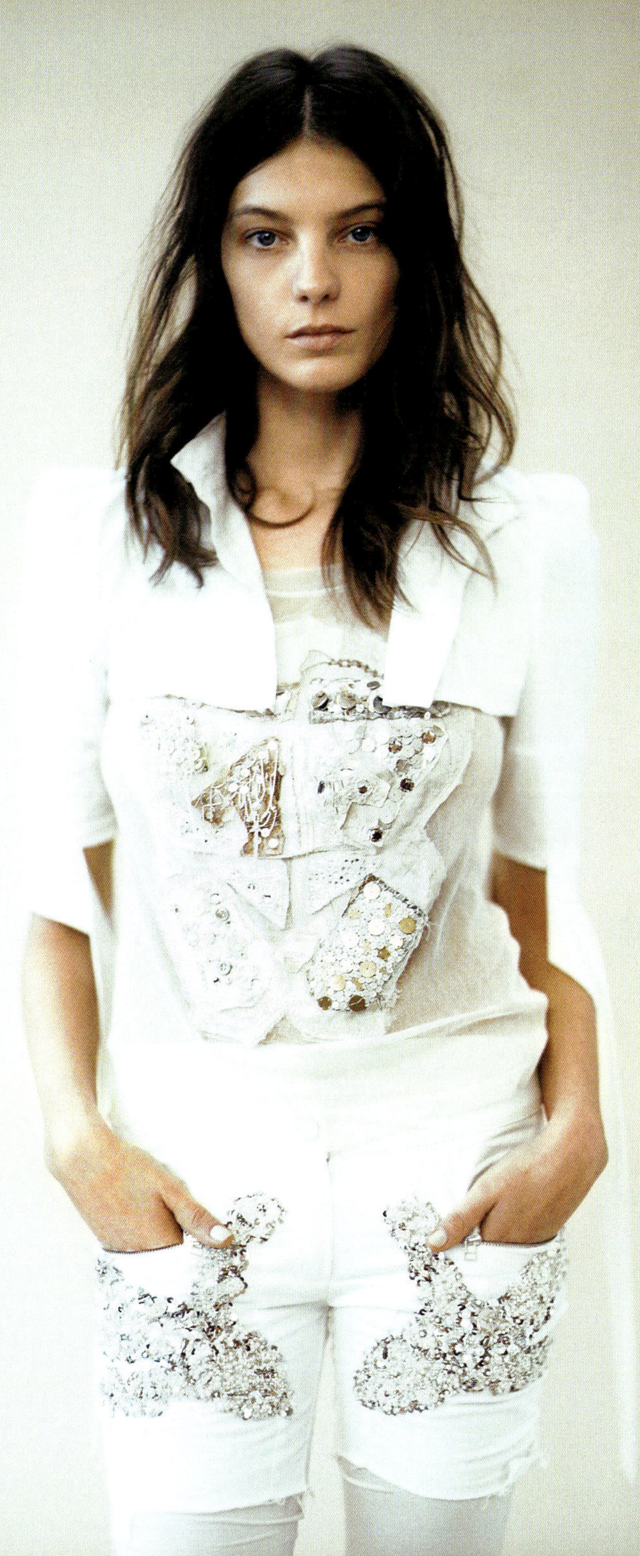

Della Oake

Fortunately, Della Oake's modelling career was more successful than her first love, the stage. Fortunately again, Cecil Beaton, whose first love was film, ventured backstage, star-spotting, on a visit to Shepperton Studios. 'I noticed a picture of misery sitting on a packing case,' he recalled. 'She was wearing tawdry finery supplied by wardrobe and a tired cotton camellia on her partly dyed head. I realised this extra had something "extra".' This indeed proved so. In London, Paris and New York, Della Oake gave 'a refinement and delicacy to every garment she wore, until she was claimed in marriage by an American tycoon'.

Beaton, as he showed, was entranced and showcased her fragile, thin-as-a-sparrow looks whenever he could. A memorable Christmas cover saw her wrapped up in a generous red bow. He also arranged her in several of his 'chamber pieces', by which he meant romantic, often ballroom settings with deep-pelmeted curtains and several models doing very little but disporting themselves elegantly. Miss Oake's laughter – she tinkled like a mountain brook in spate – and her primness hid a mischievous sense of humour and belied any frosty appearance (*de rigueur* for the times). Henry Clarke considered her a treasure and she would get the pick of the Paris collections over Bettina Graziani or Fiona Campbell-Walter, higher up the pecking order, or even Dovima, who was considered the *ne plus ultra*. She was, as Clarke clearly noticed, a couturier's dream (Balenciaga's especially) in puffed-out sleeves and a tightly cinched waist.

Miss Oake could reprise any role: soignée outside the Savoy in one-shouldered shantung; demure in a frosted gossamer tulle and lace ballgown at Versailles; elegant in a giant-balloon-cuffed Balenciaga afternoon suit, which would have defeated less confident mannequins. She was a great favourite of the perennially 'difficult' American photographer Clifford Coffin (who adored her English Rose appeal), and was there at his famous Stonehenge fashion shoot. This was aborted when he declared that the standing stones were not big enough and the wrong colour, and he was observed kicking them in disgust before heading back to London.

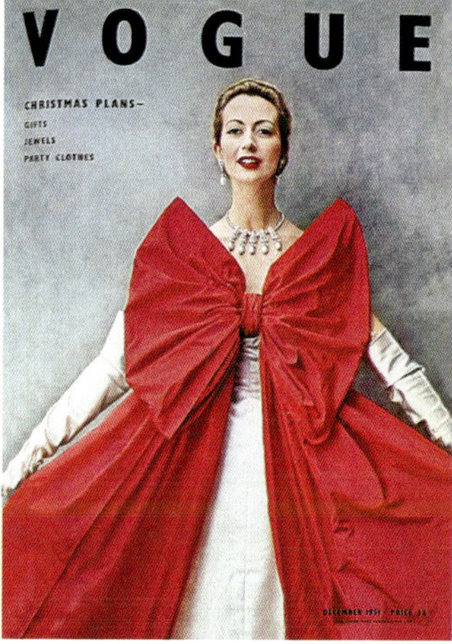

She modelled for Beaton, Clarke and Norman Parkinson with less fuss. Especially the latter, of whom she had happy memories. 'I remember one wonderful shoot – he had me running down the drive of a derelict mansion in a thunderstorm… I loved going on location with him. He made such funny remarks while driving. He thought "Stockbroker Tudor" was rather *déclassé* as we passed it by, forgetting we were in a rather ostentatious 1939 Cadillac from the United States…'

Della Oake (fl. 1946–56)

Above:
'Christmas Plans', December 1951, by Cecil Beaton. Fashion by Balenciaga

Opposite:
'Romantic Quality', February 1951, by Norman Parkinson. Fashion by Norman Hartnell

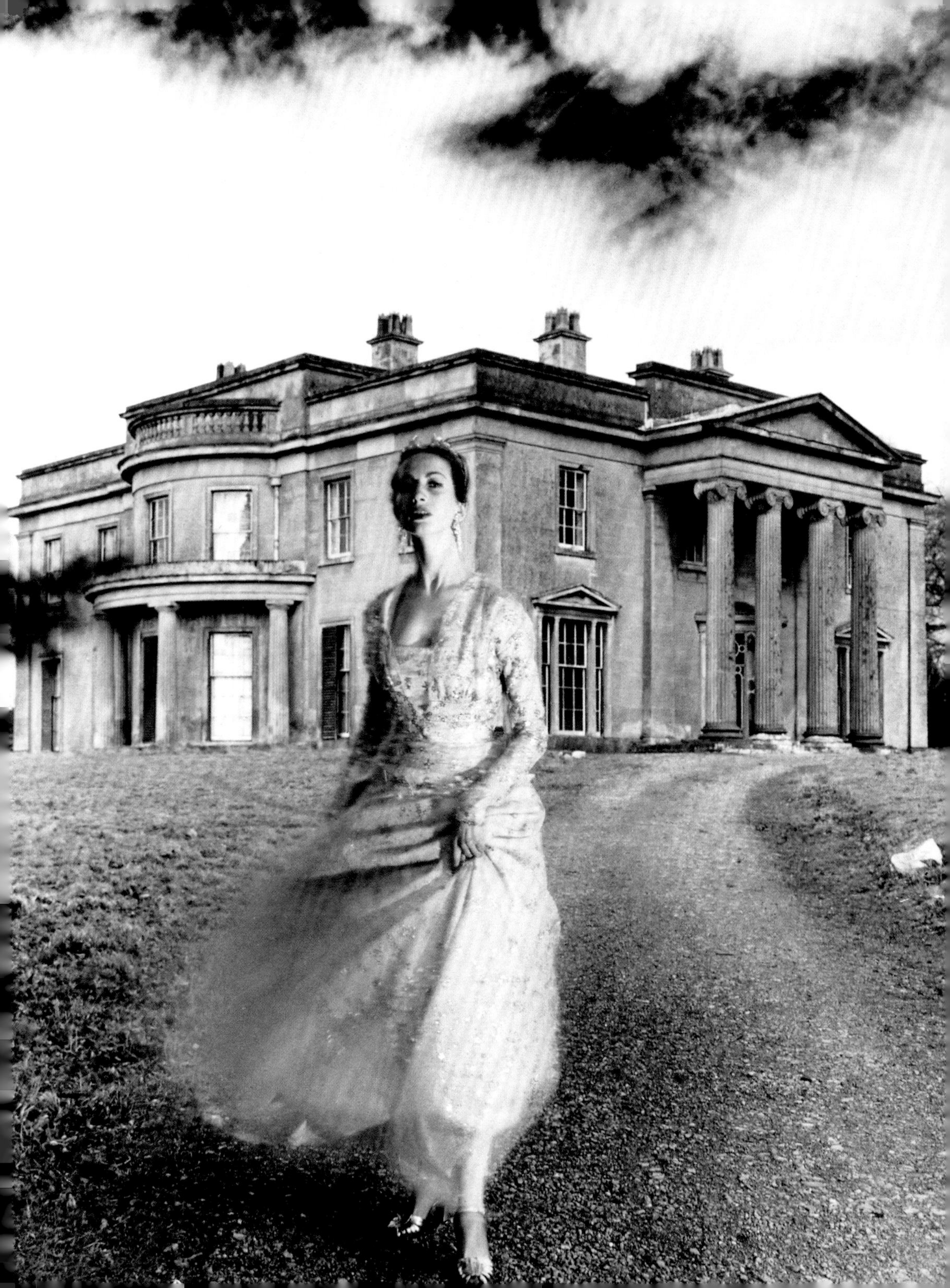

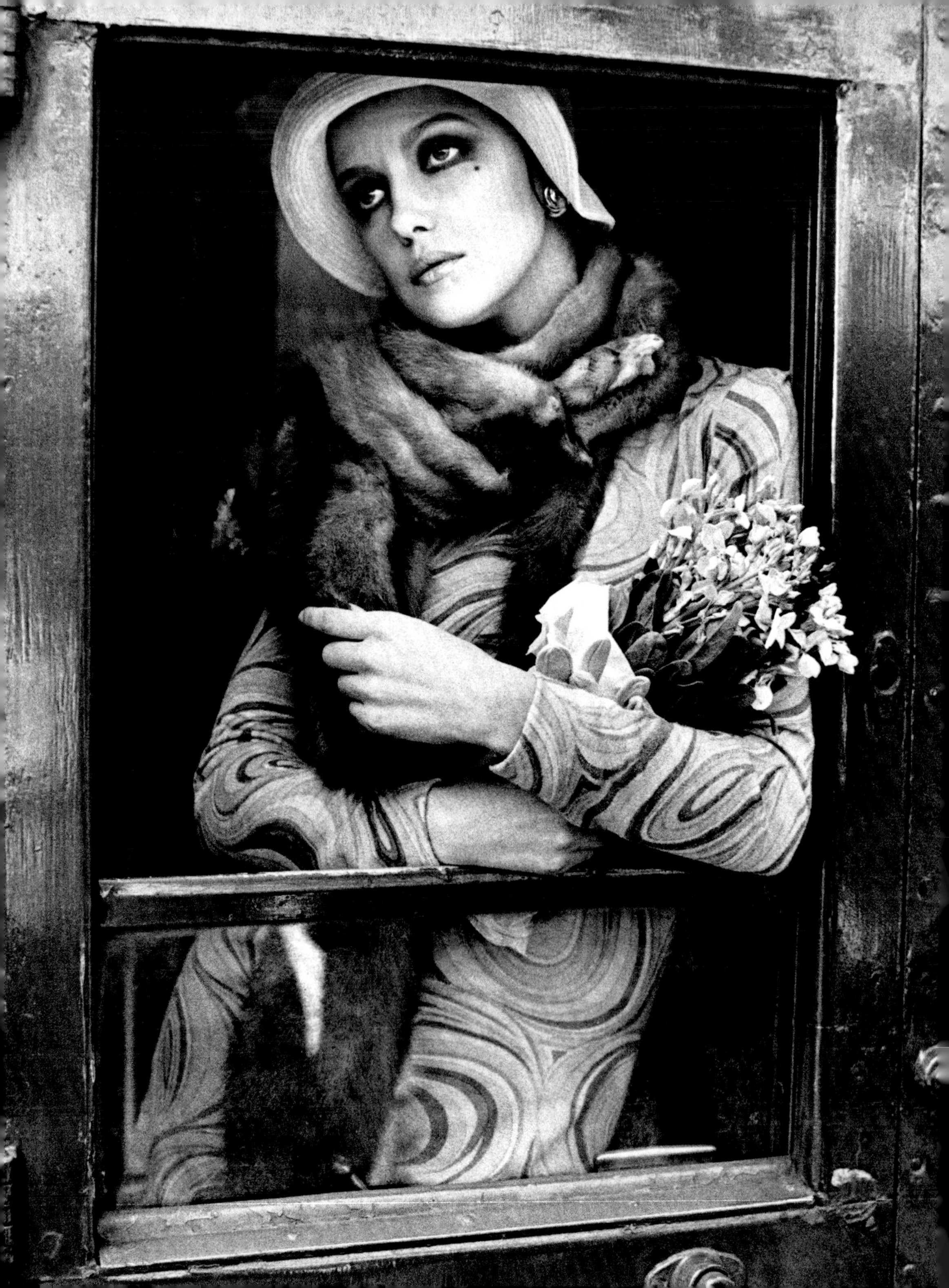

Donna Mitchell

'Donna could take the gestures of the street,' said the photographer Melvin Sokolsky, 'and turn them into the highest form of elegance. She had the knowledge of the world in her little face.' As the 1960s spun from playfulness to pessimism, she represented a departure from what mainstream fashion magazines considered acceptable; not her face, which often looked knowing, self-assured, captivating and mysterious in the space of one fashion story, but her every nuance and gesture and the unsettling mood they created.

More practically, Donna's refusal to work unless it was with her photographer of choice unsettled editors greatly. But they knew that it worked. She preferred to collaborate on photographic assignments rather than feature in scenarios of someone else's making. To this end, her collaborations with Bob Richardson led to a pivotal moment in fashion photography. Together they made sequences of photographs that tied together like stills from a movie to form a dark, richly textured narrative in, say, a dozen pages. 'They said she looked drugged and beaten,' recalled Richardson of the atmosphere created (he described it as 'a stoned ambience'). 'I thought she looked like a fallen angel.'

If anyone looked beaten it was Richardson himself: with his star in the ascendant, rebellious, difficult and egocentric; lonely, unbalanced and desperate on the way down. And his star shone briefly until drug addiction and schizophrenia made it wane. The narrative tableaux he spun for *Vogue* are still considered masterpieces. And the best of them were nothing without Donna Mitchell.

Not all photographers were in tune with Mitchell's *modus operandi*, though they recognised the magic. David Bailey, who flew on assignment to Turkey with her, said on his return that she 'is the most difficult model, a sort of "method" affair, but certainly the most rewarding. She slept most of the time, even when I was taking pictures.' To the French photographer Jeanloup Sieff she was '*Vogue*'s pure medieval moonshine girl'.

The times Bob and Donna lived through were troubled and uncertain, and their photographs, meditative and forlorn, reflected a bleak reality and a hopeless future. The outlook for Richardson – put down in black and white for *Vogue* to publish – was hazed by marijuana smoke and paranoia: 'I wanted to put reality in my photographs. Sex, drugs and rock'n'roll. That's what was happening. And I was going to help make it happen. But they didn't want that in America...' he said later.

Richardson's stream-of-consciousness reflections, written shortly before he died (in 2005), pass for the autobiography he might have written. 'Donna Mitchell was not my favourite person – she was my favourite model – she was short for a model and had beautiful breasts – she was from the Bronx – she was the best model of the 1960s – the Glamazons got the publicity – Donna got the photographers. She could act – she had a problem with speed – her hands were ice cold – the fashion editors hated her because she was the future and they clung to the past – they still do.' He ends, resentfully or maybe poignantly, 'We were never friends.'

Donna Mitchell (fl. 1966–1972)

Opposite:
'Dressing Soft',
September 1966,
by Bob Richardson.
Fashion by Chic

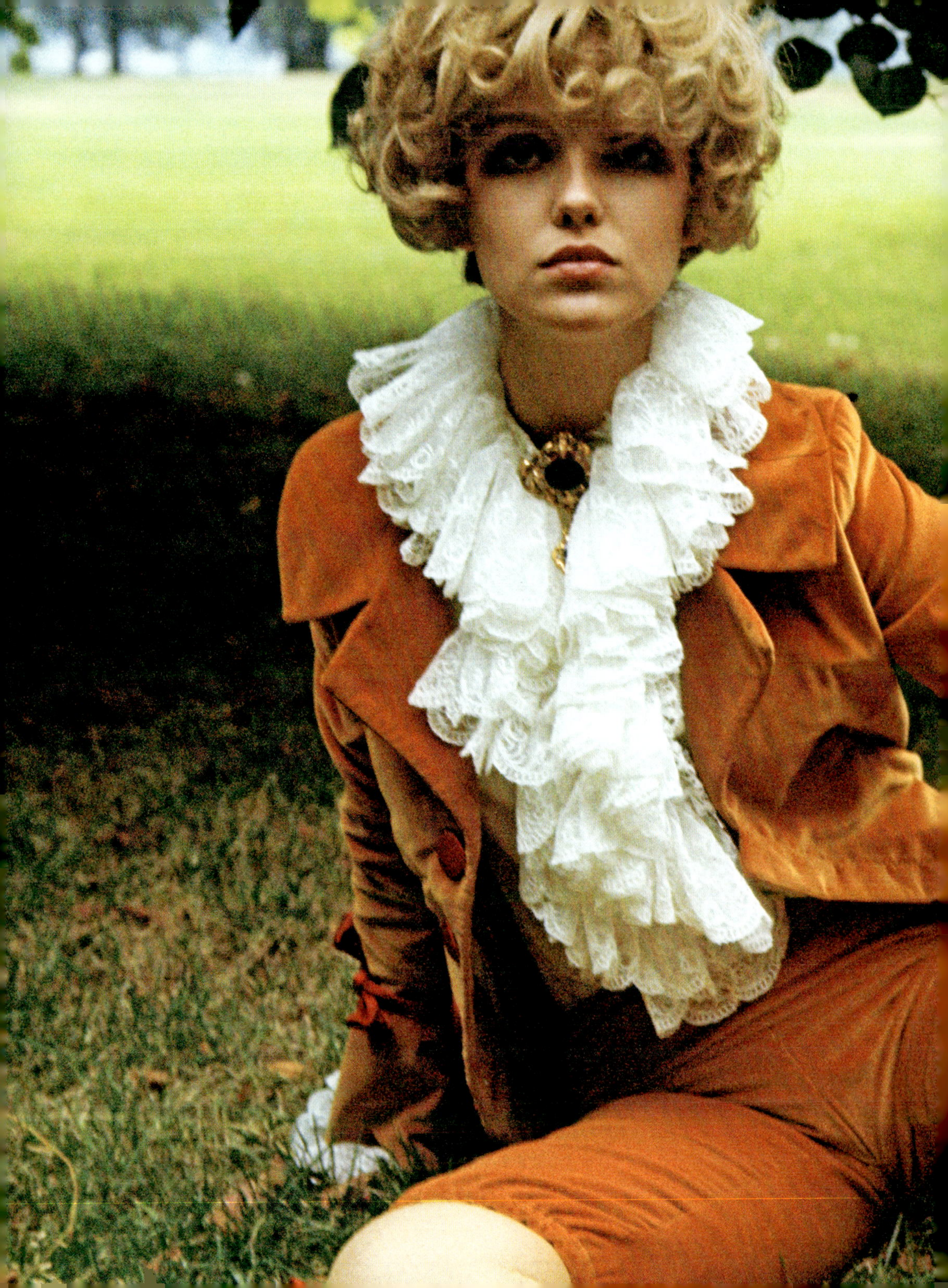

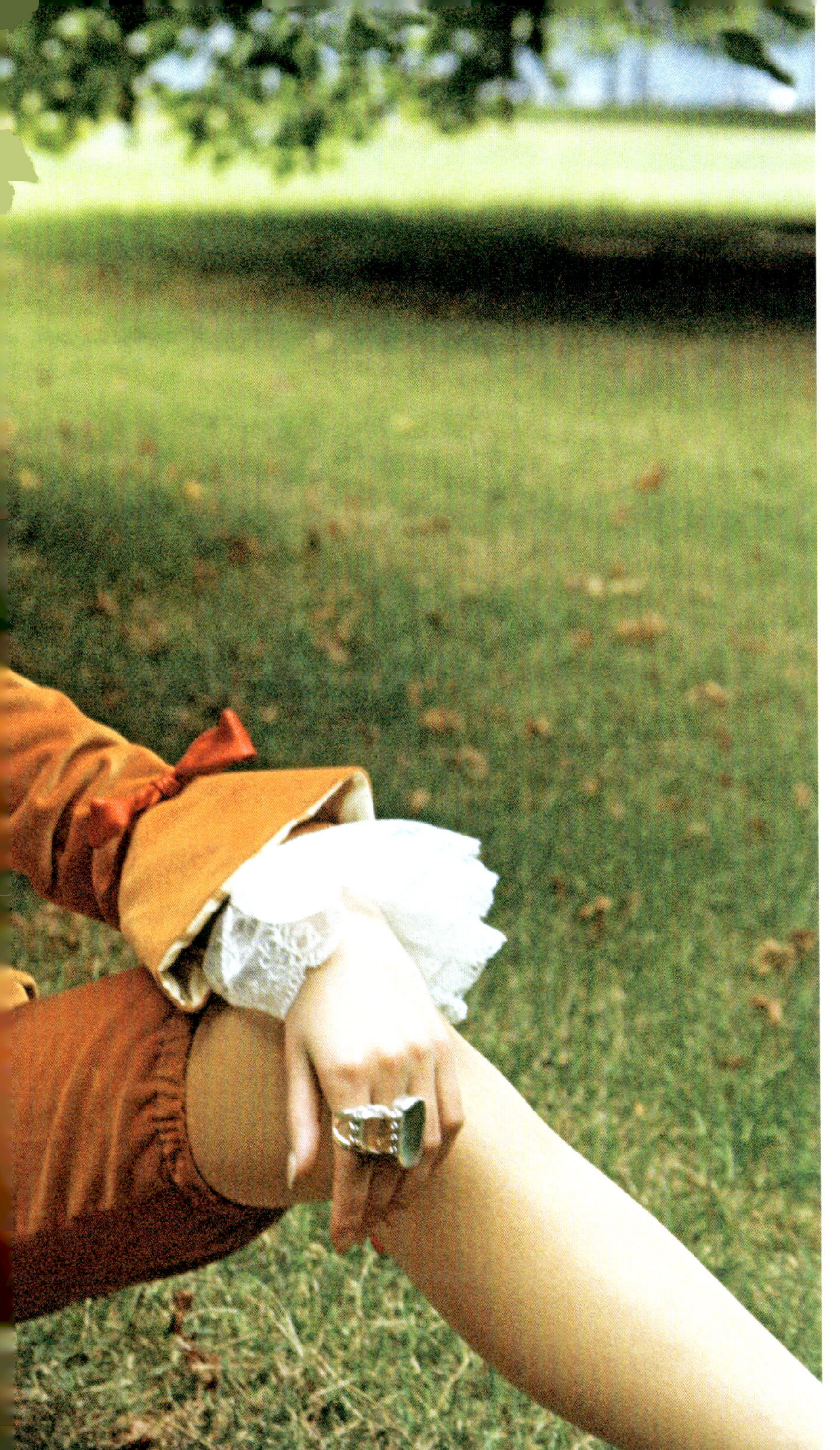

'Cameras, Lights, Shoot!', October 1966, by Bob Richardson. Fashion by Candida & Robin

Dorian Leigh

The American Dorian Leigh, born Parker, was the self-proclaimed *Girl Who Had Everything* (the title of her racy autobiography). This was not without irony, for as quickly as everything arrived, most of it towards the end had gone. Would she have changed anything in her long life? 'Yes,' she replied. 'Every single minute of it.'

A friend of Truman Capote, who called her Happy (as in happy-go-lucky), she is said – as many are – to be the inspiration for Holly Golightly, the free-as-the-wind heroine of *Breakfast at Tiffany's*. Cecil Beaton called her 'the best model with whom I have ever collaborated' – not necessarily for her looks, for he considered Leigh never strictly beautiful in the academic sense, but for her physical presence and stamina. 'She trained herself to keep still for hours on end without showing a twitch of fatigue. Dorian sensed exactly what to hide, what to project and was an inspiration… by inventing a new mood, she elevated the sitting above the level of tawdry commercialism.'

Leigh, whom more than one photographer opined you would not notice were she to pass you in the street, was skilled enough to realise that while her appeal might be a barely suppressed hauteur, she had also to delight the great American public as a whole if she were to reach the top of the pile. Ordinariness was never something she knew much about, coming from a privileged background (her inventor father had made a fortune from the chemical industry). Her mother marked her out early as a hothouse exotic to be nurtured with care. Her sister Cissie – there were four Parker girls – recalled the family seamstress sitting through a movie many times in order to reproduce accurately a dress that Dorian had glimpsed and wanted.

Before alighting on modelling, which took off for her in the mid-1940s, Dorian's life had not been without incident. She had married a college sweetheart while majoring in mathematics, and bore two children before divorcing at 19. Her studies led to an early (though ultimately thwarted) career as a technical draughtsman for the US navy, and then as a designer of aircraft parts for the Eastern Aircraft Corporation. She was offered a job as a badly paid apprentice advertising copywriter in Manhattan and, to make ends meet, joined a model agency. At 27, she was considered too old and too small and her eyebrows too zigzagging – but she exuded confidence and, having taken eight years off her age, was booked by photographer Louise Dahl-Wolfe at *Harper's Bazaar*.

She was an overnight success and, at the hurried instigation of her family, dropped the name Parker for Leigh (modelling was still not considered an acceptable pastime for young ladies). Popular with virtually all *Vogue*'s photographers – in Irving Penn's well-known 1947 group portrait of his colleagues Serge Balkin, Cecil Beaton, George Platt Lynes, Constantin Joffé, Horst P Horst and Erwin Blumenfeld, she was given a place of honour – she reached a wider public as the face of Charles Revson's cosmetics. In 1945 she had been the image of Poison Apple – 'the most tempting colour since Eve winked at Adam' – but as the Fire and Ice girl, photographed by Richard Avedon, she became a superstar and household name. The campaigns and their straplines were unorthodox and daring: 'Do sables excite you, even on other women?'; 'For you who love to flirt with fire; who dare to skate on thin ice.' She was succeeded as the Fire and Ice girl by her red-haired younger sister Suzy Parker (the family were suitably pleased with Dorian's achievements to allow the family name to stay this time). By 1950, she had appeared on the cover of over 50 magazines – seven for *Vogue* in 1946 alone.

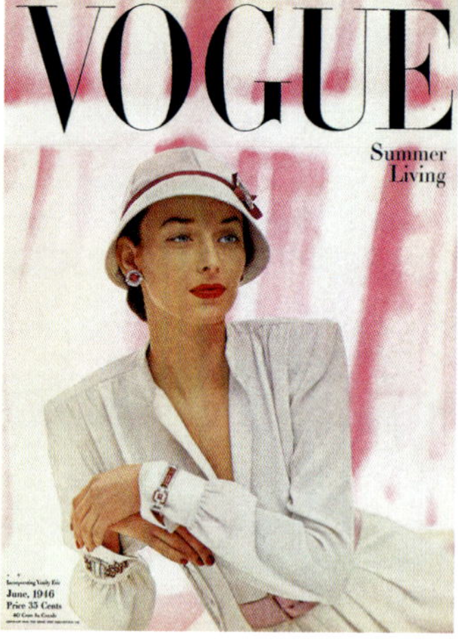

Leigh's domestic life was turbulent. She had a tendency to refuse the hand in marriage of older millionaires in favour of young, handsome men who were usually broke. 'And if I had to pay some bills to make that possible, well, it was only money…' she wrote in *The Girl Who Had Everything*. Suzy Parker, who disapproved of her sister's many liaisons, suggested as an alternative title *The Girl Who Had Everyone*. High-profile distractions included Irving Penn, Hollywood producer Sam Spiegel, calypso king Harry Belafonte, jazz drummer Buddy Rich and craggy poet Robert Graves. She married four times, mostly unhappily, but had five children, of which two predeceased her.

She had quit when she was ahead, much to the chagrin of her photographers. There were few others who could, as one commentator observed, 'conjure up the languid mood of a long June evening simply by letting her right hand rest on a cool, curvaceous cup…'

Dorian Leigh (b. Dorian Parker, 1917, USA; d. 2008)

Above:
'Summer Living', June 1946, by John Rawlings. Fashion by Henri Bendel

Opposite:
'This Half Century', January 1950, by Irving Penn. Fashion by Dior

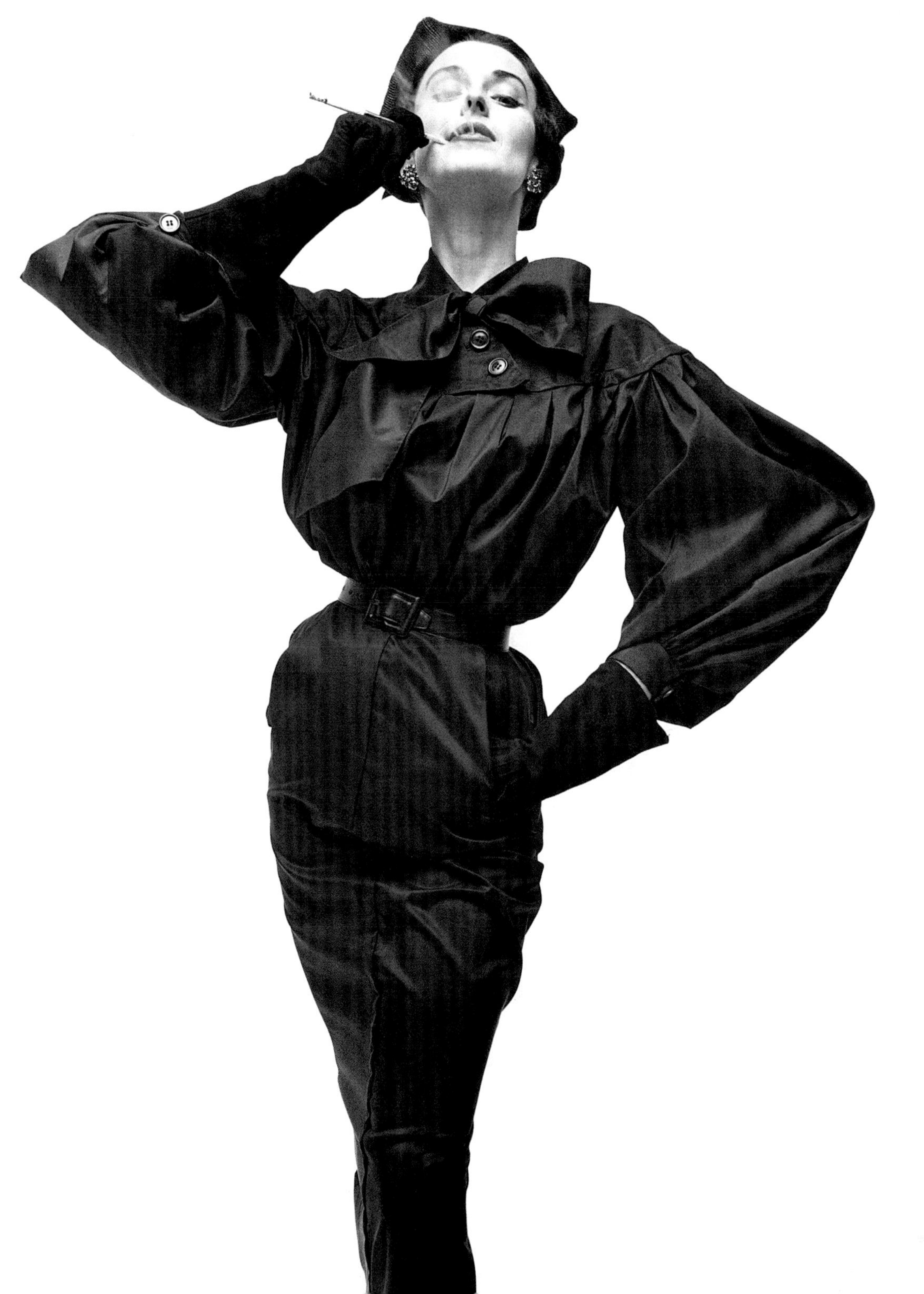

Dovima

'I think you are a super-duper superstar,' announced Diana Vreeland to Dovima in 1955 after a particularly successful Paris-collections sitting. Richard Avedon had just taken what would turn out to be one of fashion photography's most recognisable images, widely known as 'Dovima with Elephants'. With photographs such as this, shot at the Cirque d'Hiver, Avedon turned what had been regarded as a sedate occasion into a theatrical event. It also cemented for posterity the name of one of the decade's finest models, whose rise-and-fall life story mirrors the vagaries of the fashion world. Avedon called her 'the most remarkable and unconventional beauty of her time'.

Animal epithets tended to follow Dovima. Beaton called her 'a beautiful giraffe from the suburbs of New York with almond-shaped face, raven hair, turquoise eyes, her face painted so white that her teeth appeared black'. Henry Clarke described her as 'panther-like'.

Dovima (her *nom de guerre* an acronym of her given names, Dorothy Virginia Margaret) was a firm Avedon favourite – 'a brushstroke, in human form, of inspired calligraphy,' according to the writer Judith Thurman. Born in 1927 in Jackson Heights, New York, Dorothy Juba invented Dovima as an imaginary friend who would help see her through bouts of grave childhood illness. She spent seven years mostly indoors, a sickly home-tutored child raised like an exotic orchid by an anxious mother. Trapped, she dreamed of being a model; in 1949 it came true in the fairytale fashion she had imagined. Pausing outside an Automat on Lexington Avenue, she was grabbed by a passer-by and taken upstairs. It was the offices of Condé Nast Publications. 'They took some pictures; told me to come back and next day I was a model,' she recalled years later. Her keen-eyed accoster was the model agent Eileen Ford, and the next day brought a booking with Irving Penn.

Dovima, the childhood fantasy, was made flesh. She kept her mouth firmly closed as she had cracked a tooth and the resulting smile, beguiling and mysterious, became an early trademark – enough to make her within a couple of years the city's highest paid model, at $30 an hour. It went stratospheric ($60) when Avedon's gaze lit on hers. America's 'Dollar-a-Minute Girl' was worth the price tag. 'We became like mental Siamese twins, with me knowing what he wanted before he explained it.' Along with Dorian Leigh and Lisa Fonssagrives, Dovima was the epitome of wasp-waisted, fragile-wristed, etiolated mid-century Manhattan elegance. She looked, said Eileen Ford in admiration, as if she 'could freeze ice'.

The brittle beauty that Dovima projected did not square with her hard-luck upbringing in Queens. She felt she never quite deserved the fame and fortune, expecting both to evanesce as quickly as they had arrived. She drank and smoked too much and made two unsuitable marriages. In due course, fashions changed, beckoning the years of ever-diminishing returns, until there was nothing left and she was broke and exhausted.

An acting career did not work out. Then followed a series of jobs, each more poorly paid and briefer than its predecessor – model booker, talent scout, spokeswoman for a man-made fibre, department-store salesgirl – until she became a hostess at Two Guys Pizzeria in Fort Lauderdale, where she had relocated in 1984. There she found happiness in a third marriage, which lasted 12 years until the cancer which had claimed her husband claimed her too. She died in 1990, aged 63.

For a few years she had had everything, though she thought she had nothing. 'I have never thought of myself as beautiful,' she said at the height of her powers. Her friend Carmen dell'Orefice noted that with Dovima it had only ever flowed one way – out.

Dovima (b. Dorothy Juba, 1927, USA; d. 1990)

Opposite:
'The Organdie Touch',
April 1956,
by Henry Clarke.
Fashion by Jacques Fath

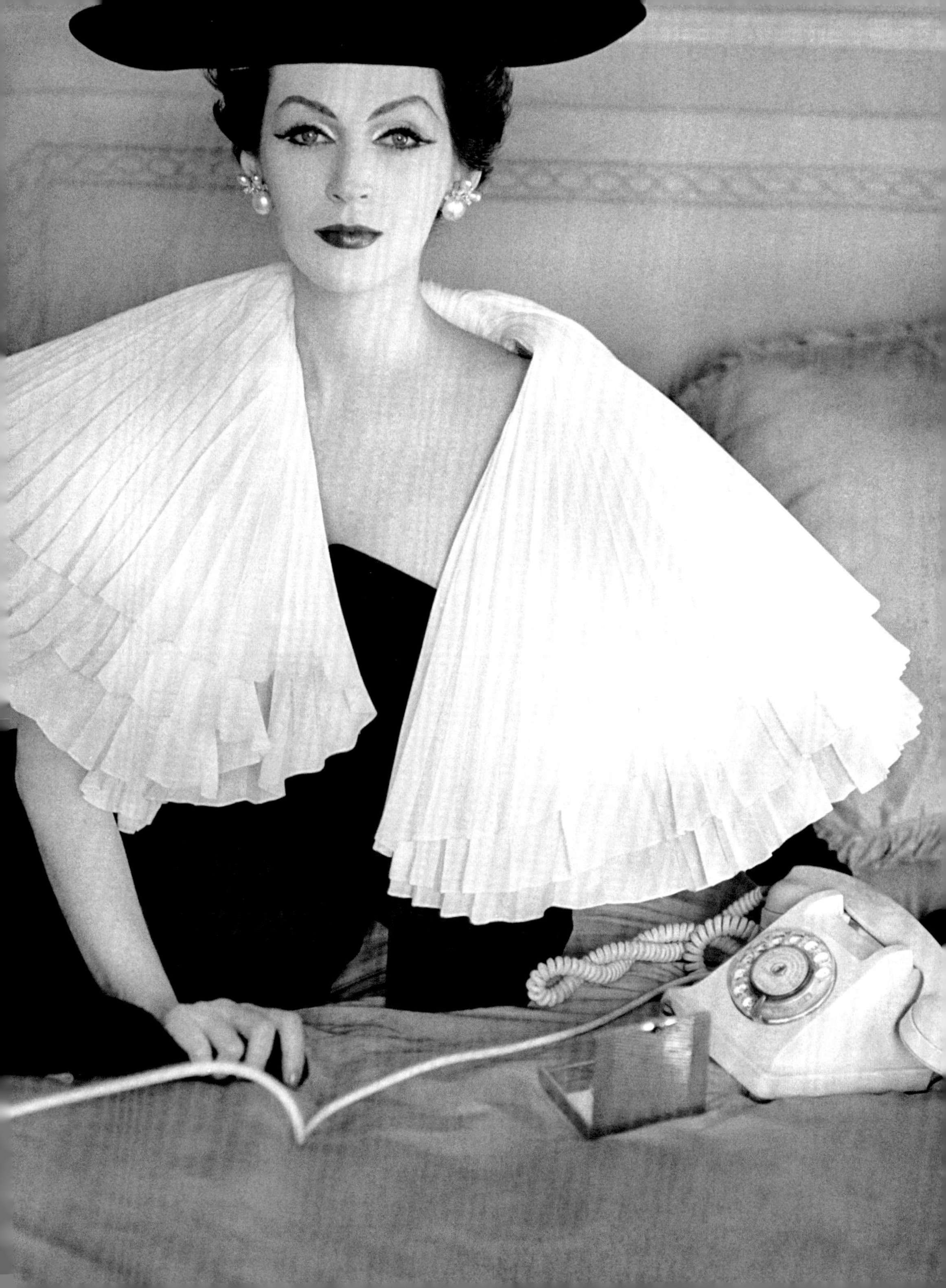

Elise Crombez

As a crop of sweet-natured, delicately featured newcomers poked their fresh-as-a-daisy faces towards the first rays of fame, US *Vogue* put it best: 'On a pierced, tattooed, dour-faced type, baby-doll-pink chiffon ruffles look either ironic or silly. But on a fresh-faced ingénue they look honest and *right*'. And they didn't come pinker, fresher or more ingénue back then than Elise Crombez from the small Walloon town of Mouscron in Belgium. Genuinely so, because Elise had been modelling for less than a year when, gathered up by Steven Meisel, she became the new face of Prada overnight. Meisel later cajoled her into dyeing her slightly mousy-blonde hair red. Then Karl Lagerfeld plucked her out for the Chanel catwalk. She was the first to admit it was all a bit baffling: 'Oh God, that's me!' she would winningly exclaim whenever she chanced upon a picture of herself in a magazine or on a billboard, both events threatening to become more commonplace by the week.

She was perhaps more winning for admitting that her most treasured compliment came from a photographer who called her 'both ugly and beautiful'. (*Vogue* discreetly concurred, noticing a 'faint Brueghel look about her features'.) More still for conceding in 2004 that 'my best friend is my Ossie Clark dress'. More winning yet for possessing a lucky Evil Eye protector from Indonesia, which she claims has prevented her from 'a major wipe-out' on the catwalk. By 2004, *Vogue* noticed that her ever-so-slightly androgynous *jolie-laide* look had turned into a womanlier one, even sensual, and that photographers and editors 'love her dancer's poise and grace'.

Apparently it started when, as a student of marketing, she was noticed at a 'Miss Mannequin' modelling competition, though there remains a question mark over whether she was actually in the running or merely an interested bystander. She assumed that the talent scout pursuing her was a stalker. She had no intention of actually becoming a model; in fact, she told *Vogue* that her ambitions were relatively modest: she wanted to be a secretary because she enjoyed 'taking down telephone messages for my dad' (he is in the pharmaceutical industry).

Both the spectacle of the couture shows and its participants entranced *Vogue*'s Christa D'Souza, who spent several days in Elise's company backstage and in the front row. At the Dior show: 'It becomes more and more of a [John] Galliano melting-pot spectacle. I've known Elise for less than a day but her combination of earnestness, bravado, fervency and swagger has completely won me over and I get an almost maternal urge to shout "You go girl!" when she passes by my section for the finale.' Asked why Elise makes such a great couture model, Jean Paul Gaultier replied, 'She's feminine, she's elegant, and she understands. She's one of those people who connects to the client.'

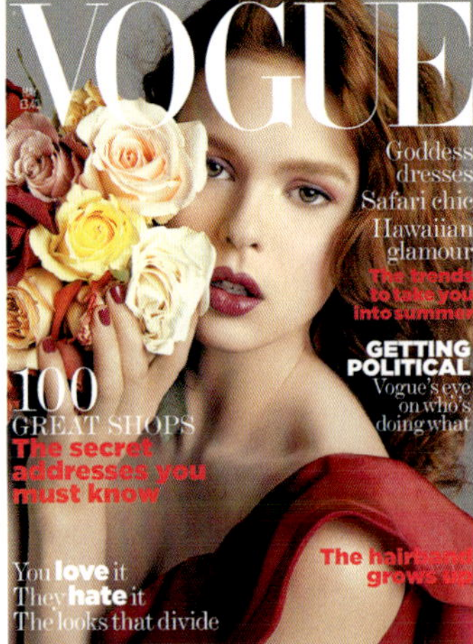

Elise admitted a while ago that she looked at the world 'as an enormous planet full of unreachable places'. In the intervening whirlwind years she must have reached a fair number of them, but her enthusiasm for her world, at least, is undimmed: 'I want it to be an enjoyable experience for people to work with me,' says the ever-affable Elise. 'Sometimes I think I give off the wrong impression and that's a shame. If only they knew. I'm *so* happy doing this.'

Elise Crombez (b. 1982, Belgium)

Above:
'Goddess Dresses', May 2005, by Inez van Lamsweerde and Vinoodh Matadin. Fashion by Yves Saint Laurent

Opposite:
'Deadlier than the Male', September 2004, by Paolo Roversi. Fashion by House of Jazz

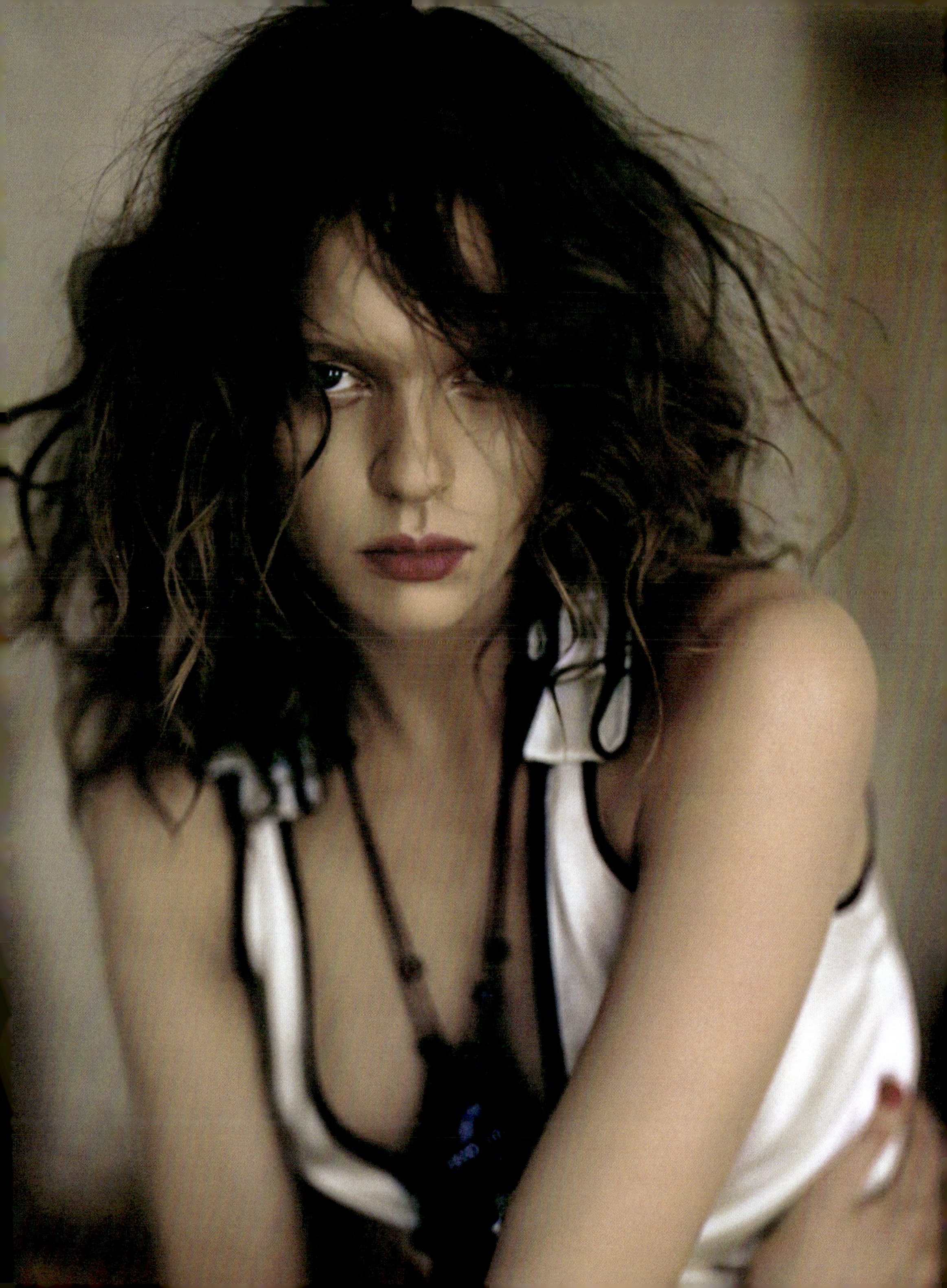

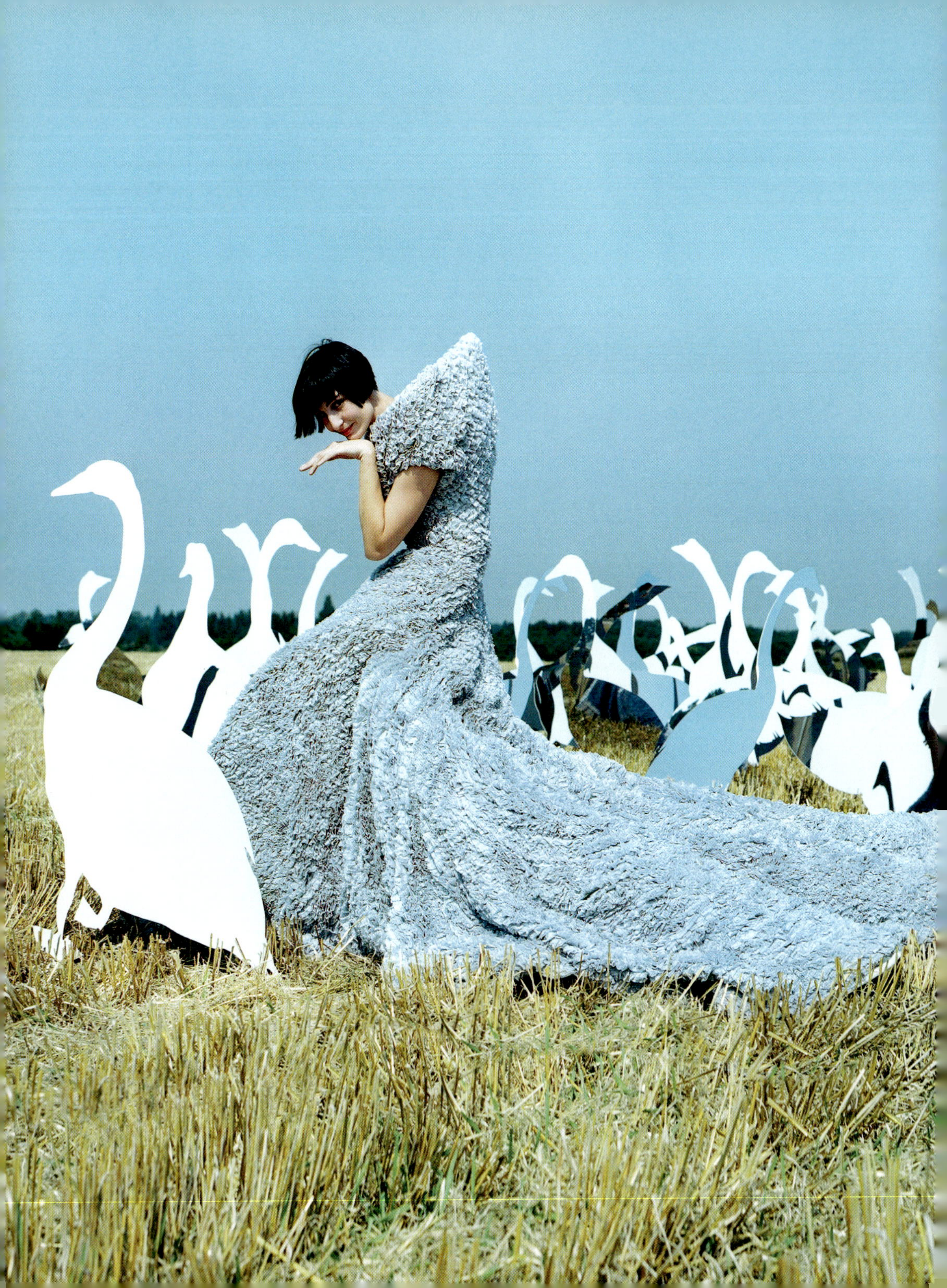

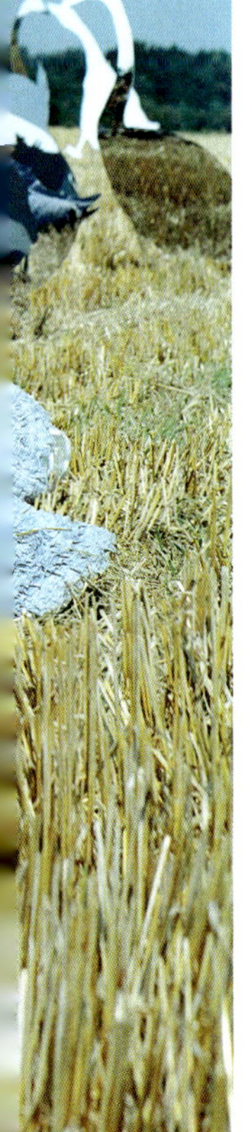

Erin O'Connor

Described by Karl Lagerfeld as 'one of the best models in the world' and by Jean Paul Gaultier as 'like theatre, an extraordinary inspiration', Erin O'Connor was discovered on a school outing to *The Clothes Show Live* in Birmingham by a scout from Models One. And a star was born. It's a well-known story and a romantic one but, as Erin explained, 'actually I was bent over a bargain bin rummaging for goodies'. The scout, she was convinced, was monitoring her for shoplifting. A delicate sense of balance mentally, as well as physically, has been her mainstay. She is renowned as one to whom the accolades have flocked like moths to a paper lantern, but who has not changed in the slightest. 'I'm not an average beauty,' she told *Vogue* with a keen sense of self-worth. 'I have to interpret charm and sexiness my way.'

She interpreted it with resounding success on the catwalk for Gaultier and Chanel: 'What's really different is the way the new girls move,' said Lagerfeld in 1997, 'much less aggressive glamour than before. They're lighter and more fluid – which makes clothes look more contemporary.' Fast-forward a few years to 2004 and the magic was being worked again at Dior. Erin famously opened as a Nefertiti in gold lamé and lapis lazuli, complete with scroll beard, headdress and 'heavy metal' 16in corset. 'Knowing I could only put one foot in front of the other,' she said later, 'made me very calm indeed. I had no other choice.'

Carrying the day with aplomb became Erin's trademark, and *Vogue* was not to let her off the hook lightly. She opened Tim Walker's '*Vogue* Pantomime' in 2004, a famously extravagant shoot: 80 white rabbits, 20 ballerinas, 250 ostrich eggs (sprayed gold), a flock of mirrored geese, a box of giant plastic hands, a room full of white umbrellas, 20 Christmas trees, a wolf's head and feet costume, a giant squishy pumpkin, fake silver armour, a horse (also sprayed gold) and hundreds of Ali Baba oil lamps. Furthermore, *Vogue* found it was cheaper to buy a vintage Rolls-Royce than to risk damaging a hired one. Erin was shoehorned into a huge lace 'swan' dress by the late Alexander McQueen: 'It was so structured,' she recalled, 'that if I passed out due to heat exhaustion at least I would have remained standing.'

Perhaps as some sort of reward, *Vogue* commissioned an Erin O'Connor hat from sculptor Antony Gormley, made out of dyed straw applied to a cast of the model's entire head: 'The idea was to make Erin a superego – a strange "other" that would sit on her head looking at the world in the opposite direction.' Gormley added – as if we would not have guessed it – that it was hard work for his sitter. 'She was very brave when we moulded her in seaweed gel and plaster: she was in there for much too long, but kept her pose beautifully.' But then again, as *Vogue* has known from the mid-1990s on, she always does.

Erin O'Connor (b. 1978, UK)

Left:
'The Greatest Show on Earth', December 2004, by Tim Walker. Fashion by Alexander McQueen

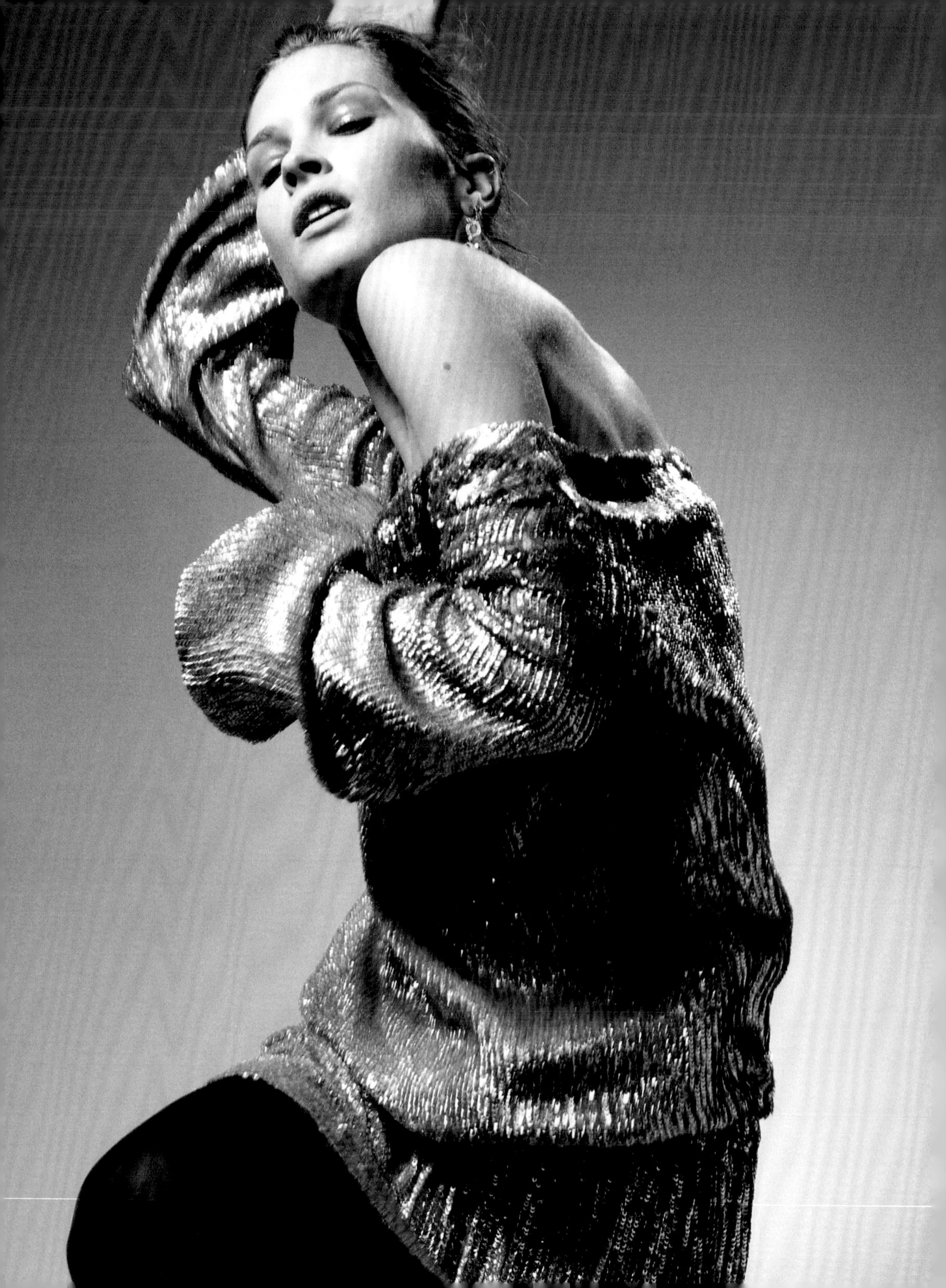

Erin Wasson

One of Texan Erin Wasson's high points at *Vogue* was in a rose-strewn set as a dazzling high-born débutante in a Givenchy strapless ballgown, a fur stole from Marni, blue topaz and diamond earrings from Garrard and an unquantifiably expensive pavé-diamond and platinum cuff from Harry Winston. This contrasted sharply with her starring role a month before in 'The Real Thing', a portfolio of nude photographs by Mario Testino (an early Wesson champion), in which Erin and her pierced navel were scrutinised. 'When the shoot is finished for the day and the clothes have been returned, back in their hotel rooms the girls' natural beauty is revealed,' said *Vogue*. It did not take away from Erin's vulnerability that she appeared to be wearing an elderly Bavarian's folkloric trilby. The theme (nudes, not alpine costume) was continued memorably in 'Playgirl', a set of delicate soft-focus pictures, again by Testino but in thrall to the soft-focus oeuvre of photographer and filmmaker David Hamilton.

Despite such persuasive evidence, none of the above is remotely true of the real-life Erin Wasson. 'I hate to say it,' she says, stopped in the street by *Vogue*, 'but my style is a bit, well, skate-girl. When I go out I try to stay comfy and wear loose, flowing dresses… usually with sneakers.' *Vogue* called it a 'fearless high/low fashion sense'. Wasson ventured that you might find her at the Manhattan designer store Kirna Zabête, and 'flea markets around the world, *obviously*'. Her natural and commendable thriftiness was enhanced when she revealed that 'believe it or not, this Balenciaga dress, the Marc Jacobs skirt underneath, the Chanel boots, the Moschino bag and Paco Rabanne belt were all gifts from designers at the shows'.

It also helped, perhaps, that Erin discovered that she and edgy designer-of-the-moment Alexander Wang lived in the same apartment block. It was therefore a short hop to her designing his catwalk show, and so successful was it that she might happily carve out a second career alongside her modelling work. Wang told *Vogue* he had striven for a 'working-woman-made-funkier look', thus Wasson dressed model Natasa Vojnovic in a boxy cherry-red blazer and accessorised the 'look' with her own jewellery. Wang was delighted: 'This collection is the most "me". Erin totally gets it!' Another look is 'hipster-dorky' and thus a touch subversive. Erin says admiringly: 'Alex's clothes are so simple and radical. I just go with my gut.'

Not having lost her enthusiasm for skateboarding, she told *Vogue* that she would love her own skate-clothing line – as she put it, 'cool streetwear with a high-fashion look'. It was a given that it would include 'wicked sneakers to hit the pavement'.

Erin Wasson (b. 1982, USA)

Opposite:
'Shades of Grey',
June 2003, by Robert Wyatt.
Fashion by
Collette Dinnigan

Eva Herzigova

'When I look in the mirror, I just don't see it,' said Eva Herzigova of her stupendous beauty, 'I just see the circles under my eyes.' But then again, for a while at least, it was neither her intense greeny-blue eyes nor her unblemished complexion that commanded the greatest attention. More than one commentator reminded us that this was the woman whose 'cleavage launched a thousand car shunts', a reference to her celebrated 'Hello Boys' Wonderbra ads. Circa 1994-5, such introductions were hardly necessary as she loomed out on the daily grind from billboards up, down and across the British Isles. She was dubbed 'the last of the supermodels' by *Vogue* – as if, like black rhinos or alligator snapping turtles, she should be encouraged to mate for the good of the species. The circles under the eyes, incidentally, have become another trademark.

A mining engineer's daughter from Litvinov (a hub of the central European oil industry), Eva was born in 1973, when the Czech Republic was still a part of Czechoslovakia. She entered a beauty contest, rather against her best instincts – she'd only gone to accompany a friend – and came out in front. She stood, apparently, a full head and a bit over the runner-up, being 5ft 10½in (she is considerably taller in heels).

Litvinov was somewhere to leave by any means possible. 'It was,' Eva recalled, 'very polluted, [with] a lot of dead trees and holes in the ground', and swimming might have proved a way out for her. She was very talented in that respect, something she inherited from her father, who had been a full-time swimmer (something of a recognised profession in the Eastern bloc). The beauty pageant led to modelling work and eventually leave to go to Paris, a month or so before the Velvet Revolution of 1989 made such legal niceties unnecessary.

Having spent much of her earlier career writhing on sun loungers in lingerie – understandably, considering what first put her name in lights – Eva's catwalk appearances are remembered with fondness, tending as they did to zero in on her best assets. ('My grandfather told me if you drink beer, your breasts will grow,' she joked, possibly. 'I've always drunk beer.') She made full use of her early training: another line of Eva Herzigova lingerie and beachwear is expected soon.

In 2002, Eva lost the curves that made her famous, and thereafter any lingering Bardot comparisons dropped off, too. To a casual viewer, the transformation – she also cut her hair short – seemed more dramatic than it really was, leading to speculation of eating disorders and drug addiction. She had to remind the world that in pre-glamazon-era schooldays she had been known as 'the Cigarette' on account of her straight-up-and-down-ness. And in any event the Wonderbra was not called 'Wonder' for nothing (her vital statistics are, by the best accounts, a relatively modest 34-23-34). Among her many and considerable achievements, she has managed effortlessly to bridge the chasm between lads' mag and upmarket glossy, each happy with the Eva they know and love. She considers her greatest triumph to be that 'I still haven't gone mad.'

Eva Herzigova (b. 1973, Czechoslovakia)

Right:
'Summer Beauty Special',
June 2002, by
Enrique Badulescu.
Fashion by Chanel

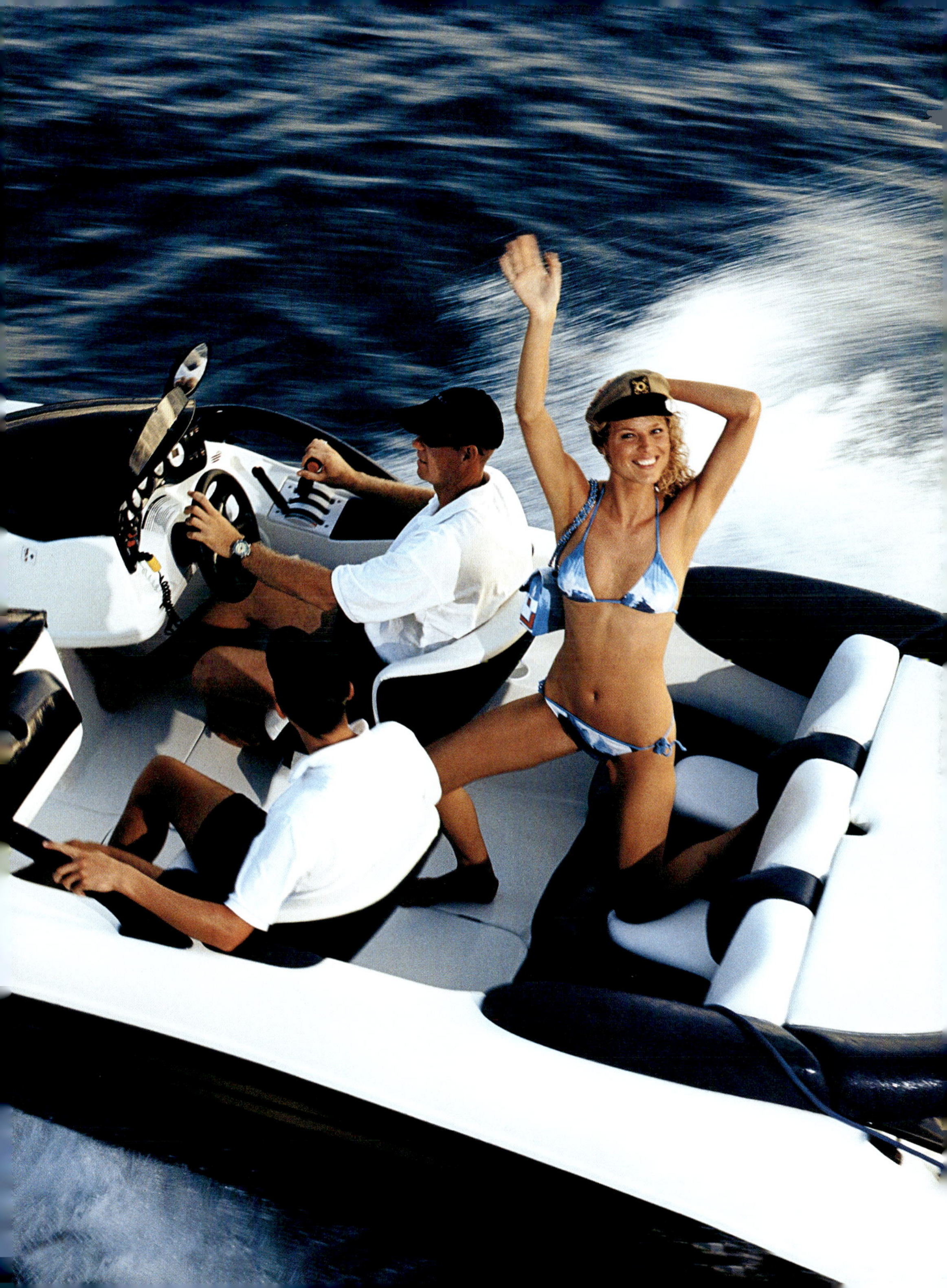

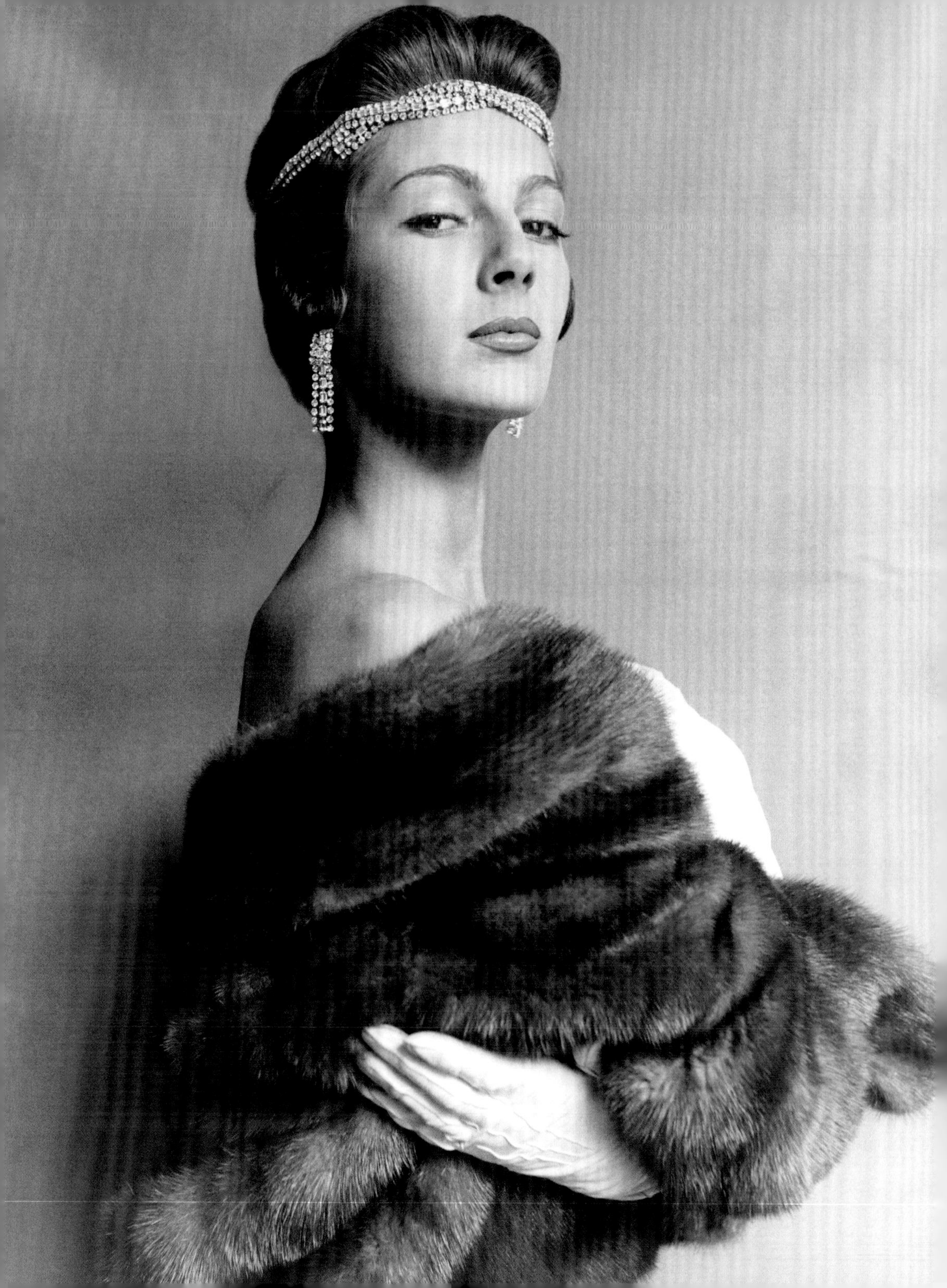

Fiona Campbell-Walter

By the early 1950s, British models had become noticeable on the world stage. Cecil Beaton followed their every move, 'to Berlin after a Paris stop-off and then ricocheting across the Atlantic'. In the person of Fiona Campbell-Walter, the British model became indispensable. She was one of the great beauties of the era, one that made the camera lens more eager and avaricious. *Vogue* was moved to breathless admiration: 'the richness of her tawny hair and eyes against pale skin, the delicate nose and chin, the proud Pharaoh's carriage of her head, the humour that will suddenly flick out of her still perfection and make her both a tireless model and a stimulatingly audacious actress.'

The daughter of a rear admiral, born in New Zealand – though Scottish through and through – Fiona Campbell-Walter could tramp through the mud in a mackintosh and wellington boots ('magnificently, majestically', according to *Vogue*) or wrap herself in a bizarre extravagance of jewels with a gaze that, Cecil Beaton considered, tinted 'the outrage with genius'.

She was discovered by Henry Clarke, a peripatetic American who captured the rarefied world of postwar haute couture more consistently than anyone else. His pictures of Dovima, Della Oake, Anne Saint-Marie, Suzy Parker and Campbell-Walter, all high-cheekboned mannequins of impenetrable hauteur, are now considered masterpieces of extravagance, tempered by good taste. Like all the best fashion photographs, they were removed from reality, but not unimaginably so. Clarke was entranced on his first meeting with Campbell-Walter: 'She was so young that the make-up wouldn't stay on her face. She was so fresh, so beautiful and so lovely. She had great style and great allure – she was a girl with almost a woman's body.'

Campbell-Walter's modelling days were brief. She retired in 1956 to marry the heir to a steel, armaments and chicken-wire fortune, the art collector Hans Henrik Agost Gábor Tasso Freiherr Thyssen-Bornemisza de Kászon et Impérfalva – usually abbreviated to Baron Heini von Thyssen. The marriage lasted nine years; they divorced in 1965. But during those years, the Von Thyssens were a fixture in *Vogue*'s social pages: ten-pin bowling with Dominican playboy diplomat Porfirio Rubirosa in St Moritz, skiing in Gstaad and thence to Knightsbridge for hairstyling.

Campbell-Walter went on to have a well-documented affair with the Greek shipping heir Alexander Onassis, who was 16 years her junior. His father, Aristotle Onassis, did not entirely approve of the relationship, which came to an abrupt end when Alexander died in a plane crash, aged 24.

Vogue continued on an almost monthly basis to be in thrall to Campbell's Celtic moorland beauty and easy grace. One contributor to the magazine remarked on her quizzical eyebrows and her strongly chiselled profile of 'almost piercing clarity, thrust forward like a ship's figurehead'. And for a few brief years, the flame-haired, leonine, green-eyed Scotswoman coming through the rye was unstoppable.

Fiona Campbell-Walter (b. 1932, New Zealand)

Opposite:
'Model Contest',
August 1954,
by Cecil Beaton.
Fashion by Calman Links

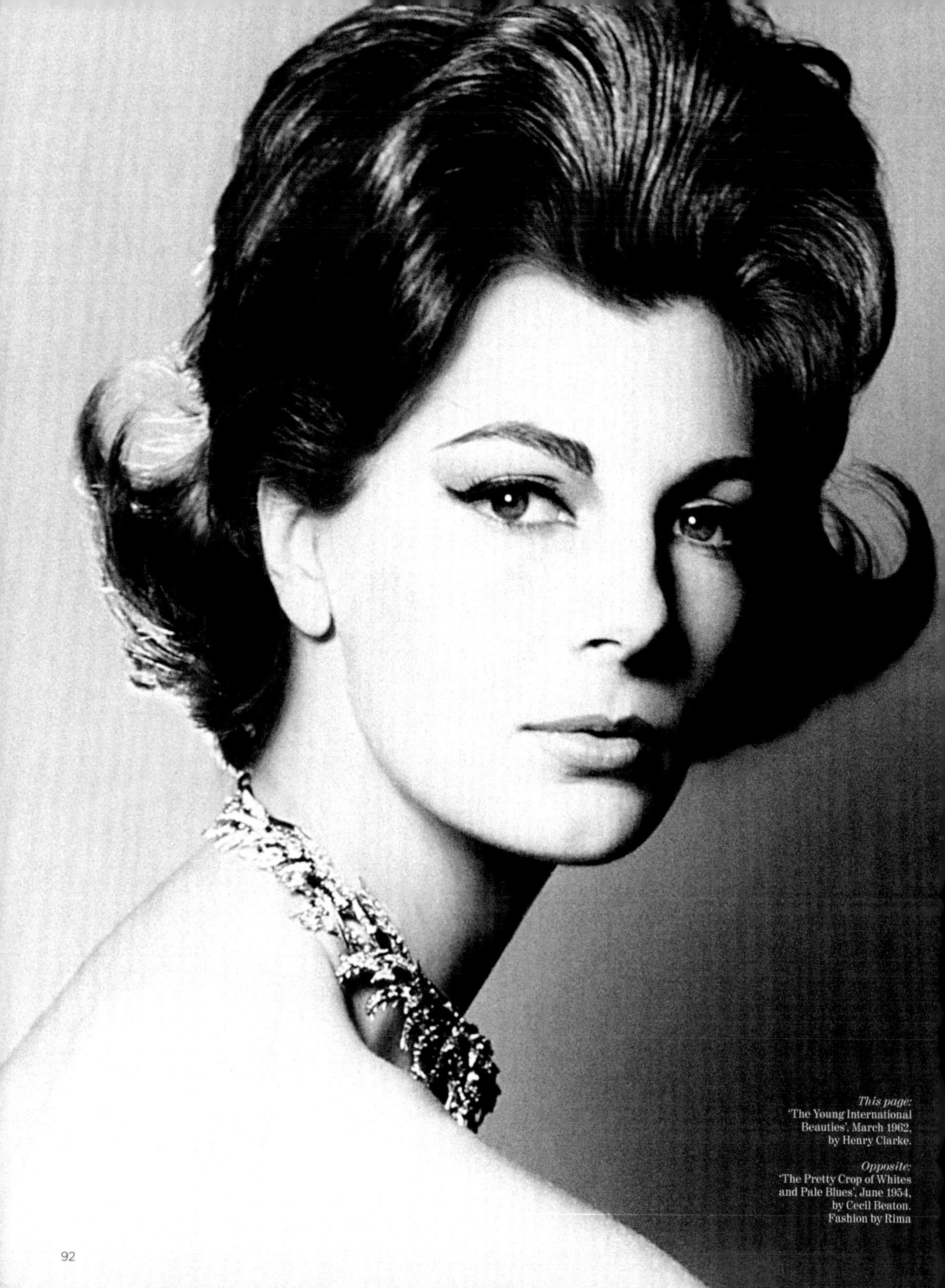

This page:
'The Young International Beauties', March 1962, by Henry Clarke.

Opposite:
'The Pretty Crop of Whites and Pale Blues', June 1954, by Cecil Beaton. Fashion by Rima

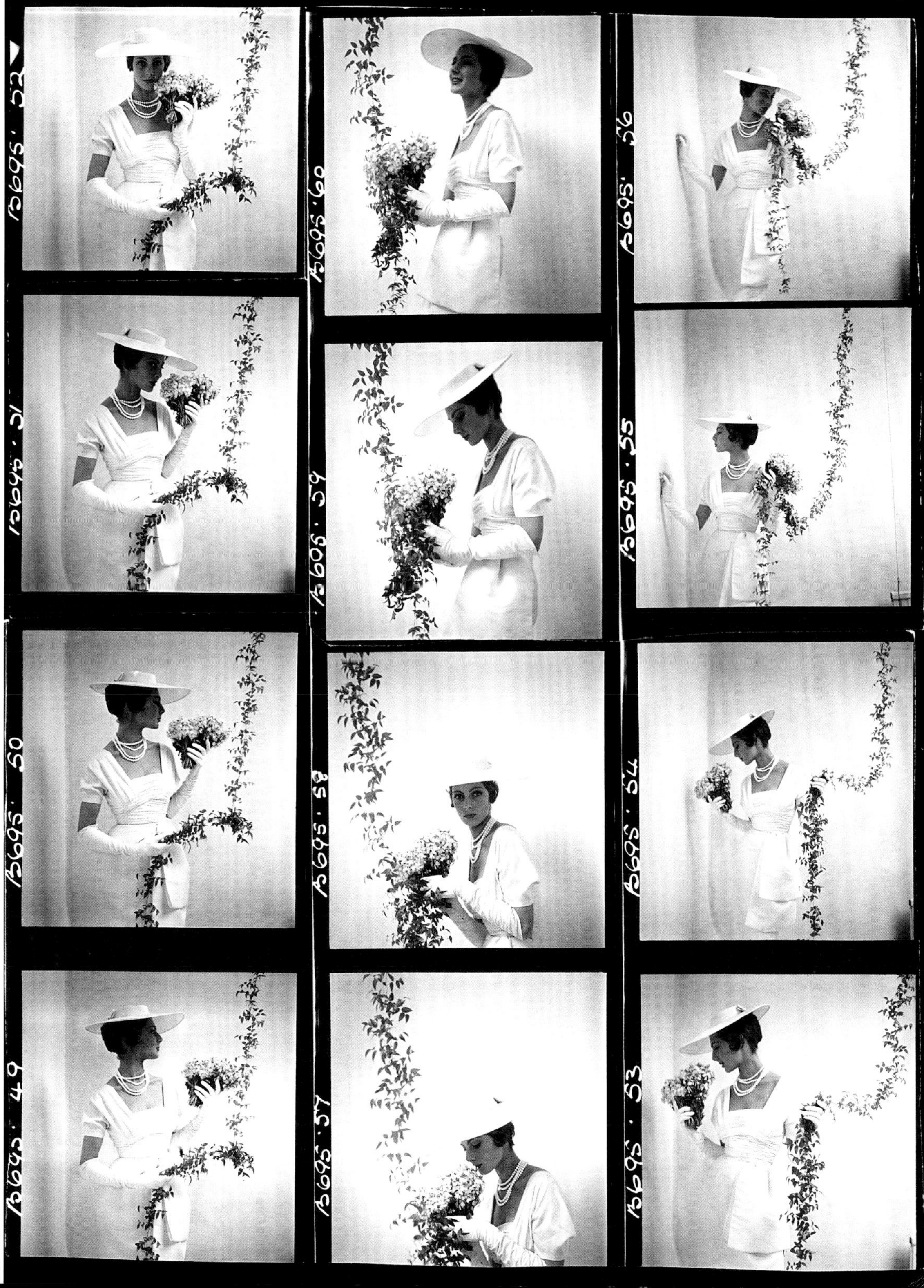

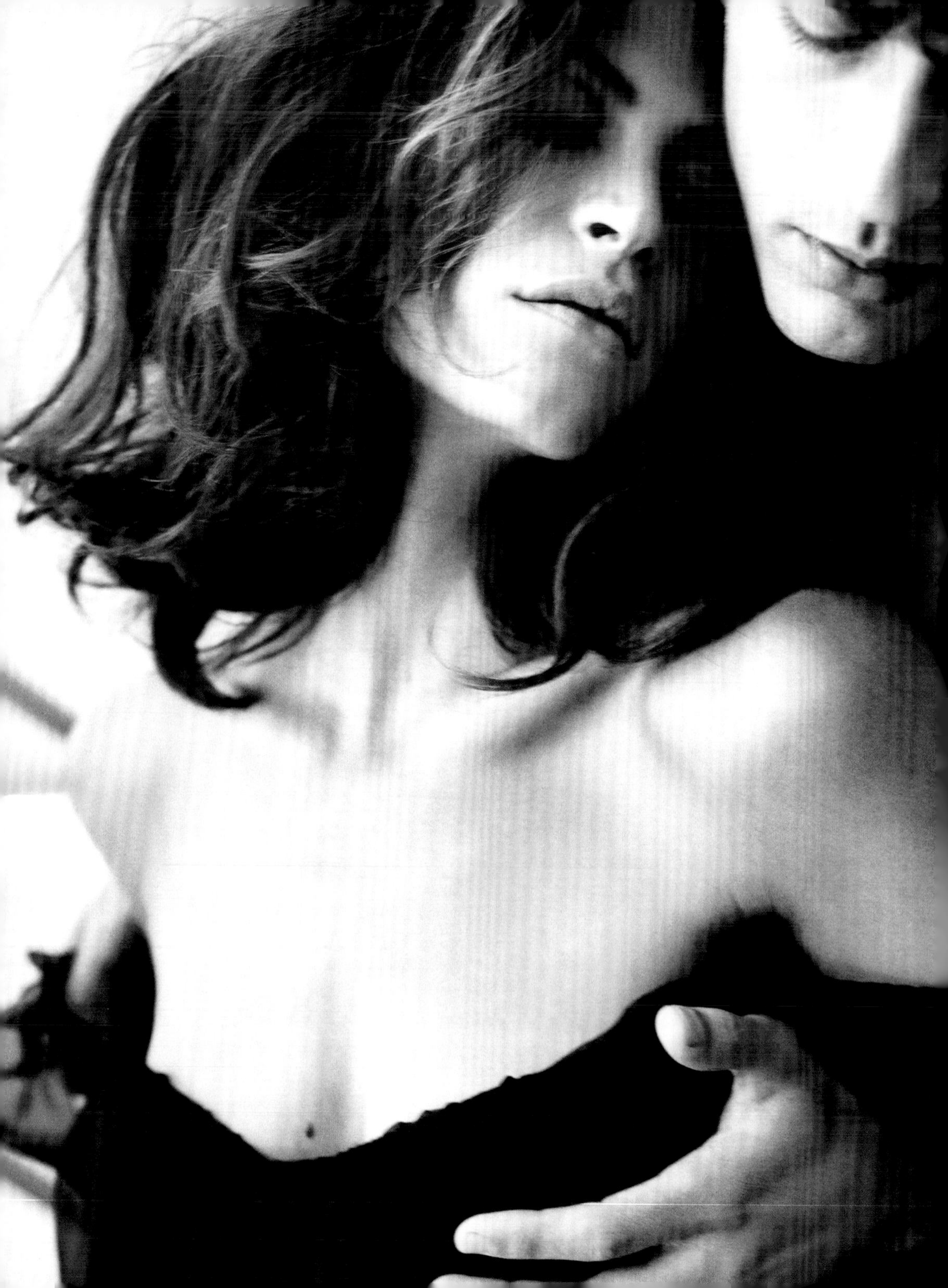

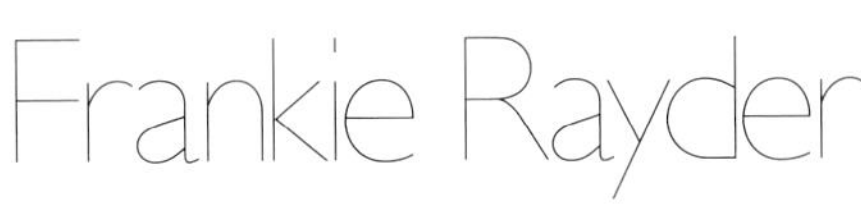

Frankie Rayder

By 2002, *Vogue* was delighted with Frankie Rayder's rapid progress, her innate sense of chic and her London credentials: 'She's best friends with Kate [Moss] and Jefferson [Hack, father of Kate's child], goes out with film director Roman Coppola and, after only five years as a model, has notched up glitzy ad campaigns for Versace, Tommy Hilfiger and Gucci.'

Rayder described her own personal style as 'Chanel bag lady', which did her few favours other than to highlight an endearing self-effacing nature. She was – and remains – an astute sifter of the thrift-store rack, an early exponent of the craze for vintage. She was, though, not shy of adding her own idiosyncratic twists. Caught on the street by *Vogue*, she wore an old but vibrant red Carolina Herrera coat she had picked up in New York, an older and more worn pair of Levi's, and a shirt 'specially monogrammed for me' (by Albertelli, the Roman tailors). She was fond of sporting her trademark argyle-patterned socks. American *Vogue* picked up on her individuality too: 'I have so many clothes,' she told the magazine, which noted that a recent acquisition was a Louis Vuitton dress, short with long sleeves, which she planned to wear one day with 'big, dirty high-heeled boots'.

The girl from almost unpronounceable Oconomowoc, Wisconsin, betrayed an admirable sense of perspective in a high-pressure world. On the eve of the prestigious VH1/*Vogue* Fashion Awards 2000, in which she was nominated as Model of the Year, she deadpanned: 'I mean, I must have done some really good modelling this year…' (Her colleague Carmen Kass was the eventual victor, to no hard feelings.)

At school Frankie, whose given name is Heidi, excelled on the track and field (400m especially, and the one-mile relay) and was, according to *Vogue*, a whizz at basketball too. The interest in sports continued into her early youth, when she took a job at a golf clubhouse. Her modelling career began early in nearby Minneapolis; within a couple of years she came to the attention of Steven Meisel. The upward trajectory remained unchecked; she first took to the catwalk in 1997 and was an instant success. More Meisel shoots followed (she was a feature of Gucci, Versace and Dolce & Gabbana advertising for several seasons).

Her younger sister Melinda 'Missy' Rayder embarked on a modelling career too, and it flourished in tandem with Frankie's. The Fabulous Rayder Sisters became an it-girl sensation – 'the most delightfully distracting sister act in recent memory,' according to one aficionado, who added, 'Frankie may well be the most attractive person ever to have been born in Wisconsin.' They starred together, and with a third sister, Molly, in a notable campaign for Gap clothing, 'Put a Little Love in Your Heart', in 2003. (There is, in fact, a fourth sister, and a brother too.)

Rayder's relationship with Roman Coppola faltered and she announced her engagement in 2005 to Michael Balzary, known simply as Flea, bass player of the Red Hot Chili Peppers. After a break from modelling to look after their daughter Sunny Bebop, Frankie returned to the fold in 2009, to a rapturous welcome.

Frankie Rayder (b. Heidi Rayder, 1975, USA)

Left:
'How Do You Want Me?',
September 2002,
by Mario Testino.
Fashion by Valentino

Freja Beha Erichsen

A little unfairly perhaps, the reputation of Freja Beha Erichsen, from Roskilde in Denmark, rests on a rather mannish appeal – she is the first stop for any fashion editor and photographer compelled to style masculine tailoring or to riff on *The Man Who Fell to Earth*, or some other otherworldly androgyne. This does not appear to overly perturb Freja. In fact, an occasionally 'disconnected' appearance reinforces the notion that nothing has ever perturbed her, nor is it likely to soon. This sets her apart from most of her contemporaries, together with an ineffable coolness and disdain for what might pass as industry norms.

It is usually a given, for example, that models do not sport tattoos – for obvious reasons. Or, if they must, then the tattoos are placed somewhere discreet (the ankle is a favourite). Freja's nonchalance has manifested itself in around a dozen tattoos, possibly more. These comprise some small and pretty – circles and hearts – but the most visible are aphoristic: 'serendipity is life' (the outside of her upper right arm); 'float' (on the side of her neck); 'this too shall pass' (the reverse of her upper right arm). 'Nobody has minded so far, I don't think,' Freja told *Vogue*. 'I did make a deal with my agent: she said I could get as many tattoos as I wanted, as long as I didn't cut my hair.' Though no time limit was specified, strictly speaking Freja did not keep her end of the bargain – 'I just felt like it,' she said as *Vogue* admired her new schoolboy crop, 'and so I cut it myself.'

Such disinterest manifested itself early on. Her modelling career appeared to be spontaneous: a talent scout glimpsed her in the street from the window of a taxi. 'When I was 15, I did a little modelling as a summer job,' she told *Vogue*. 'I didn't think it would become anything serious, but the little jobs led to bigger jobs and two years later, I was walking down the catwalk for Prada.'

Freja's undeniable allure has led to several fashion items made in homage to her: initially, the Jill Stuart Freja handbag, which, one expert opined, 'has a slightly geometric, slightly boho feel to it, as if Frank Lloyd Wright and Jack Kerouac cared about purses.' Then there was the Chloé Freja clutch of 2008 and the Freja lace-up stiletto boot by Alexander Wang.

Her enthusiasm for tattoos has continued unhindered, occasionally underscoring the tougher side to her character. On her revolver tattoo: 'I like guns,' she confided to *Vogue*, adding: 'and the design is pretty.'

Freja Beha Erichsen (b. 1987, Denmark)

Opposite:
'About a Boy', April 2008,
by Nick Knight.
Fashion by Luella

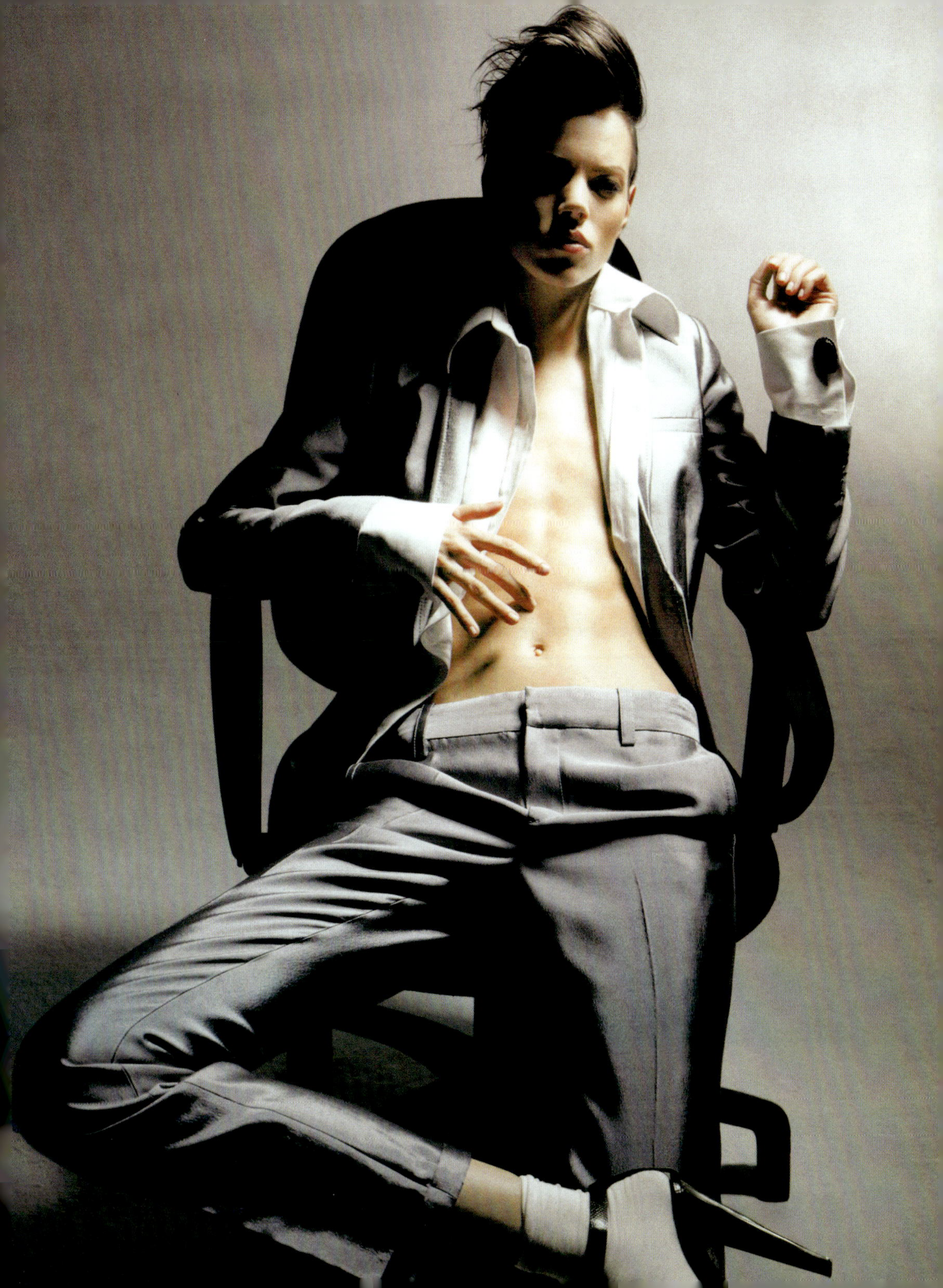

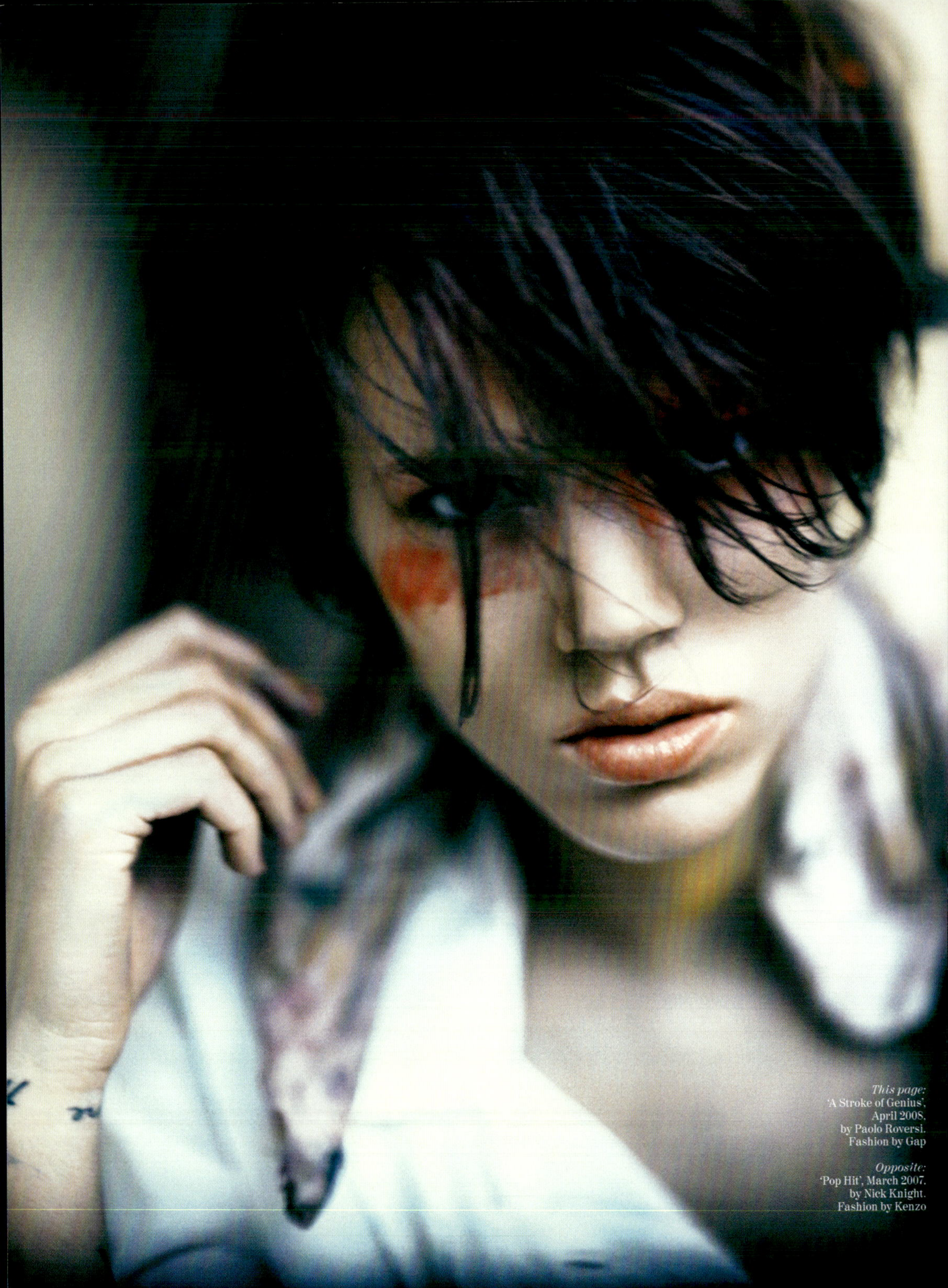

This page:
'A Stroke of Genius',
April 2008,
by Paolo Roversi.
Fashion by Gap

Opposite:
'Pop Hit', March 2007,
by Nick Knight.
Fashion by Kenzo

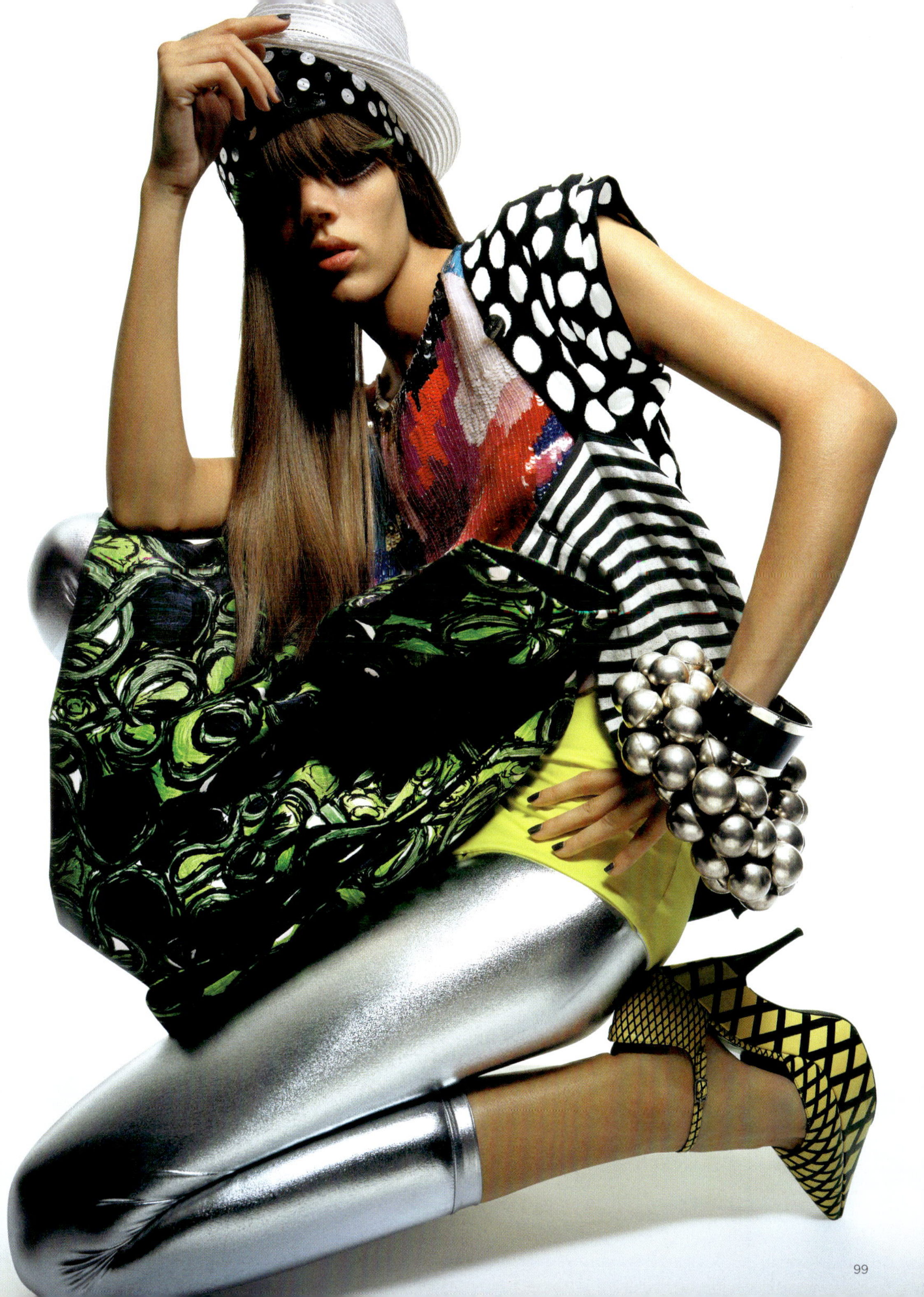

Gemma Ward

'With her wide forehead and otherworldly gaze,' remarked *Vogue*, 'Gemma Ward brings to mind an exquisitely formed alien dropped to earth for us to admire…' With regret, the truth was more prosaic – though not without a twist. Gemma grew up in Perth in Western Australia, the middle child of a doctor and a nurse, and sibling to younger twins and an older sister, who modelled before her. It was not a choice she had made for herself: 'I thought I'd become a comedian,' she told *Teen Vogue*.

However, accompanying some friends who wanted to try their luck in a modelling competition, she ended up being noticed herself. It was an unlikely scenario but, as Gemma recalled it, 'I had come straight from my auntie and uncle's farm, and I was wearing this big grey barn jacket with mud over it…' Her accomplices pushed their reluctant friend in front of the camera. She duly failed to win. However, the fairy tale continued inexorably: she gained an agent and another in New York – somehow – glimpsed her and sent a picture to Prada. The ethereal, winsome blonde was cast, sight unseen. 'She really was the model of the moment,' recalled Karl Lagerfeld. The baby-faced porcelain doll was also that rarity, 'an exotic blonde', according to photographer Michael Thompson; according to another, Nick Knight, 'Gemma is particularly graceful and fine in her movements. I do find her one of the most extraordinary models…' Prada was followed by Versace, which was followed in turn by a $1.5 million contract for Calvin Klein's perfume Obsession Night. A hiatus from school was all but inevitable. 'I'm doing things in my own time,' she told *Vogue*. 'I've learned that you have to take risks in life. That's what makes it exciting. You learn so much more from your mistakes than just being safe and sorry.'

Vogue's Lucinda Chambers had spied Gemma at catwalk shows for Prada, and cast her in a shoot with Nick Knight, ostensibly with a circus theme. It also made her, along with co-star Lily Cole, the youngest model to appear on a *Vogue* cover. The shoot was involving: 'I can feel the weight of the Gucci dress digging into my shoulders… The glare of the light keeps me warm as I stand against the green backdrop. The studio is in darkness but the light is blinding me and all I can hear is Nick's voice giving me directions.'

'I work with lots of different models,' says Knight, 'who are all very good in different ways. It's a bit like working with actresses. You cast the best actress for the right role. When she walked into the studio, this was the first time I'd met her – not often do you take a step backwards… I was very surprised by her beauty. She had a kind of beauty that was then slightly "otherworldly", slightly not quite of this planet. There's such a fragility about her.' The fragility was tested *ad extremis*. Knight put Gemma in a room full of mirrors and asked her to behave as if she hated her reflection. 'She beat her fists against the mirror until they bled. And she screamed screams that came from somewhere very deep. I do think she's fantastic. She's very, very bright.' US *Vogue* concurred: 'Those bedroom eyes, those lavish lips, one of the youngest in the vanguard, she knows how to create drama.'

Gemma Ward (b. 1987, Australia)

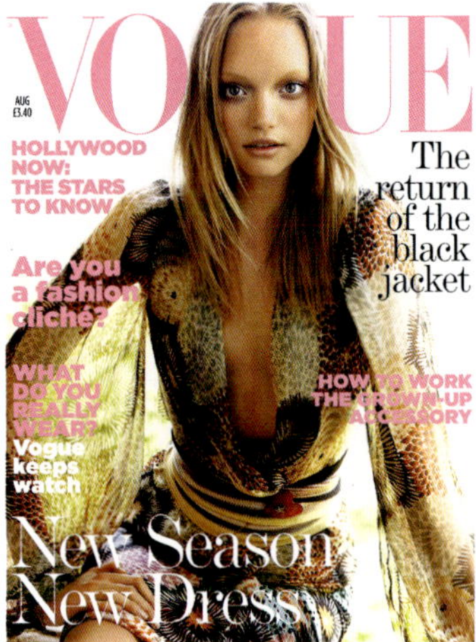

Above:
'New Season. New Dress', August 2005, by Mario Testino. Fashion by Missoni

Opposite:
'Roses', March 2004, by Paolo Roversi. Fashion by Stephen Jones Millinery

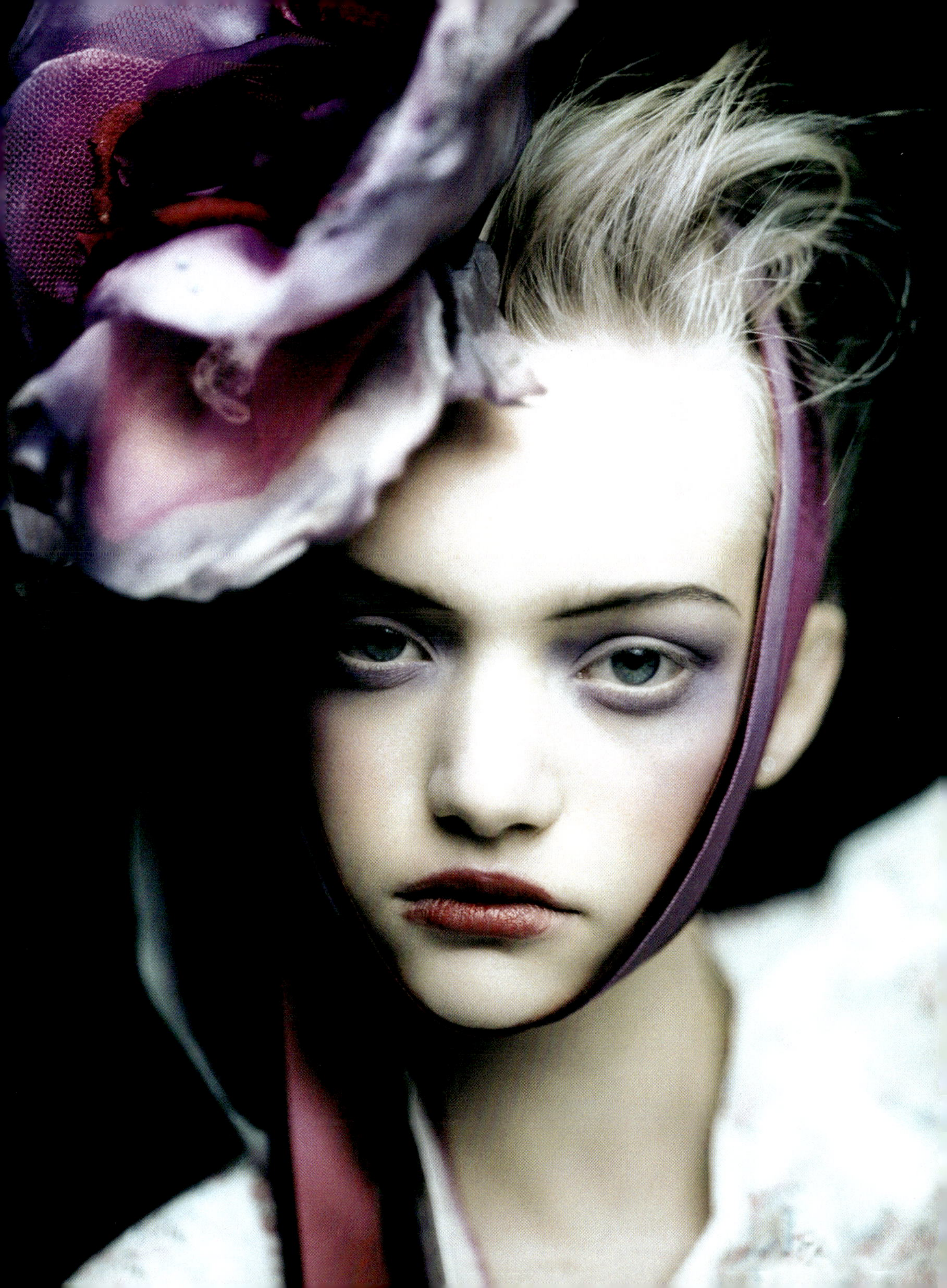

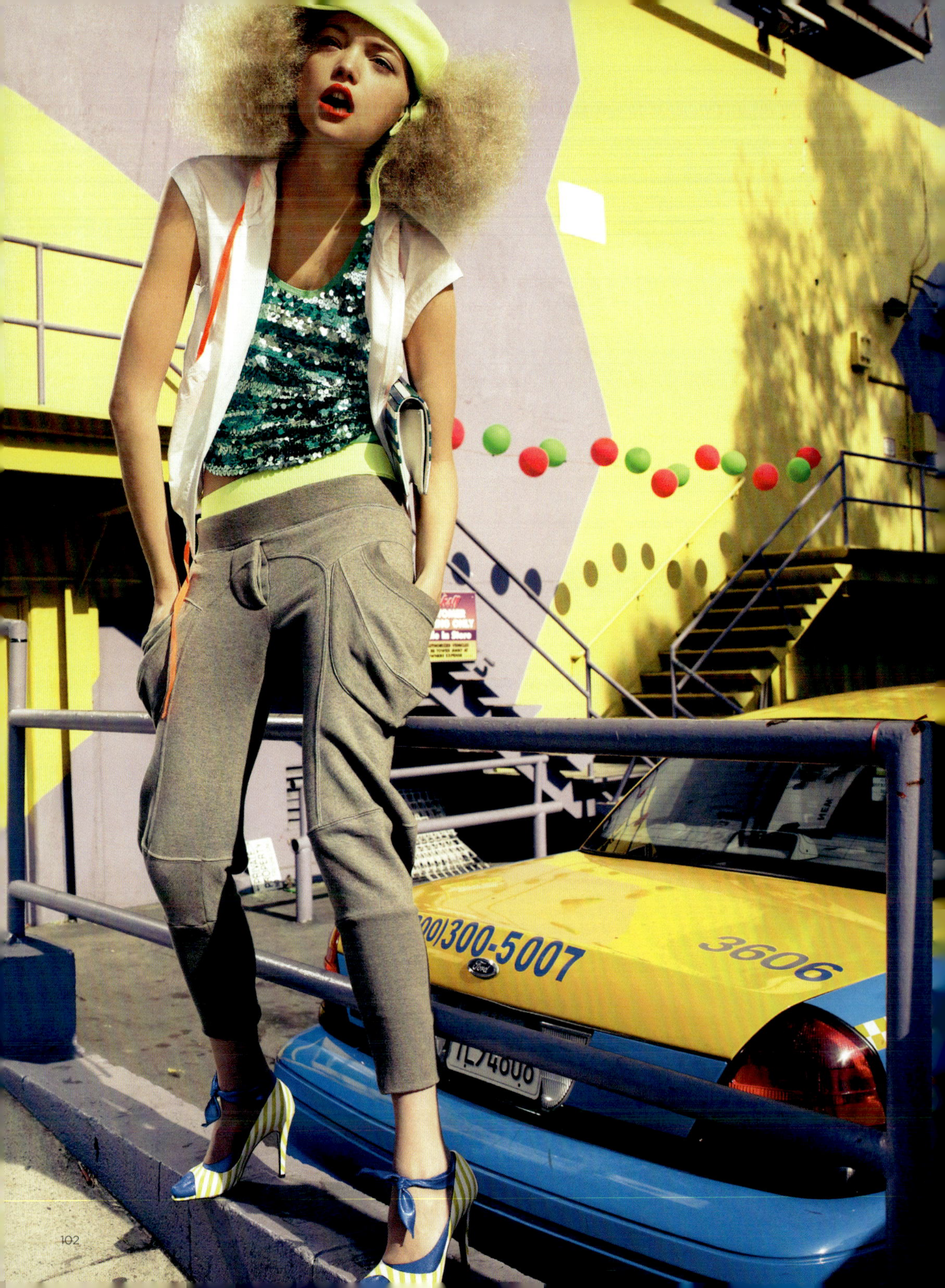
00)300-5007
3606

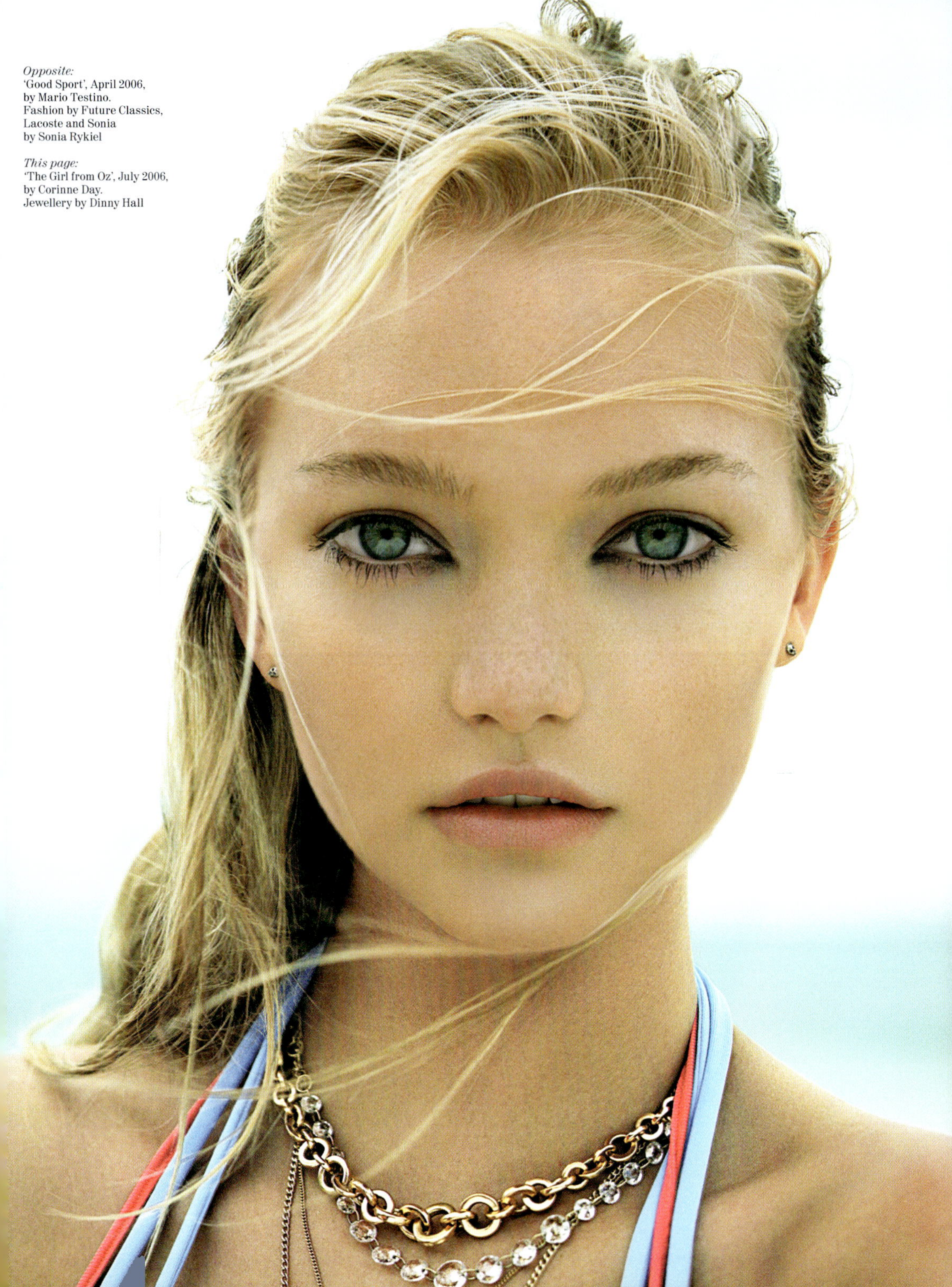

Opposite:
'Good Sport', April 2006,
by Mario Testino.
Fashion by Future Classics,
Lacoste and Sonia
by Sonia Rykiel

This page:
'The Girl from Oz', July 2006,
by Corinne Day.
Jewellery by Dinny Hall

Georgina Grenville

Backstage at the Chanel show, *Vogue* reported, 'the stylists go into a huddle... they huddle with the designer to discuss the length of a skirt. They are in a huddle again to decide whether Georgina Grenville's navel tattoo clashes with the diamond on her Chanel belt buckle.' For South African-born Georgina Grenville, the projection of an image was key to her *modus operandi* and that could be hard work. She confided to *Vogue*: 'It can be stressful and quite lonely. And it's difficult to make plans when your schedule changes so much.' She concluded on a more hopeful note: 'There's a lot more that I like about modelling than I dislike about modelling. It's a great job.'

She revealed further that in the more intimate catwalk shows – for which she was much coveted – the models would overhear the audience's asides: 'Sometimes they'll say "Oh, she's put on weight" or "She looks good", but you never know whether they're talking about you or the girl in front.' Although at these twice-yearly rituals of the fashion calendar, designers were allowed to act insanely, Georgina played the game shrewdly – by attending at least two key parties each season. 'It's expected. The magazines and designers like to think they're getting a personality.'

Georgina found fame as the original 'Gucci Girl', an early ornament of the designer Tom Ford, for whom she regularly appeared on the catwalk. She closed his final show for Gucci. In an acutely observed and knowing slice of art imitating life, Georgina appeared again as 'Gucci Girl' in a special episode of the television sitcom *Absolutely Fabulous*, a satire on the inner workings of the fashion and fashion-magazine industries.

Bearing in mind all the hard work, *Vogue* professed to be shocked to hear 'that one of the sultriest, sexiest models *du jour* prefers to hang out on her father's ranch in Kenya than at the coolest metropolitan nightspots', but it conceded cheerfully that that just makes her so much sexier.

Georgina Grenville (b. 1975, South Africa)

Opposite:
'Sunny Delight', June 2000,
by Regan Cameron.
Fashion by Moschino

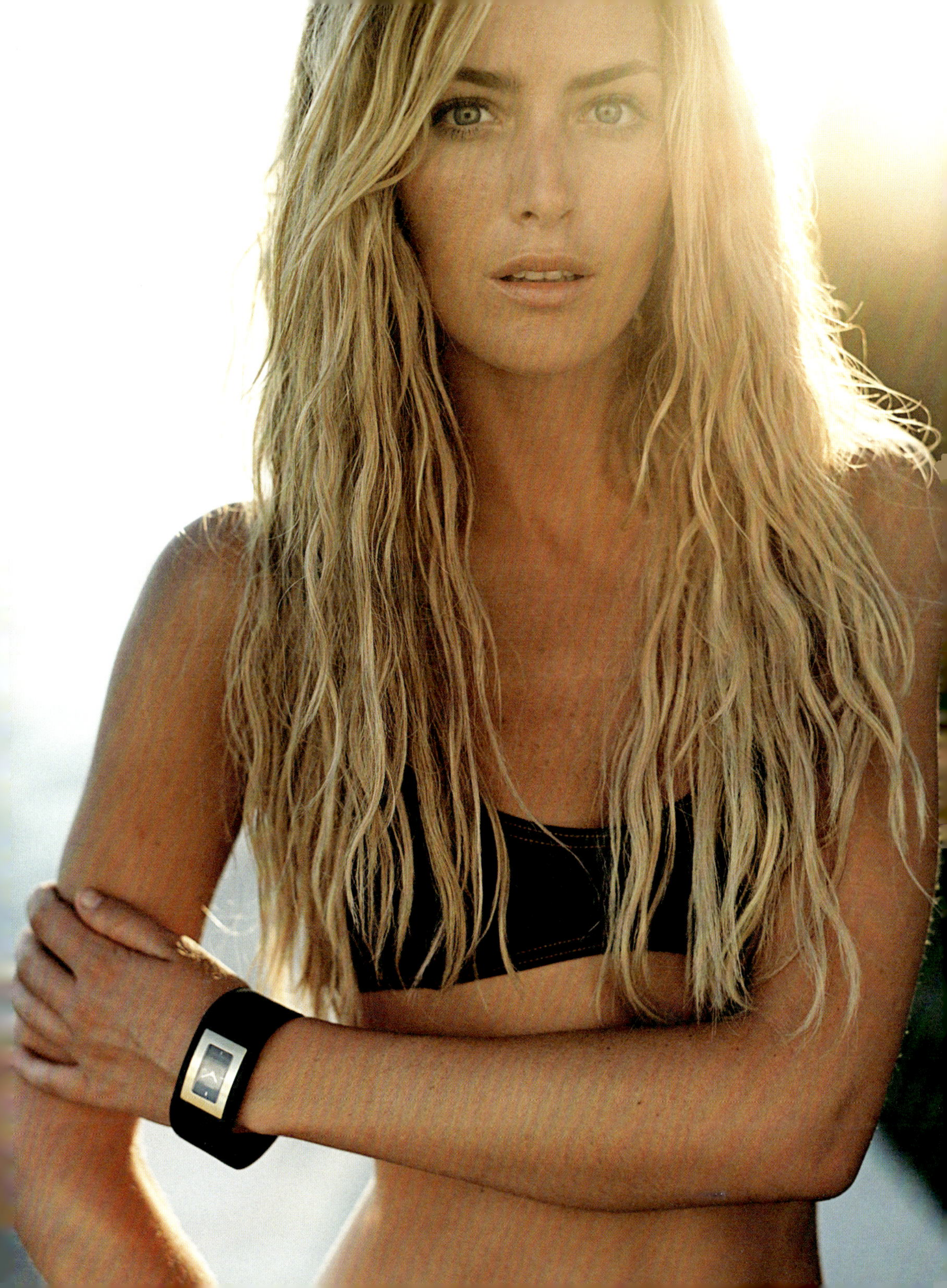

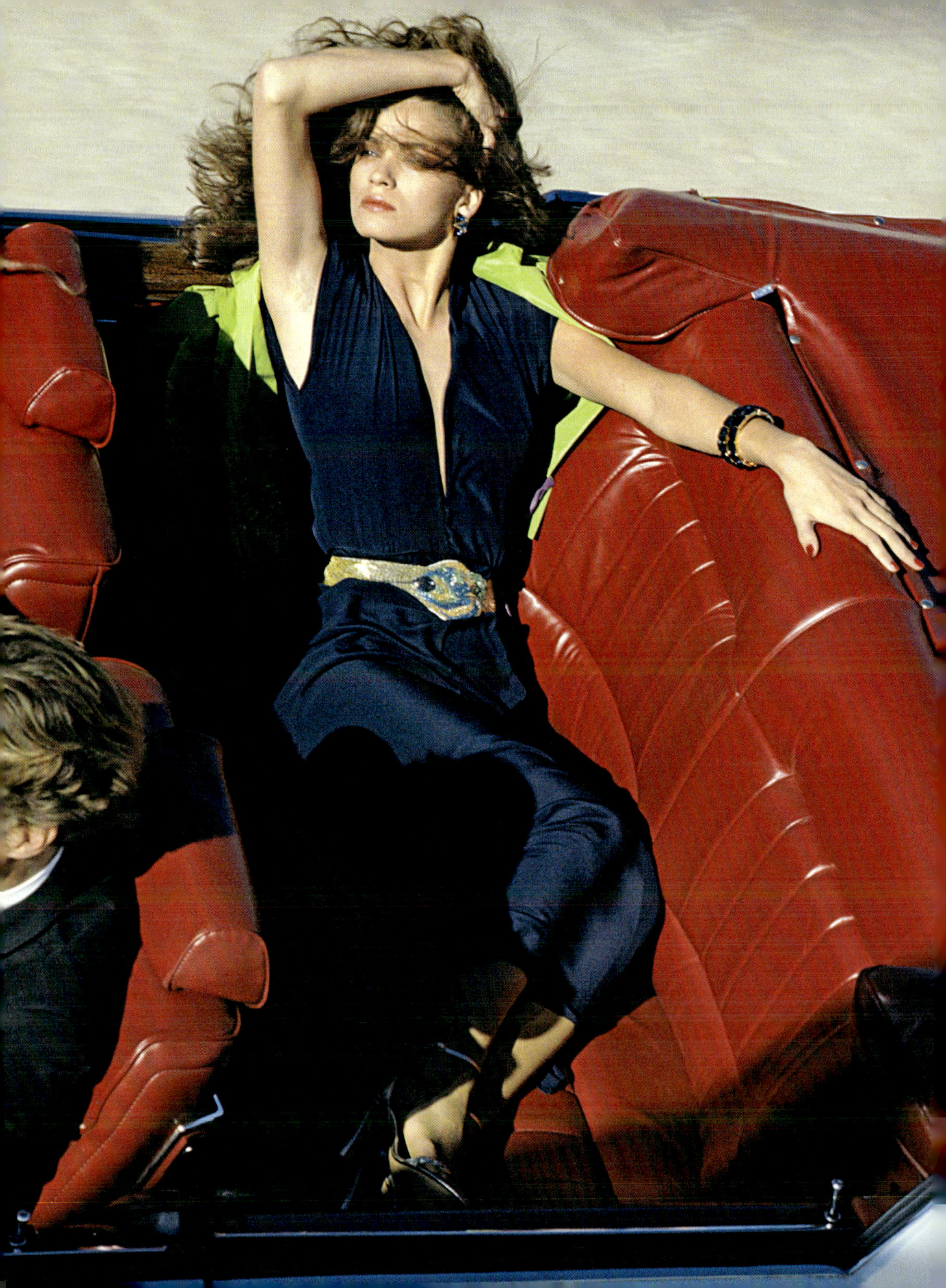

Gia Carangi

'Gia was fantastic when she hit [town],' recalled *Vogue*'s Polly Mellen. 'I thought instantly, "Oh wow! Boy? Girl?" I've always been fascinated by Garbo and the way she looked in men's suits. Gia had that same androgynous quality...'

No photographer, it was said, could resist Gia from Philadelphia – half Irish-American, half Italian-American. Her mere presence made them reach for their cameras and fire the shutter straight off. Chris von Wangenheim refused to let her leave his studio – she was there on a speculative go-see – until he had exposed some frames. And from then on he wanted her entirely for himself. She laughed, and he failed. Arthur Elgort had seen her the previous morning: 'She was tough and streetwise. But I just thought she was such a special face, extremely beautiful, sexy and cool... She was scooped up fast.'

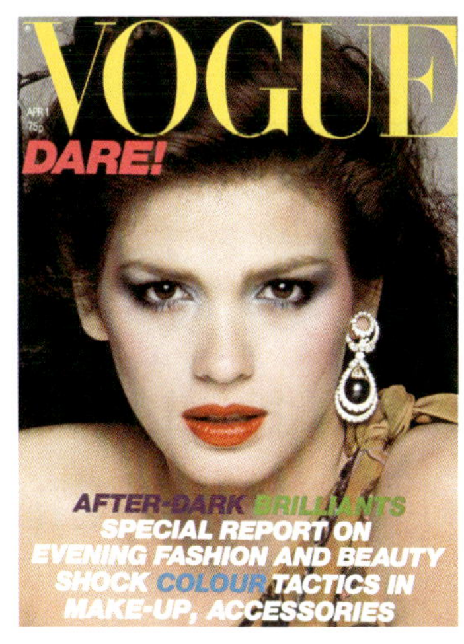

Gia's career was short. It began in 1978, lasting barely four and a half years (intermittently towards the end) until she slid from *Vogue*'s attention around 1983. By then she was in thrall to heroin addiction, somehow still working, but her most prestigious clients were deserting her fast. Raw photographs would show needle tracks up and down her arms. She slid further in a downward spiral; in 1986 she died, aged 26.

Her fall from grace was part of fashion-industry folklore, her example waved as a warning in front of recalcitrant newcomers. Cindy Crawford, who shared her dark and sultry looks, was known in her early career as Baby Gia. Only fashion insiders knew who Gia had been. Not until 1993 and a harrowing biography, *Thing of Beauty* by Stephen Fried, did Gia's name became known to a wider public. Later she was the subject of a TV biopic, *Gia* – Angelina Jolie took on the title role – which recounted her life story for a prime-time audience in 1998.

When it was all fresh and new and fun, the pictures were superb. As her career accelerated, and a dark star began ever so slightly to occlude her beauty, the pictures became gripping. 'She was about melancholy and darkness,' said a fellow model, 'and that made great pictures.'

Helmut Newton selected Gia for a suite of pictures taken in the Hotel George V in Paris. Cecil Beaton commented that Newton liked to 'play tricks on his audience' and this was one of the best. A female model, hair slicked back, dressed in a YSL suit, towered over Gia while lighting her cigarette for her, tip to tip. The eroticism burned on the page – the more so to aficionados as Gia's bisexuality was a well-known industry secret.

Then there was the Chris von Wangenheim oeuvre – colourful, to say the least. He became known for single-handedly making a model's career – chiefly Gia's. Her figure, he said, was unbeatable, any pictures he took of her 'page stoppers'. Most page-stopping of all were his homoerotic pictures of her and another rising star, Juli Foster. They eschewed the cool eroticism of Helmut Newton for something colder and harder. In one shot, Juli's high heels pressed into Gia's naked hips; in another, Juli and Gia, wearing only high heels, were locked in a fierce embrace.

When Gia shone, she made an unforgettable impact, but as drugs took hold of her she became increasingly unreliable: arriving late; having to leave early; not showing up at all; stumbling in, unable to work. A watershed was reached when she walked out of a sitting with Richard Avedon (usually career suicide). She worked sporadically again, but the inexorable decline accelerated. Arrests, rehab, clean periods, rehab again. Finally she became HIV positive. For the last few weeks of her short life she was hospitalised, all but unrecognisable as the exuberant, streetwise kid from Pittsburgh, a *Vogue* cover model and disco-era hands-in-the-air catwalk sensation, who had hit the ground running barely a few years previously.

Gia Carangi (b. 1960, USA; d. 1986)

Opposite:
'Evening... A World Apart', February 1979, by Chris von Wangenheim. Fashion by Bill Blass

Above:
'Dare!', April 1979, by Alex Chatelain. Fashion by Genny

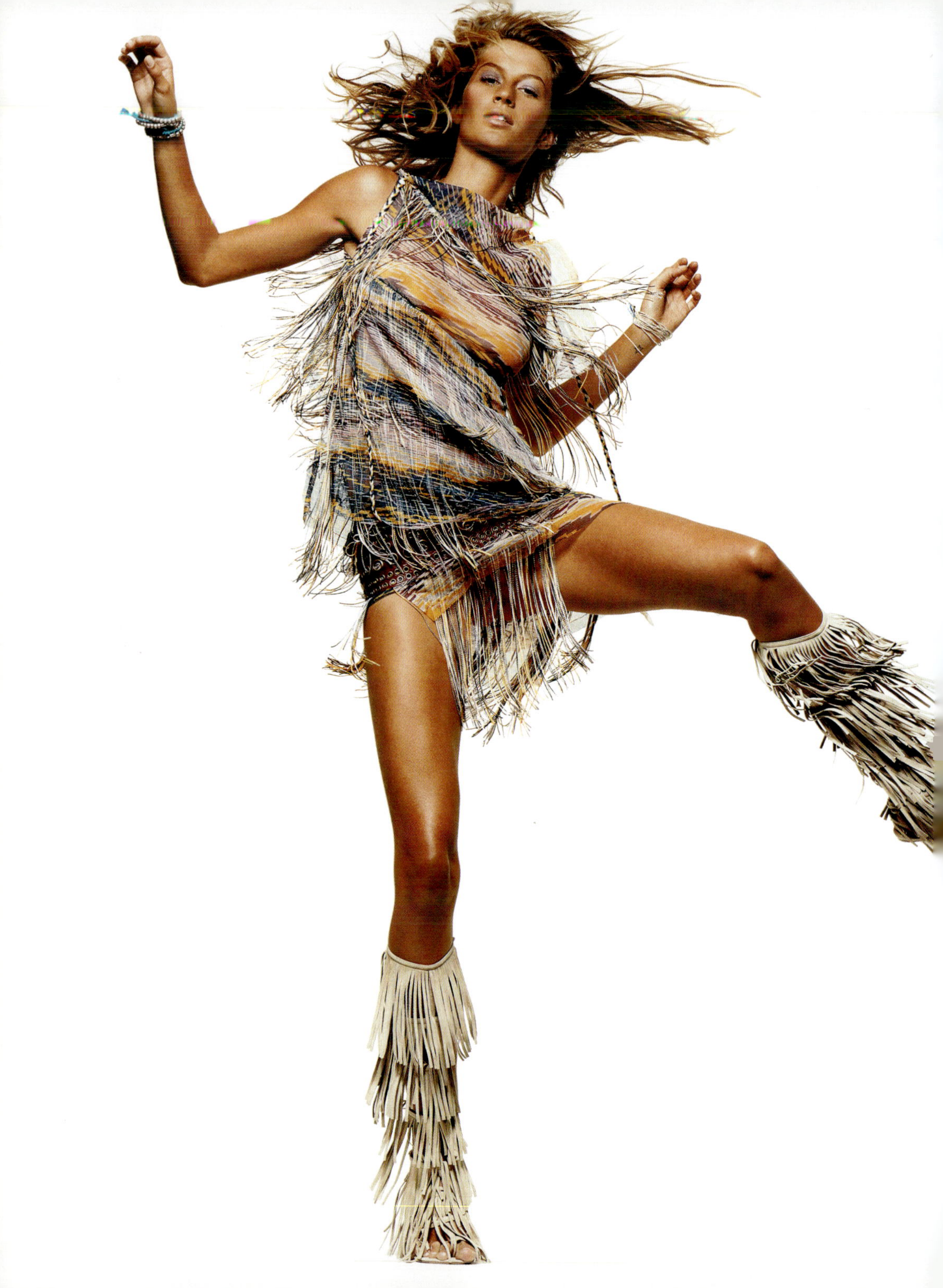

Gisele Bündchen

'They've tried pushing intelligent and weird before and it doesn't work,' one stylist opened up to *Vogue*. 'Women in America want to be Gisele. That's just how it is.' The world's highest-paid model of several years (fortune estimated, conservatively, at $150 million and rising) has also sold the most Brazilian flip-flops in the world. This is her own line, the Ipanema Gisele Bündchen. In a worldwide poll carried out by the International Society of Aesthetic Plastic Surgeons, it was revealed that the most desirable abdomen and hair, as chosen by potential patients, belonged to Gisele (she came second in the breasts category). On the same theme, Gisele topped an *Elle* magazine poll for 'best hair in Hollywood', despite having appeared in only one leading role (as a bank robber in 2004's *Taxi*). The grace of her deportment also moved the fashion correspondent of the *New York Times* to neologism: 'She has this instinctive thing where you just go… *schwing!*'

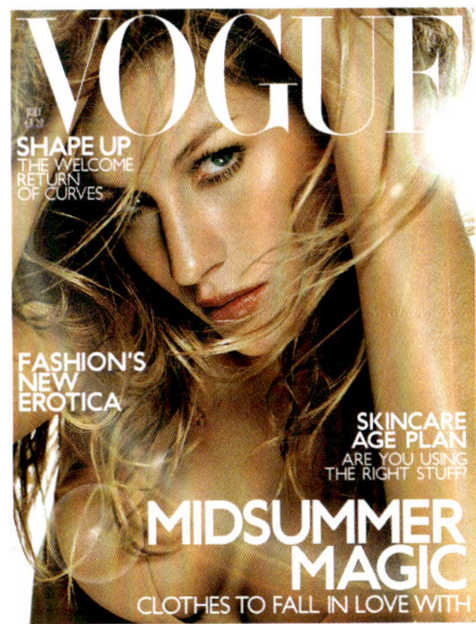

She has come a long way from the village of Horizontina, 28 hours by bus from São Paulo – relatively close by, in Brazilian terms. There it began, as all great modelling success stories do, with the boys at school teasing her for her height and skinniness (she was called Olívia Palito – Portuguese for Olive Oyl). 'I was like the ugly duck,' she confirmed. 'It was horrible.' She thought she might make it as a professional volleyball player. She is 5ft 10½in and weighs around 115lb – every single one, according to American *Vogue*, in precisely the right place. 'The return of the sexy model,' it proclaimed in 1999, with Gisele as its poster girl. This physique, all tanned curves, muscle and light freckling, is honed to perfection. It has come to redefine the way people want to look (and not just the clientèle of the world's cosmetic surgeons).

Ironic, perhaps, that Gisele was, as is now fashion folklore, discovered by a modelling scout among a dozen almost identically clad 14-year-old schoolchildren in a São Paulo branch of McDonald's. She did look slightly taller than the rest. It was her first Big Mac and her first trip to a big city. There was little hesitation, although she had never seen any fashion magazines: 'I was so happy about this, so thrilled. What lay beyond São Paulo was Rio!' There were parental obstacles to overcome, but by 1996 her persistence had paid off and Gisele travelled to New York, able to speak only a few words of English – enough, she said, to get her to assignments and that was it. (She now speaks it, and several more languages, fluently.)

Patrick Demarchelier saw her in 1997 and made a few exposures of the burgeoning Brazilian beauty. 'She was so different, so healthy. At the time, models were all edgy, with the look like drug addicts, and no-one was interested in Gisele. And then eight months later *everyone* wanted Gisele.' The catwalk put her on the map (a McQueen extravaganza, a show-stopping turn for Dolce & Gabbana), but her photographic break came on a chance go-see to fellow South American Mario Testino's studio. 'He holds a special place in my heart,' she says. 'He's been there with me from the beginning. But more than that we understand each other… He's a little bit *safadinho* – you know, a bit naughty and mischievous.'

Also a little bit naughty and mischievous is Gisele's little dog Vida, the best accessorised Yorkshire terrier in the animal kingdom (a dog necklace/collar from Chanel; a Vuitton dog bag by Marc Jacobs). 'I just want my dog to be normal. I would not like my dog to be a model. No way, and that's it.'

Gisele Bündchen (b. 1980, Brazil)

Opposite:
'Nature's Child',
January 2002,
by Thomas Schenk.
Fashion by Missoni

Above:
'Midsummer Magic',
July 2001,
by Nick Knight.
Fashion by Versace

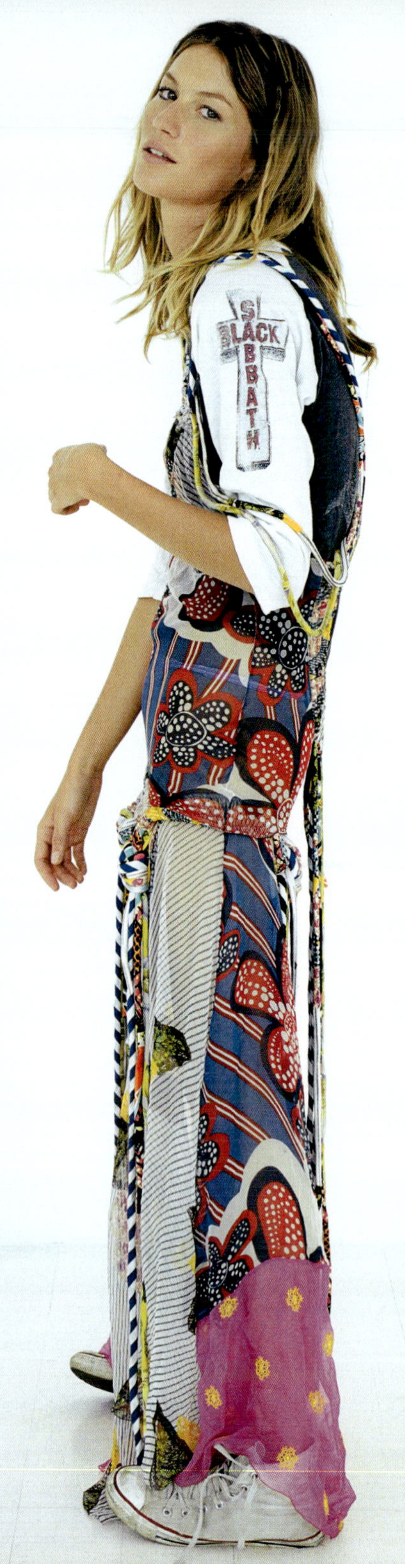

This page:
'The Long Story', June 2002,
by Corinne Day.
Fashion by John Galliano

Opposite:
'High Summer', June 2004,
by Carter Smith.
Fashion by Calvin Klein

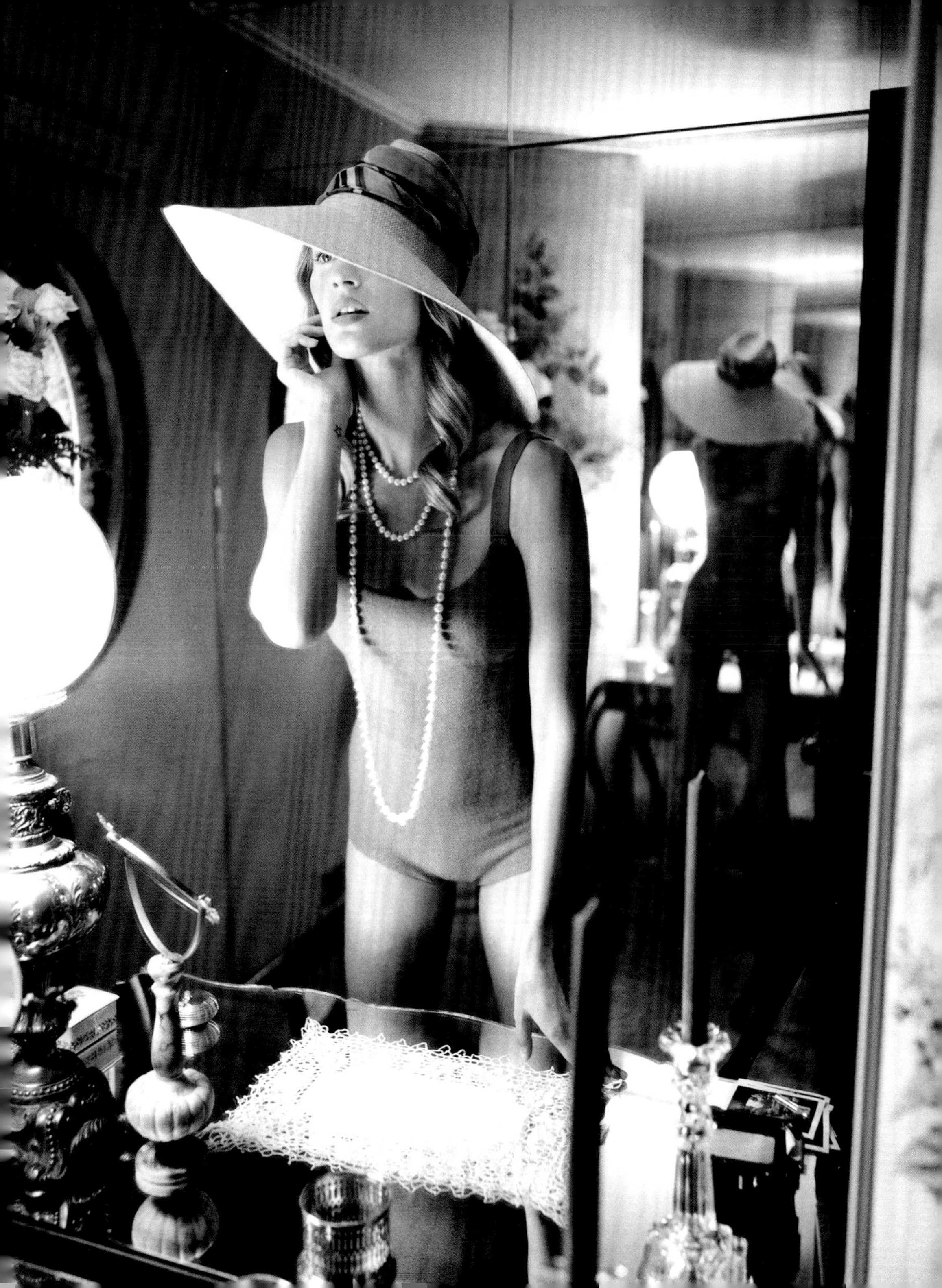

Grace Coddington

The creative director of American *Vogue*, which she first joined in 1988 after 19 years as a fashion editor at British *Vogue* and a spell at Calvin Klein, Coddington has edited some of fashion's most inspirational and inventive pictures. 'She is a Merlin, who could magic the best from a given set of circumstances,' says Barry Lategan, with whom she produced exotic pictures fit for the whimsical 1970s. However, her work ethic, extraordinary planning and attention to detail ensure that nothing is left to chance. She would, as her collaborator Bruce Weber has said, 'climb any mountain, fall out of any tree for a picture'. Or – scarcely believable but true – attempt to dye the sea a deeper blue for Guy Bourdin.

Born and raised on the isle of Anglesey, she suspects her subscription for *Vogue* was 'probably the only one in a 100-mile radius'. In late-1950s London, while working as a waitress in a Putney coffee bar, she enrolled on a modelling course. The Cod first made her mark on *Vogue*'s fashion pages by winning its model contest in 1959. Sporting a signature Vidal Sassoon asymmetrical cut, she learnt about fashion by wearing it and watching the great photographers at close hand: Helmut Newton, David Bailey, Terence Donovan and Norman Parkinson. Since then she has given photographers strengths they never knew they had and immortality to those who might not otherwise have deserved it.

Norman Parkinson was the first to see the potential, arranging a shoot which involved, among other things, Coddington running naked through a farmyard. 'It didn't occur to me that this wasn't an everyday occurrence. I thought, well, maybe that's what models do…' Parkinson taught her, too, that great fashion photographs are the product of teamwork. 'It's really all about people. The fashion is almost incidental,' she has observed. He taught her, she says, 'everything I know, to understand a country, not just to whip in and take from it…'

Even a car crash did not stop her, though she made the change from in front of the lens to behind it. 'I always had an opinion,' she said. 'As I now know, I'm one of those models you don't want to work with. I'm incredibly stubborn and I just nag on till I get what I want.' She has aided the careers of many: Manolo Blahnik, whose wooden platform shoes she championed in 1973, and Calvin Klein, who was all but unknown in Britain before she took him up.

Her own style, focusing on her tumbling auburn hair, has been equally influential: one moment a languid St Tropez athlete, the next a pale aesthete in baggy cardigans. For nearly 40 years, she has pushed *Vogue* to do more, to give it an even greater sense of style. 'It's not just frocks,' she once remarked, 'it's how we do our houses, our gardens, how we eat and drink.'

She is, as her colleagues have discovered, a perfectionist. To Anna Wintour, US *Vogue*'s editor-in-chief, 'Grace has the best eye in the business and can sense a trend even before the designers have an inkling. She's also persistent: if Grace has an idea she will grind me down until I accept it – and she's usually right.' As viewers of the 2009 documentary *The September Issue* will have seen for themselves, the quietly forceful, eminently self-deprecating and genuinely deadpan-funny Grace Coddington is still, after half a century in the fashion business, a creative whirlwind, her collaborations enviable and photographs endlessly ripe for copying. In the meantime, as the writer Georgina Howell observed, she is immune to the more ostentatious elements of her chosen business: 'It gives her authority not to be bowed by flattery or bought by every kiss.'

Grace Coddington (b. 1941, UK)

Opposite:
'Top Coats', September 1966,
by David Bailey.
Fashion by Harvey Gould

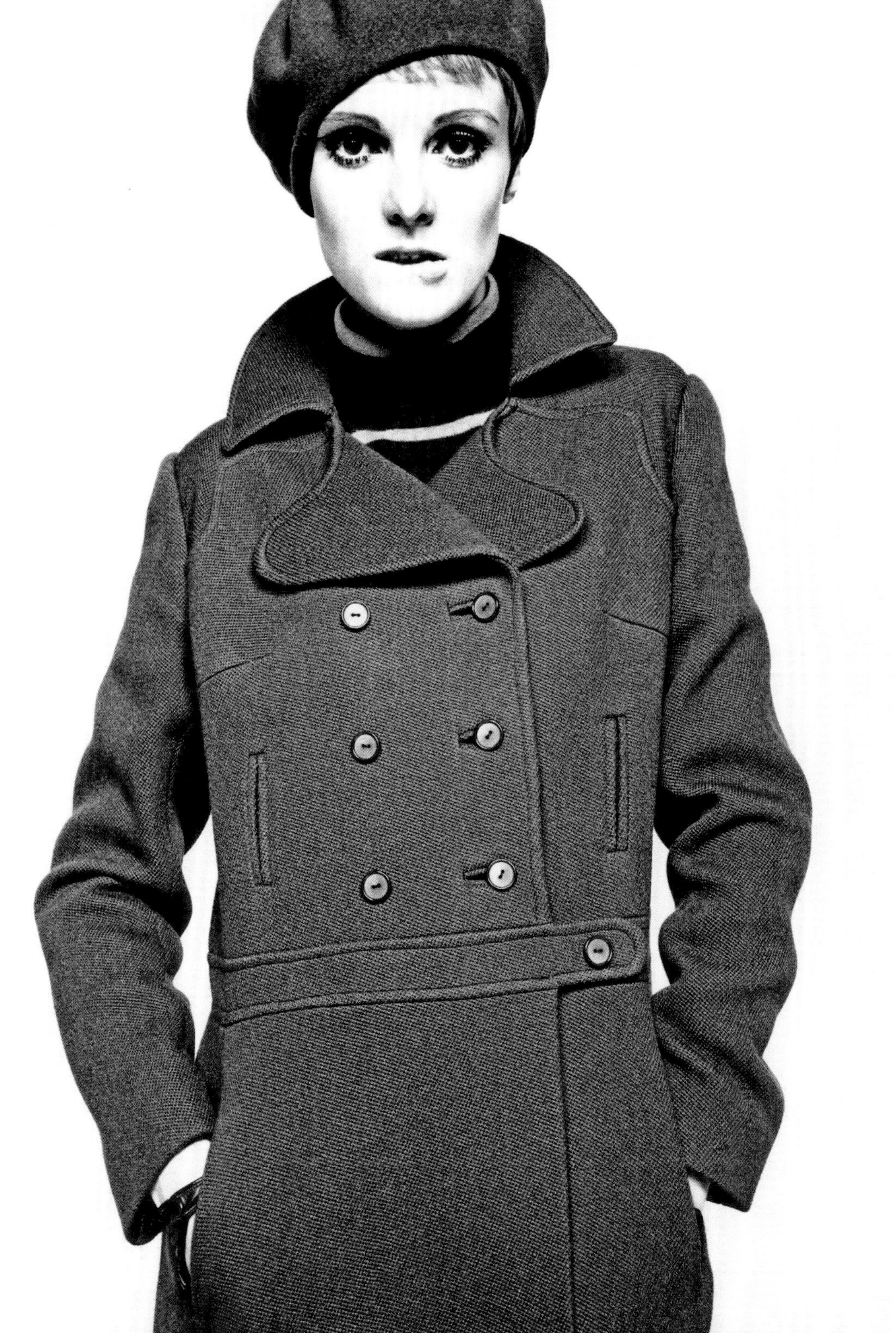

Guinevere Van Seenus

Vogue has praised the 'darkly seductive allure' of Guinevere Van Seenus and she remains an inspiration to many in the industry, but it was not always the case. In 1995, admiring greatly the 18-year-old refugee from Washington, DC (via Santa Barbara), the magazine singled out her 'dreamy eyes' for praise. It did, however, mention in passing her 'leading man's square jaw', which might not have been an asset even in the last flickering days of the supermodel phenomenon.

In fact, Guinevere had recently been dropped by the Elite agency but another, Storm, had picked her up. She made no pretence to being anything other than she was, though it was not initially the most favourable calling-card. *Vogue*'s Lisa Armstrong takes up the story: 'She arrived at Ben de Lisi's Soho studio to audition for his catwalk show... She had the confidence to trust her own instincts. She didn't sashay up and down in front of the designer or twirl at the end of an imaginary catwalk or demonstrate her deftness with jacket buttons. She didn't get the job, either.'

Her time, *Vogue* predicted, would come; it came sooner than either might have imagined. Fortunately for Guinevere, the 'glamour is back' revival of 1995 did not last much beyond the end of the year and athleticism, once decidedly in, was rapidly going out. Stella Tennant's nose-ring was attracting attention and the alien otherworldliness of Kristen McMenamy was playing to packed ateliers. 'Clients,' *Vogue* reported, 'had stopped asking for the next Cindy, Christy or Helena and were booking girls who expressed a fresh set of qualities...' Mario Testino booked Guinevere for French *Vogue* and the particular fresh set of qualities she brought was fostered further by younger and less established photographers, such as Juergen Teller, David Sims and Craig McDean, who tended to bypass the traditional casting in favour of something more ad hoc. The face of Jil Sander, Nicole Farhi and Sportmax by 1996, she was at once beautiful and edgy. 'When we used Guinevere we got so many letters,' Jil Sander told *Vogue*. 'People either loved her or hated her, but it was very important to try to challenge standard concepts of what's beautiful.'

Some 15 years after her debut, Guinevere was more in demand than ever, not least because of her ability to be whatever anyone wanted her to be: folksy traveller on the austere plains of Hungary for Tom Craig, nipple-tasselled burlesque showgirl for Javier Vallhonrat, and simply, though never plainly, nude for Paolo Roversi.

A mid-career apogee: Tim Walker's 'England's Dreaming', a story set in a rurally secluded country house. Here Guinevere was chatelaine of all she surveyed, a sort of postmodern Miss Havisham. 'We tried to imagine the upholstery and furnishings of an English country house as the folds of the couture,' explained Tim of his all-but-indescribable tableaux, 'so we tried to make a chair look like the waist of a bustled dress. That took two days and it didn't work. [Set designer] Andy Hillman made a "Charles James" dress out of curtains, its tassels a sash. That took him a whole afternoon. We posed Guinevere in a Rochas dress and she piped up: "I'm going to be the curtain that fell off the rail." At that point the sun came out...'

The sitting was marked by further absurdity: two vintage Wolseleys were clad in Aran knitwear, a feat that required 300 winter jumpers in June in Suffolk. Next, for a scenario inspired by Delaroche's painting *The Execution of Lady Jane Grey*, 80 buckets of lilacs were required: 'We cut down the entire lilac tree belonging to a neighbour,' said Tim worriedly.

Whenever the pressures of the modelling world become too much to bear – and surely they must, after all the role-playing – Guinevere always goes home. In these peripatetic times for models, 'home is wherever I can hibernate with my dog'.

Guinevere Van Seenus (b. 1977, USA)

Opposite:
'What Lies Beneath',
September 2008,
by Javier Vallhonrat.
Fashion by Emporio Armani

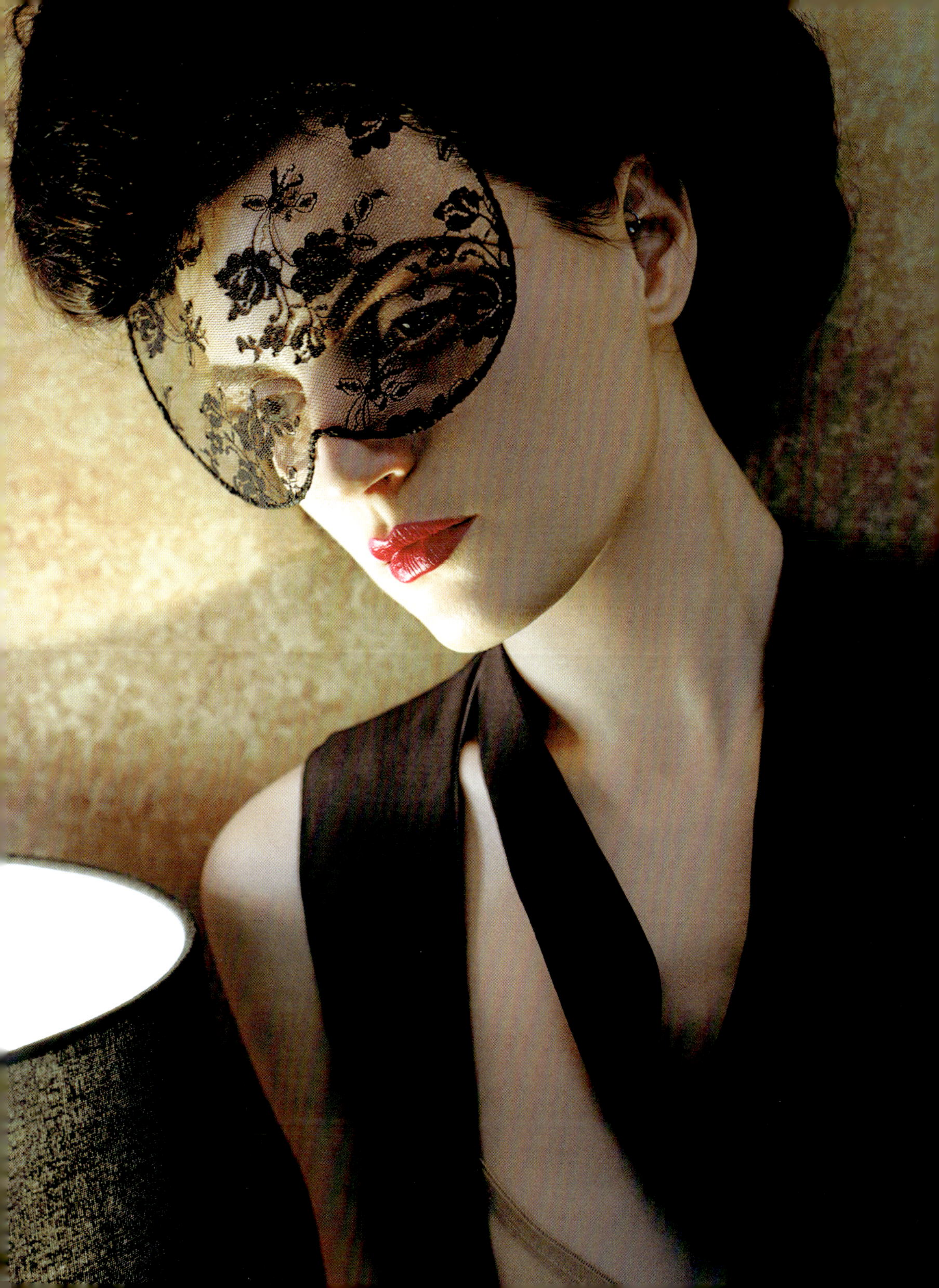

Helena Christensen

The smouldering eyes of model Helena Christensen, and her generous cleavage, added a certain *Dolce Vita* charm to *Vogue*'s early photographs of its favourite Scandinavian goddess. Truth to be told, *Vogue* was always a little bit in awe of 1987's Miss Denmark, whose 'implausible physical advantages' marked her out significantly from her colleagues. On the subject of those physical advantages, she has never been overly inhibited – 'I never mind being photographed nude. I think bare breasts are beautiful, whether they're large or small' – and never minded doing so for *Vogue*.

She was also mistress of the pertinent aperçu: 'How do you get to the top in this business? It helps if you're blonde, have big tits, and sleep with all the photographers,' she remarked to one such, Arthur Elgort. 'Just kidding!' she added. Another photographer, Max Vadukul, told *Vogue*: 'It's obvious the moment you see her. She's a sex bomb…'

Helena is also something of an eccentric, which has always endeared her greatly to *Vogue*. She confided that cheese means a great deal to her, and her devotion to the foodstuff was much chronicled. 'I love all cheese,' she told *GQ*. 'French cheese, Italian cheese, even British cheese. I've seriously thought about getting a cheese tattoo. A nice Edam on my shoulder, maybe…' The British Cheese Board has added her name to its roster of well-known 'cheesaholics', along with Prince Charles and television presenter Donna Air. Helena's impeccable Danish credentials also led her to a stint in 2002 as the Carlsberg Export girl (a successor of sorts to the Lamb's Navy Rum girls of the 1970s).

Outside the fashion and advertising pages (she was formerly the face of Sonia Rykiel and Karl Lagerfeld), Helena was still a feature of magazines, not least for her ability to juggle all kinds of things apart from modelling, such as photography and magazine work – she helped launch *Nylon* magazine – as well as writing. Helena was an acute observer for *Vogue* of the circus surrounding the Sundance Film Festival. Also keeping her in the headlines were her romances and friendships with rock stars and actors. The father of her child, Mingus, is the actor Norman Reedus. In 1992, she was photographed for *Vogue*'s 'Rock. Fame. Fashion' special at the Provençal farmhouse of her then boyfriend, the singer Michael Hutchence (*Vogue* was in thrall to her 'goddess body'). She was also close to the ill-starred actor Heath Ledger, whom it was thought she was on her way to visit when his body was discovered.

On her days as a supermodel – she was up there with Linda, Christy, Naomi *et al* – Helena looks back and says 'It was great,' adding, 'I look back at it and it just fucking blows my mind! I would do it all again if I had the chance. It was so cool to be part of it when things were exploding. Every day something weird happened that you couldn't believe was real. I had a couple of lifetimes' worth of experience crammed into 10 years…' And with modelling calling her back again, there may well be more lifetimes still to experience.

Helena Christensen (b. 1968, Denmark)

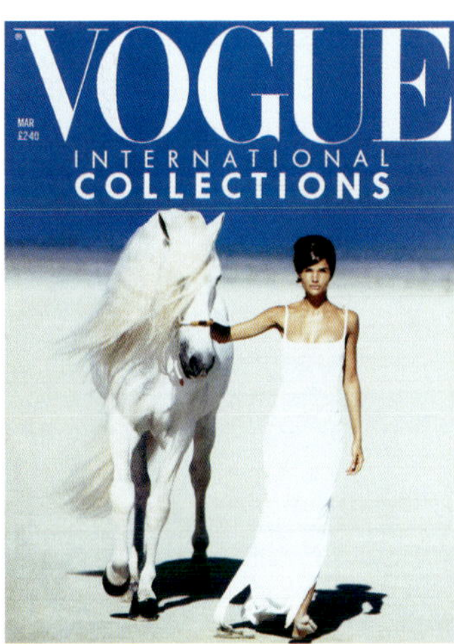

Above: 'International Collections', March 1990, by Peter Lindbergh. Fashion by Giorgio di Sant'Angelo

Opposite: 'Saving Faces', October 1993, by Nick Knight

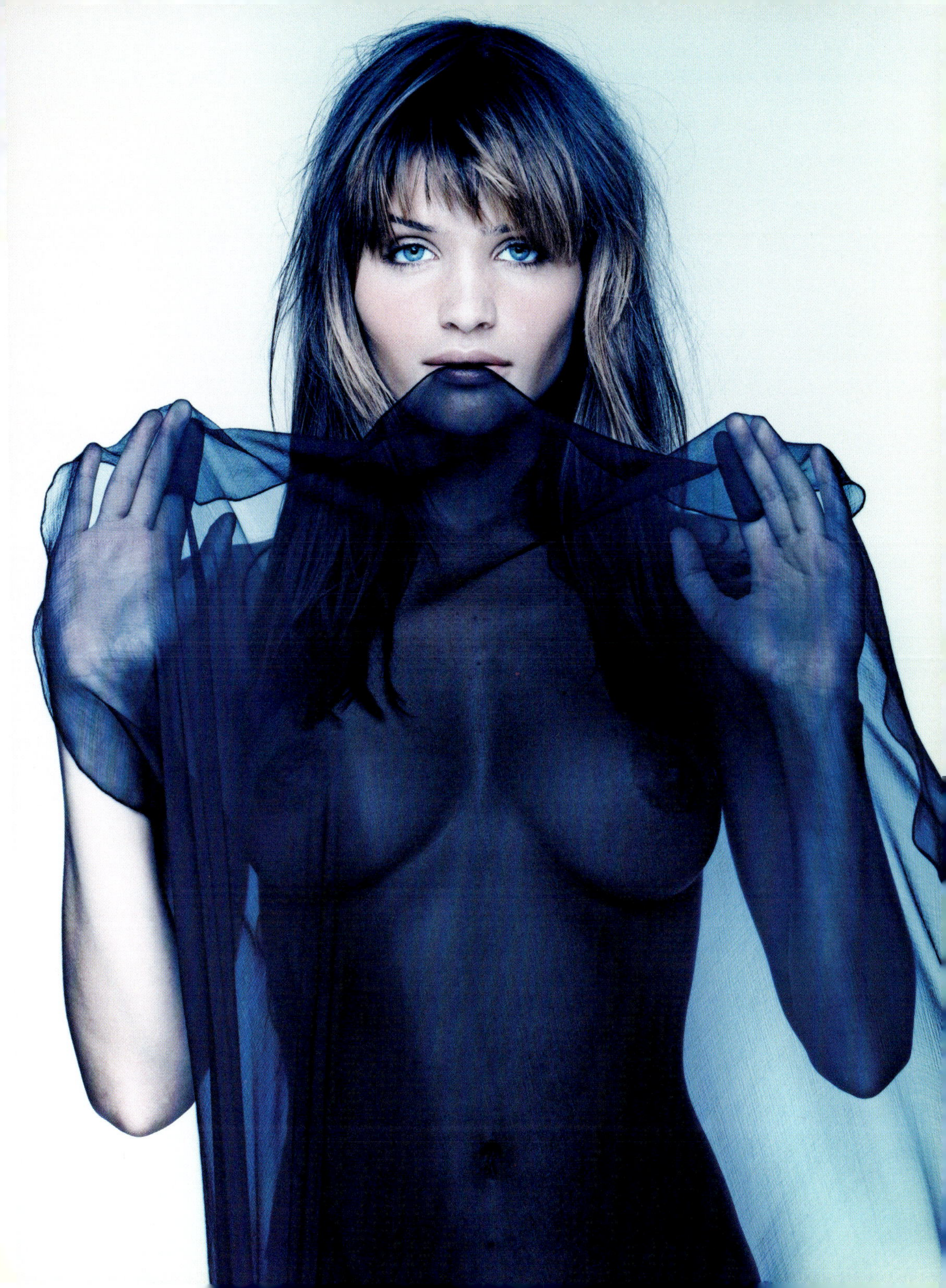

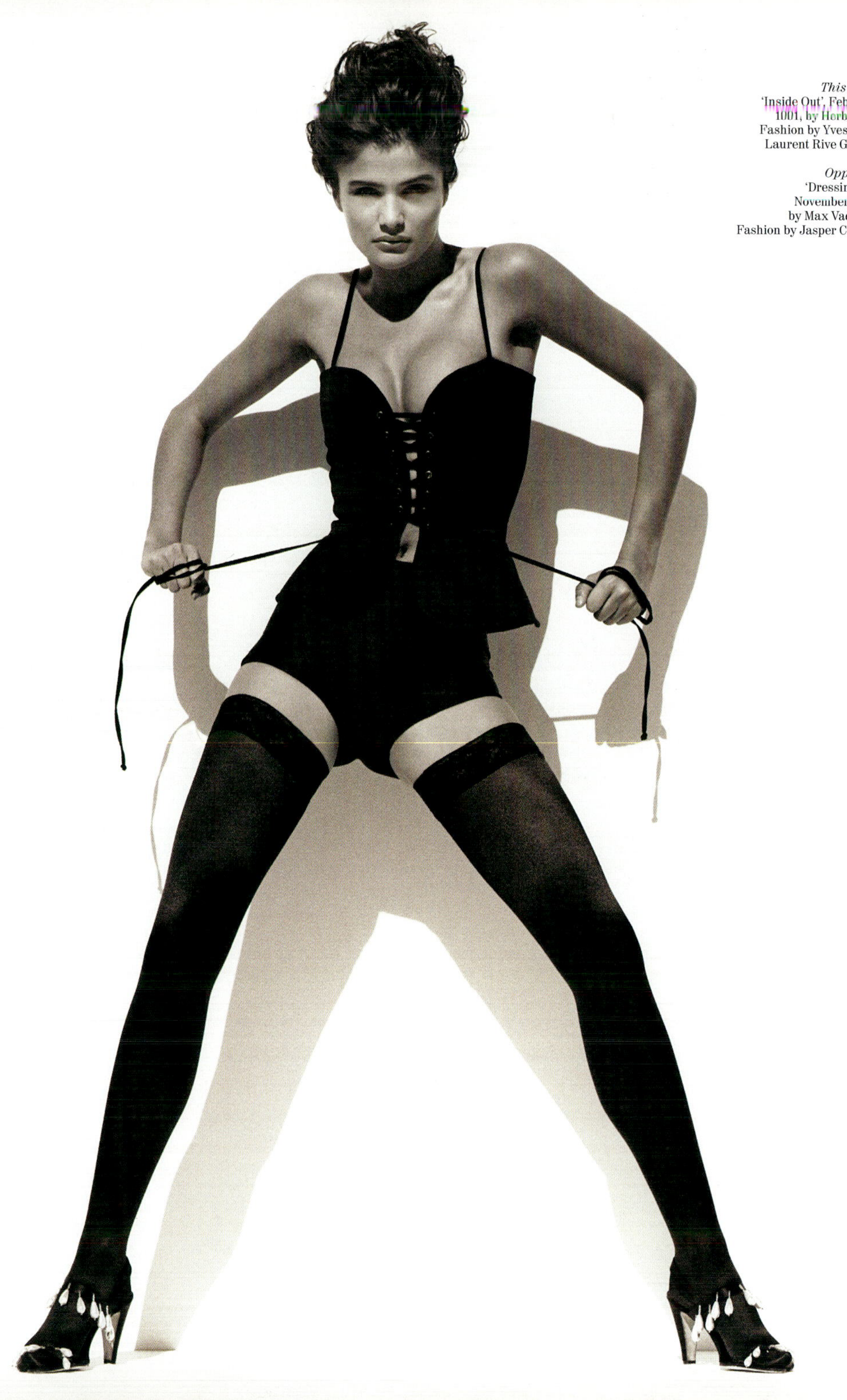

This page:
'Inside Out', February 1991, by Herb Ritts. Fashion by Yves Saint Laurent Rive Gauche

Opposite:
'Dressing Up', November 1992, by Max Vadukul. Fashion by Jasper Conran

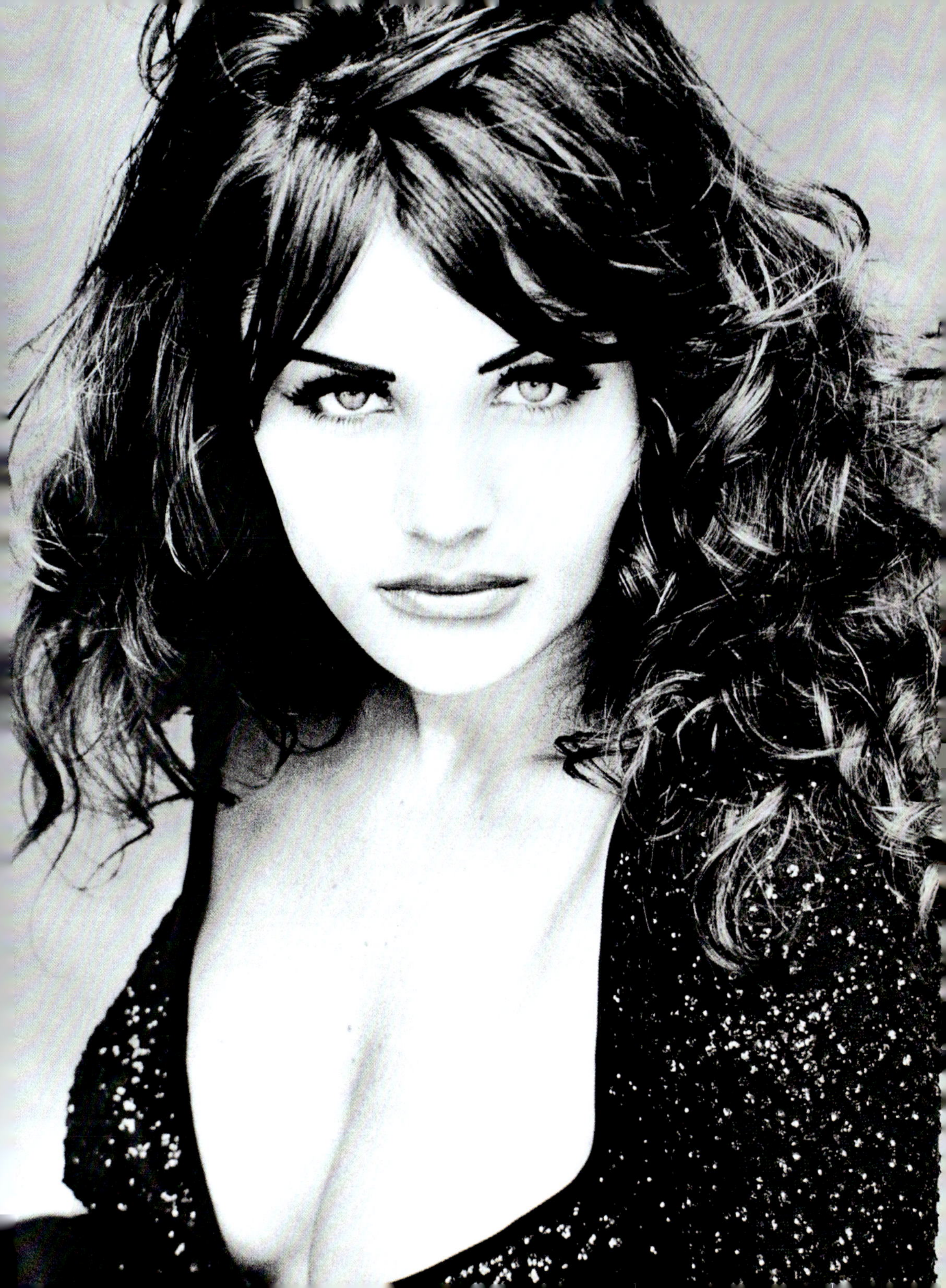

Iman

'Quite simply,' wrote Norman Parkinson in his own distinctive way, 'this Somali leopard reigns supreme among the long-legged, long-necked girls so generously stained by the sun.' There was always some dispute as to who discovered Iman, *Vogue*'s 'impala of elegance', but the magazine conceded that she would probably have made it in her own way under her own steam sooner or later. Such was her presence – statuesque, lithe, not a little imperious – that 'she made the other girls feel underprivileged *not* to be from Africa,' recalled photographer Eric Boman. The accepted history, one that *Vogue* fosters, is that it was photographer Peter Beard who found 20-year-old Iman Mohamed Abdulmajid, while filming on Kenya's northwestern frontier. He played up the exotic mystique – she was either a shepherdess or a princess – and played down the truth: Iman was the daughter of a former teacher turned Somali ambassador to Saudi Arabia, and her mother a nurse.

Vogue was not immune to the hype. 'A new beauty message from Africa,' it announced in 1976. 'Iman, 21 years old, has arrived in New York to all the razzamatazz of an instantly successful modelling career.' And it did appear to happen almost overnight. Iman, tall and effortlessly chic, was her own best advertisement. Designer Mary McFadden embraced her as muse. Meanwhile Yves Saint Laurent called her 'my dream woman', dressing her in buttercup silk gazar with cartwheel sleeves and a flounced train, and a peacock-lined flame-red satin dressing-gown coat.

Never one to fight shy of credit, Norman Parkinson claimed that he was the first to photograph Iman. The shoot in Tobago did not go entirely well: 'I had removed from my sitting-room wall, where it is usually majestically suspended, an antique dugout canoe; I carried it to a nearby bay and placed it on the black sand and waited for Iman to change. We were to photograph a simple white one-piece swimsuit. It was totally modest, but plead as I might Iman refused to put it on. The sun went in, the sun came out. She remained adamant and I remained desperate. For the first time in my life, I fell on my knees in the sand and prayed, my hands palm to palm…' The session ended up a great success (Iman had no qualms about wearing a pair of cheesecloth curtains from a Tobagan haberdashery) and launched her career.

The rewards came quickly. By the end of 1980 Iman was fast becoming a veteran of the fashion stage, a high priestess of catwalk showmanship with, as *Vogue* put it, 'real regal African mystique'. The photographer Marcus Leatherdale presented it differently: 'She was this black widow, ball-biter sorceress… If Iman wasn't in the show, you'd feel cheated.' The year before, in 1979, she was the face of Revlon's Polished Ambers, the first black African model to be given a major cosmetics contract. Her modelling career lasted a decade or so before beginning to falter; five years after that, she gave it up altogether. She tried to reignite it with a fashion line, mostly African-inspired 'blanket' dresses, but they failed to spark much interest.

What did work was a film career. Her first outing was in Otto Preminger's *The Human Factor* (1980). Her understated performance led to Oscar speculation and more parts, including a role in 1985's *Out of Africa*, though few since have tested her considerable skills or provided her with much to relish. Instead she has found success with a cosmetics line.

When Iman came to America in 1976, Peter Beard organised a press conference to show off and introduce his discovery. The assembled journalists directed all their questions to Beard, on the assumption that the shepherdess princess could not understand English. She spoke it and four other languages fluently, but engagingly remained, she said, 'fascinated' by this rather than furious. She played the long game better than anyone back then supposed she might.

Iman (b. Iman Mohamed Abdulmajid, 1955, Somalia)

Right:
'Go Tobago', May 1976, by Norman Parkinson. Fashion by Shuji Tojo

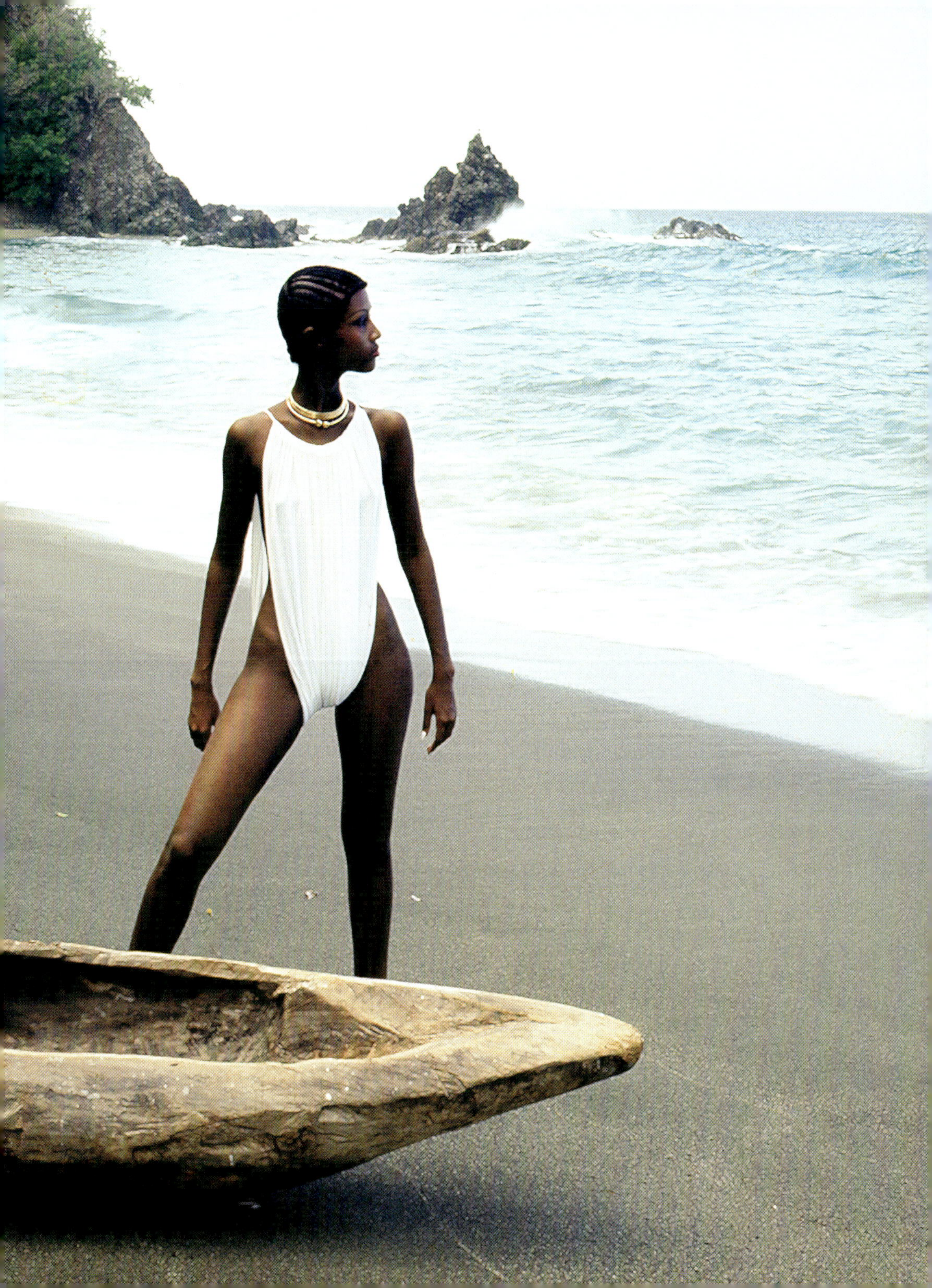

Iya Abdy

Diana Cooper considered her 'someone from another world' and Cecil Beaton that she 'invented size', while Diana Vreeland put it in general terms: 'There's nothing better-looking than a good-looking Russian woman.' Dressed head-to-toe in Chanel, who gladly gave her clothes for free, Iya Abdy always turned heads – sideways, certainly, for she was famed for her almost perfect profile, perfectly arched eyebrows and her signature hairstyle of two 'macaroons' framing her face; and upwards, too, for she was well over 6ft tall and made no concession to appearing slighter. In fact, noted Beaton, she did everything she could to 'make herself even more enormous'.

An exotic émigré aristocrat in the vein of Natalie Paley, her friend and rival in *Vogue*'s pages, she was the focus chiefly of George Hoyningen-Huene's gaze and then of Horst and Beaton, all of whom photographed her regularly for *Vogue*. Man Ray, meanwhile, photographed her for the fashion pages of *Harper's Bazaar*. Born Iya Grigorievna De Gay in Russia, she was the granddaughter of the popular painter and friend of Tolstoy, Nikolay Gay. Her father, Diana Vreeland explained, was 'a great dramatic actor, known from one end of Russia to the other. One night he was Boris Godunov, the next Ivan the Terrible, and he travelled in caravans with parrots and leopards and cheetahs and tigers. That's how Iya was brought up.' By 1921, she was the first wife of the English baronet, soldier and antiquarian Sir Robert Abdy, keeping his surname and her courtesy title when they divorced in 1928. (Confusingly for *Vogue* historians, Sir Robert went on to have several more wives, all similarly beautiful and all bearing the name Lady Abdy.)

Linking the haute monde of fashion and the demi-monde of bohemianism to great mutual benefit, Iya Abdy was close to Russian nobility in exile, as well as to struggling artists such as the young Balthus. She was widely admired for her independence of spirit, her flouting of conventions and her etiolated frame, upon which she could drape anything at all – and frequently did. *Vogue* much admired her looks, often described as 'Balinese', and her idiosyncratic personal touches: a necklace of small shells from Tahiti, a peasant straw hat from Provence. She also helped popularise the Alice band as a hair decoration. Based on John Tenniel's illustrations for *Through the Looking-Glass*, her version was a narrow hoop of pliable gold. When she made her stage debut in the 16th-century-set tragedy *Les Cenci*, as imagined by the opium-addicted experimentalist Antonin Artaud, she sparked a minor rush on Renaissance-style berets.

Abdy was famed for her dramatic entrances to costume balls. At one, Le Bal Oriental, she played up the Balinese aesthetic and dressed as a Far Eastern Mata Hari; among the attendants fanning her with giant ostrich feathers was her admirer Horst. At another party, *Vogue* reported, 'Mrs Jay O'Brien, Lady Abdy and the Baron de Rothschild milked a *papier-mâché* cow whose head disappeared into a haystack'. Another costume, in 1933, was more esoteric still: 'large amber-coloured balloons shrouded in a cloud of grey and green tulle rise from the waist and float about the silver cockleshell headdress'. Lady Abdy had come as 'sea mist'.

Possessing a touch of the *froideur* that so enchanted the public in Greta Garbo, Lady Abdy briefly tried her hand at the family trade, but her casting in the hospital melodrama *Norah O'Neale* (1934) was not an inspired one. Soon she returned to the pages of *Vogue*, where she seemed happiest – the consummate 1930s mondaine.

Iya Abdy (b. Iya De Gay, c. 1898, Russia; d. 1993)

Opposite:
'California Flowers', April 1937, by Cecil Beaton. Fashion by Altman

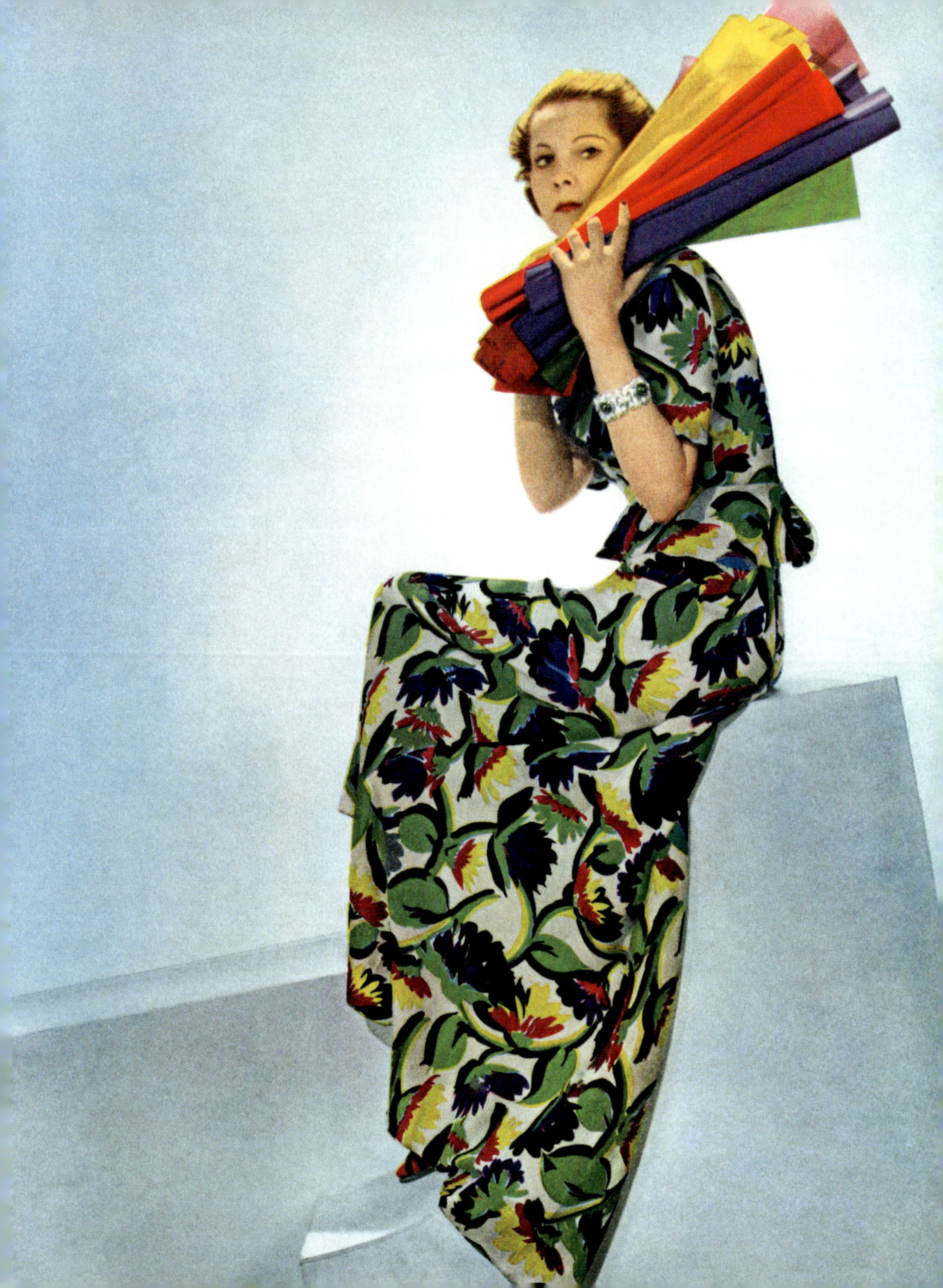

Janice Dickinson

Janice Dickinson is the great survivor. Despite her best efforts, she did not end up a high-profile casualty of the 1970s, the decade of excess and fashion cliché: 'Hot, hot, smiling hot. Now sparkle. Beautiful, *beautiful*....' Her appetite for self-destruction was enormous – but so was her staying power, and the latter overcome the former. She also possessed a larger-than-life presence and a mouth to match. (Her observations on the modelling industry are pin-sharp but mostly unrepeatable.) This has given her a late-flourishing career as a television star, often on reality-TV series and model-search shows, in which she has a tendency to speak plainly.

She is the self-proclaimed 'first modern supermodel' – this is not without justification. If, as well as catwalk glissando and fashion-magazine ubiquity, supermodeldom is quantified by star power, charisma and headline-grabbing activities, then Janice Dickinson qualifies, a prototype for those who followed in her wake. 'I could never forget staying up all night with Janice Dickinson,' said Yasmin Le Bon. 'She was very, very funny and hey, she looks great!'

It was Janice's initial misfortune to be brunette and fiery at a time when fair-haired and frolicsome were what *Vogue* really wanted. Blondes, such as Patti Hansen and Lisa Taylor, had all the fun and all the jobs. Janice's look was considered too, well, ethnic – her parents were Belorussian in origin. Her eyes were considered 'the wrong shape' to sell magazines, ditto her lips. She worked furiously and vengefully to prove them wrong: 'You create an illusion,' she told *Time* magazine as the decade wore itself out. 'I have no breasts, but by holding my body a certain way I can create a cleavage...'

Initially the illusion fooled no-one in New York; doors closed firmly in her face. They didn't like, she recalled, 'my exotic, big lips, small eyes and my... I don't know what you call it, my Lolita sexy-sexy look.' After a one-way ticket to Europe, however, Paris was wowed by that Lolita sexy-sexy look. Now Janice's express aim was to get the jobs and the experience, and go back and show those who had sneered at her in New York just how good she was. She did this in considerable style between 1975 and 1977, by entrancing photographers such as Guy Bourdin at French *Vogue*, Peter Knapp at *Elle*, Mike Reinhardt, then a *Vogue* journeyman, and fledgling *Vogue* stars Alex Chatelain and Patrick Demarchelier.

Dickinson created mini-typhoons wherever she went. And she was going far, despite being, as American *Vogue*'s Polly Mellen put it, 'totally, totally, totally nuts'. By this time the drugs were inescapable ('Everyone took them. Everyone was late. Everyone had fun,' Janice told *Vogue*), but still she was in demand and never looked anything short of sensational. It also helped that the photographers she had met in Paris were taking New York by storm; it helped too that she was tough and smart and was, according to her agents, 'a dream' – despite these agents becoming, as one of them put it, 'a sort of 24-hour attendant. You are like the little cage where the puppy goes to spend the night.'

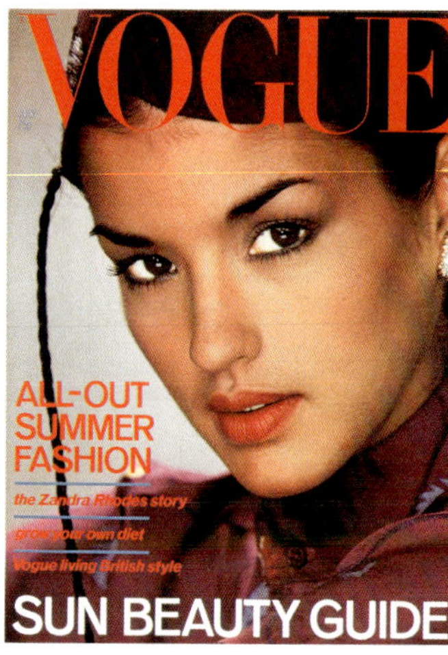

Rehab beckoned in 1982; by that time, according to Reinhardt, 'nobody could mistake Janice for sane'. But it had worked: he took his best photographs of her, and he was the best photographer she ever had. And, in a golden era for fashion magazines, their joint audience was huge. As Reinhardt admitted ruefully to the writer Michael Gross: 'I didn't know we defined our moment. I wish I had, but I was too involved with drugs. I looked down on the business. I didn't realise what I had...'

Janice Dickinson (b. 1955, USA)

Above:
'All-Out Summer Fashion',
July 1978,
by Mike Reinhardt.
Fashion by Jap

Opposite:
'Something Dramatic',
December 1978,
by Mike Reinhardt.
Fashion by Piero de Monzi

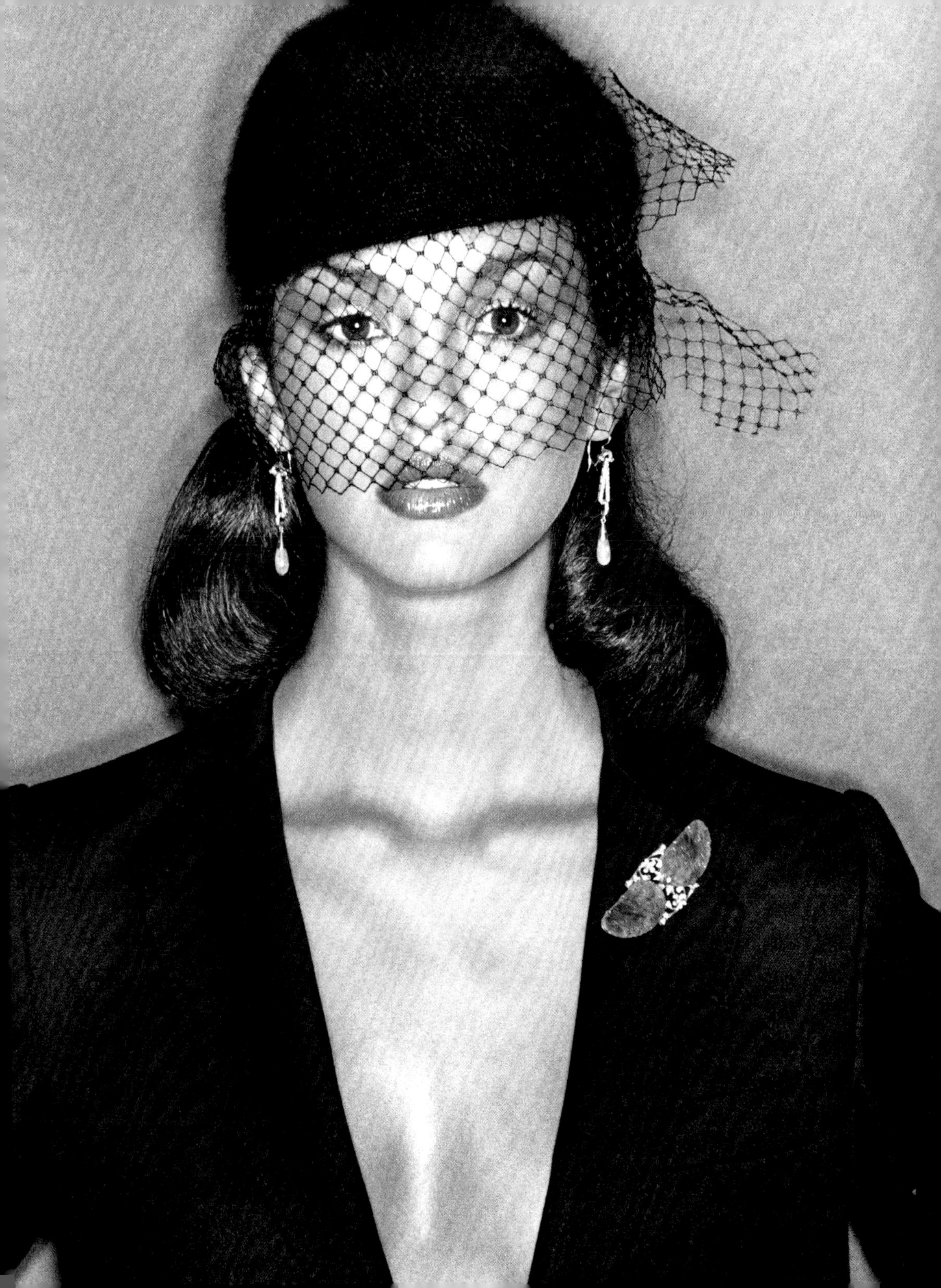

Jean Patchett

In the optimistic, early postwar years, wholesome Americanness was in demand – mostly by optimistic, early postwar American magazines. Photographers sought girls who projected scrubbed-clean freshness, radiant cheerfulness, a carefree sophistication and *soi-disant* elegance. These were not entirely impossible demands, and none came sunnier or more chirpy than Jean Patchett, straight out of Preston, Maryland. 'I'm Jean Patchett. You don't darn it, you patch it!' was her dainty icebreaker, but it belied her chic. She was, to Irving Penn, 'a young American goddess in Paris couture', the link between pre-war hauteur and new-era *joie de vivre*.

Patchett was defined by her mole, her made-up doe eyes, her arched eyebrows tweezed to implausible arches, and her mouth shaded a vivid crimson. Rarely did photographers engage her face entirely, just these ciphers: one made-up eye peered from behind a striped burnous for Clifford Coffin or a veil for John Rawlings, from beneath sunhats and a crooked elbow for Norman Parkinson, and she was invariably in profile or *profil perdu* for Penn. This reached an early apogee in January 1950 – the cover celebrating the mid-point of the 20th century. For this, *Vogue*'s art department took a Blumenfeld portrait and bleached out her face altogether, paring it down to the now-iconic essentials: mole, lips and one kohl-lined eye.

Penn's *mise-en-scène* allowed her to improvise a narrative. 'He let me use my head,' she recalled, years later. 'He always gave me a story that I would then enact. I mean, we could be at Tiffany's buying jewels or at the theatre – something. And I played the part.' Their Peruvian journey in 1949 allowed her to look anxious while chewing her pearl necklace in a café, look wistful while her boyfriend's shoes are shined in the street, and look defiant – with one eye, naturally – from behind a veil.

Sometimes the apprehension was not put on. A session was arranged for *Vogue* in Havana with Ernest Hemingway. Arriving at the Finca Vigia, the team found it empty of inhabitants but littered with discarded champagne glasses. Hemingway, vastly overweight and clad only in a pair of brief shorts, appeared at length with a drinking companion, a priest who attached himself to *Vogue*'s fashion editor Babs Simpson. The writer's natural suspicion of *Vogue* and fashion cooled when he met Patchett, but his gaze was somewhat informal. In fact, the published picture was a seamless composite of two negatives: one showing Hemingway at his least predatory and the other Patchett at her least appalled.

Never short of wealthy admirers and handsome beaux (she was a decorous adornment to the Stork Club's Friday lunches, thrown for models), Jean Patchett married and gave up modelling in 1963. It had been a busy and happy 15 years. 'I loved my career. I think that's what I was put on earth to do. Luckily I sort of backed into it,' she told American *Vogue*. 'We were the white-glove era. It was a very elegant time, and the clothes were very chic – long gloves, evening gowns and lots of fur. Oh, it was a wonderful era and wonderful fun. I couldn't wait to get up in the morning… I've been lucky. Yes indeedy, I certainly have.'

Jean Patchett (b. 1926, USA; d. 2002)

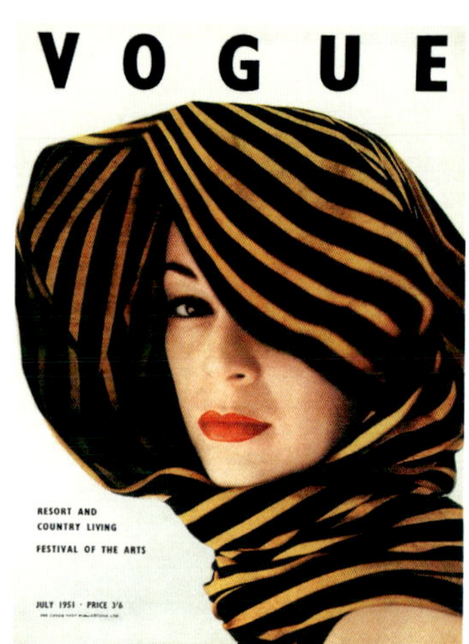

Above:
'Resort and Country Living', July 1951, by Clifford Coffin

Right:
'Vogue Patterns Go Travelling', April 1949, by Irving Penn

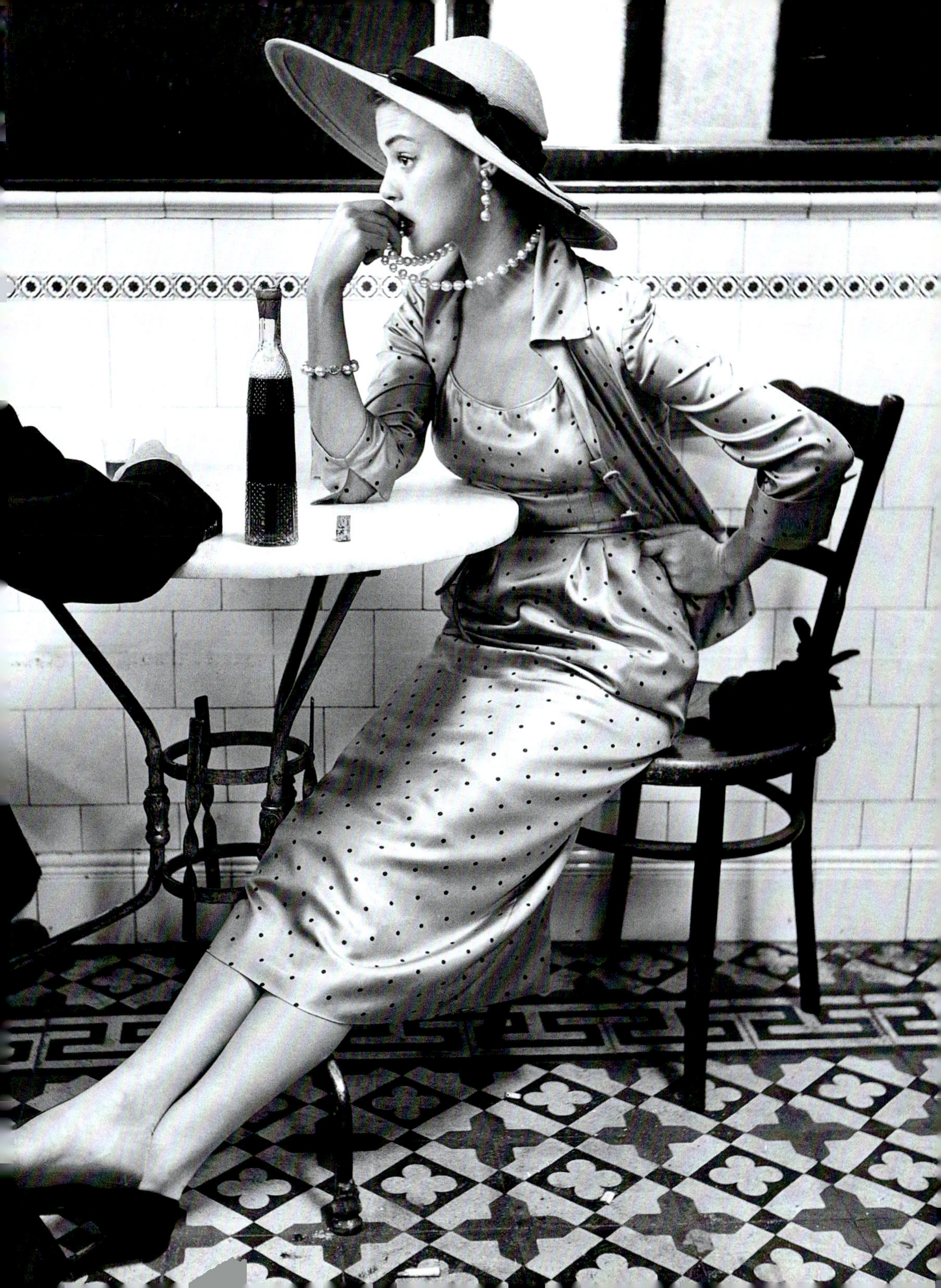

Jean Shrimpton

New York, early 1962. Before the miniskirt and the invasion of the classless popocrats, the Beatles and the Stones, there were David Bailey and Jean Shrimpton. Their significance did not go unnoticed, at least not by the arbiter of contemporary American taste, *Vogue* editor Diana Vreeland. Turning up tired and cold in her doorway – having failed to flag down a cab – these twin ciphers of a new cultural paradigm made puddles on her carpets, and Vreeland proclaimed: 'But they are *adorable*! England. Has. Arrived.'

Back home in England, the partnership of Bailey and Shrimpton was fast becoming the stuff of legend. At 24, Bailey was an outsider, brilliant and irascible. His cockney background and upbringing did not prepare him for a career in photography, far less fashion photography, which remained even then the milieu of a privileged elite. For the path he chose, his father considered him 'queer as a coot'. Meanwhile, 18-year-old Jean Shrimpton from Buckinghamshire, a graduate of the Lucie Clayton modelling school, put it more airily: she was, she declared, 'as green as a spring salad'.

Bailey and Shrimpton first worked together in 1960, hitting it off immediately; from then on, Bailey fought for her. Still irascible, but now stubborn, he nearly jeopardised a big chance at *Vogue* – 14 pages of celebrity-led fashion for September 1961 – by insisting on Shrimpton as model. Clare, Lady Rendlesham, the equally stubborn and alarmingly forbidding fashion editor, refused. Bailey dug in. A stalemate ensued. In the end Rendlesham gave in. 'I was intent on delivering the goods,' Shrimpton recalled. 'We wanted to prove Lady Rendlesham wrong.'

The sitting made Bailey's name. 'All I wanted was Jean. She was just about everything to me then. I put everything of me into her. She was my total muse – I didn't want to look at another model. There was a sort of magic there. She had a democratic kind of beauty, one that no-one could possibly object to. Kate Moss has it. Other supermodels can just scare you. They are too beautiful. But everybody loved Jean.'

The collaboration that Bailey and Shrimpton played out on the fashion pages of *Vogue* mirrored a personal relationship played out everywhere else. The tall Home Counties girl and the scruffy urban iconoclast captured the popular imagination; they were catalysts for London's emerging youth culture. Bailey had become *Vogue*'s star photographer, displacing those who said he would fail because 'I didn't have my head in a cloud of pink chiffon.' He now had an enviable shop window, hijacking nearly every issue of *Vogue* from 1962 to 1966.

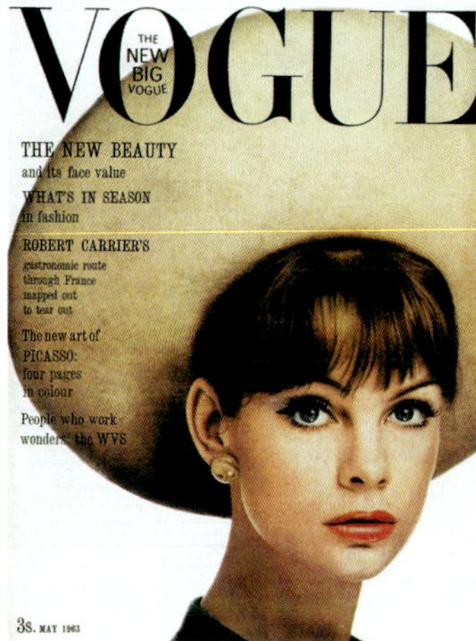

In November 1965, they threw in the towel and gave over an entire issue to him, with a portfolio of portraits of Jeanne Moreau, Claudia Cardinale, Catherine Deneuve, Elsa Martinelli and many others. 'Here are,' it trumpeted, 'the most Bailey girls in the world…' There have been many since, but when the world was young, the most Bailey girl in the world was only ever Jean. 'One of the things I loved about Jean,' the photographer remarked years later, 'was that she took to modelling with a bit of dignity. Honestly, I don't think she really cared if she did it or not…'

Jean Shrimpton (b. 1942, UK)

Above:
'The New Beauty', May 1963,
by William Klein.
Fashion by Dior

Opposite:
'Top Coats', September 1966,
by David Bailey.
Fashion by Sylvia Mills

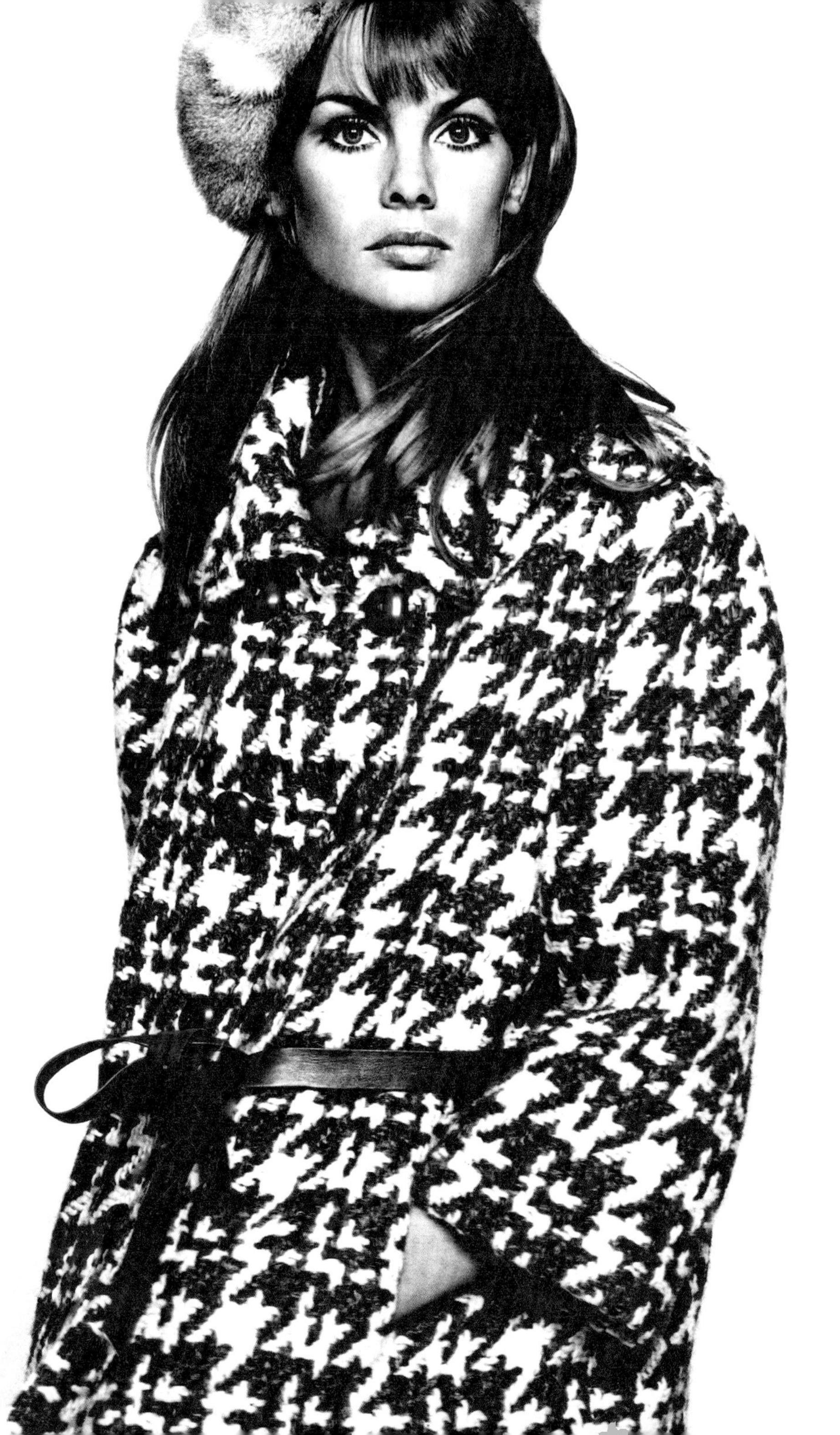

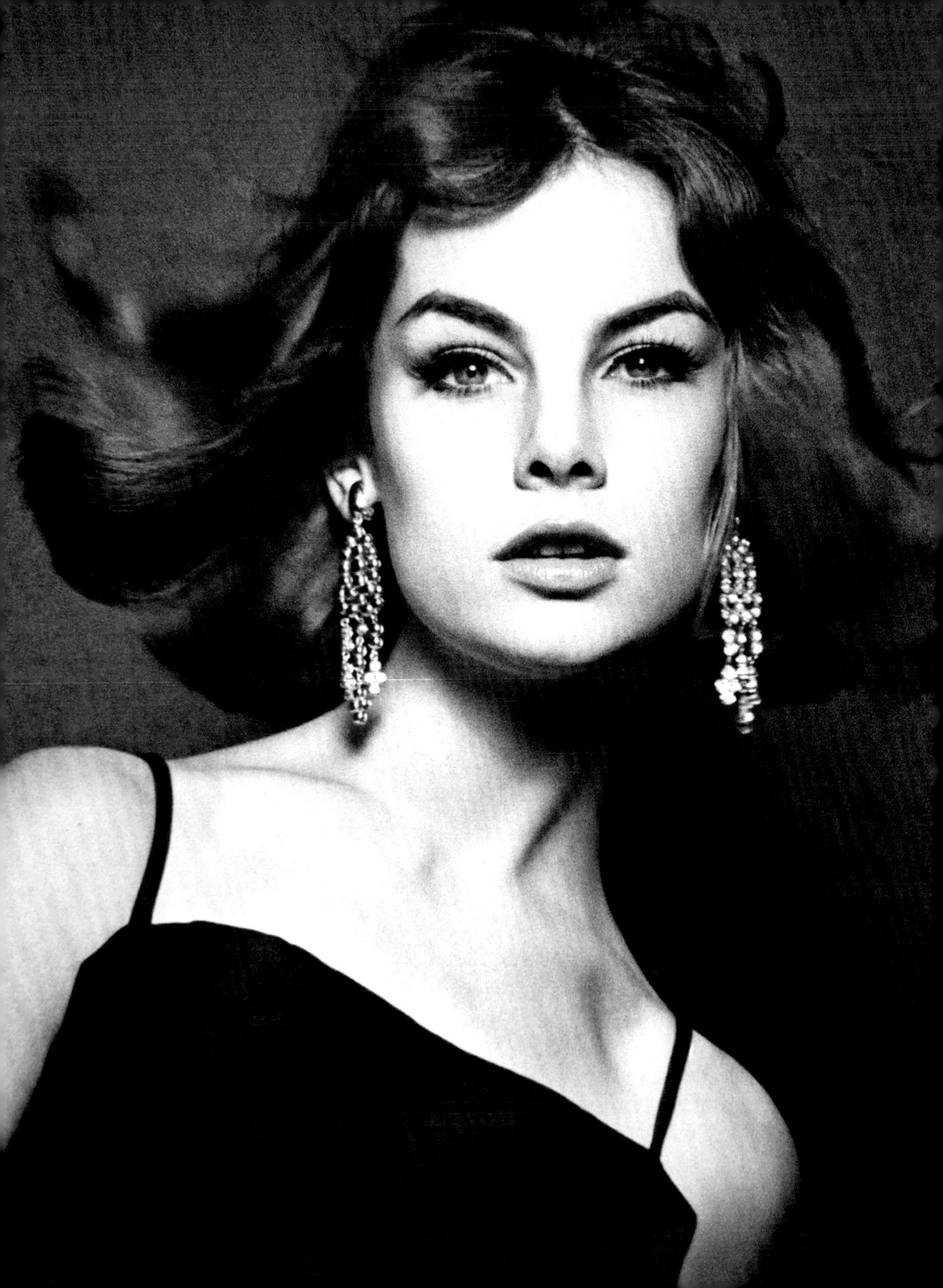

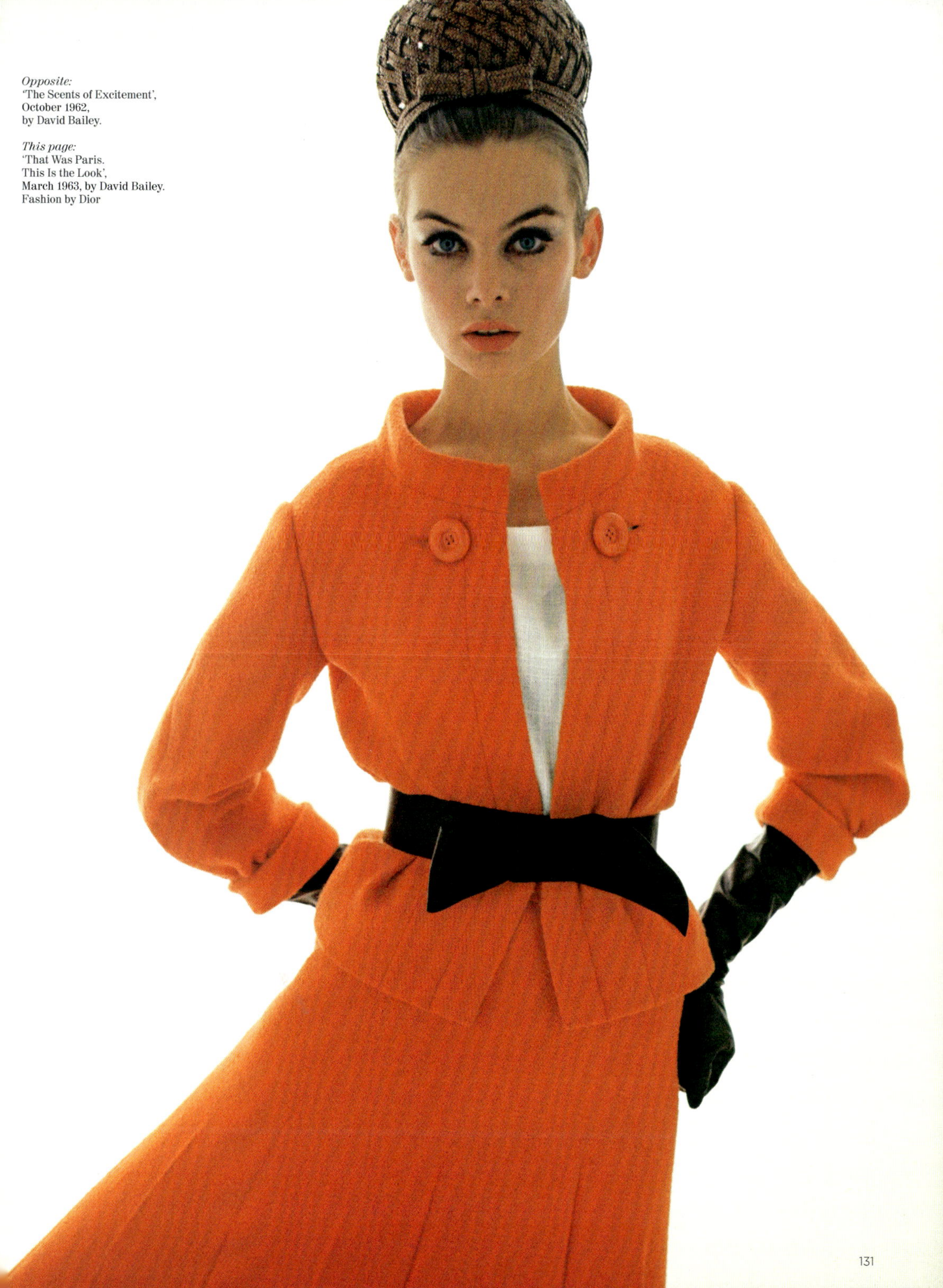

Opposite:
'The Scents of Excitement',
October 1962,
by David Bailey.

This page:
'That Was Paris.
This Is the Look',
March 1963, by David Bailey.
Fashion by Dior

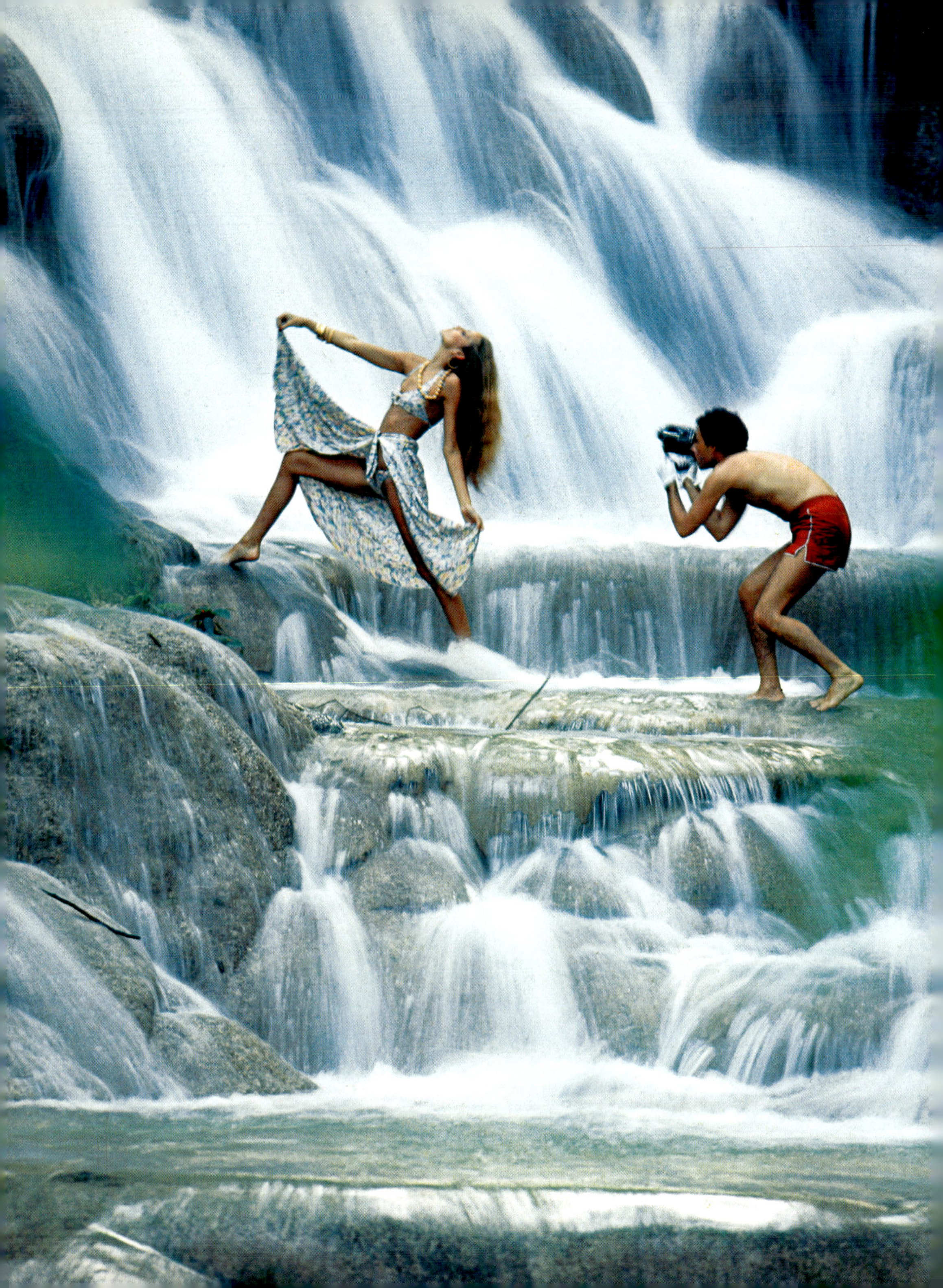

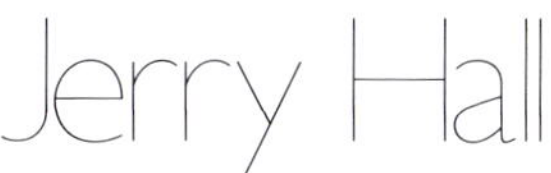

A key figure in the fashion world of the 1970s, the fashion illustrator and boulevardier Antonio Lopez is credited with discovering Jerry Hall. 'Beauty,' recalled his friend Karl Lagerfeld, 'was the only thing he desired. He lived for beauty, his vision of it and his *idée fixe* of it.' His *idée* fixed on the blonde, blue-eyed beauty fresh from Mesquite, Texas. She had recently received compensation for injuries sustained after a road crash and used it to finance a trip to Europe. At length, she moved into Antonio's Paris apartment after living for a time with fellow model Grace Jones (the statuesque duo made occasional and startling cabaret appearances).

Although many photographers would work with Jerry, from David Bailey to Richard Avedon, Horst to Helmut Newton, it was Norman Parkinson who introduced her to *Vogue*. On location near Ochos Rios in Jamaica, their first assignment together was not without incident, her career almost stalling before it started. The set of pictures was to have been equestrian-themed. Having asked her how she was with horses, Parkinson recalled that her reply was 'Parks, I was born on a horse. My sister and I have broken horses for a living. I have yet to meet a horse that I can't ride.' 'From walk to canter to gallop took exactly two seconds,' continued Parkinson, 'and my own terror was reflected in Jerry's face as she dashed away right down the beach across my line of sight. The horse turned right, jumped a couple of gulleys and stopped dead in front of a barbed-wire fence as Jerry flew over its head like some blue ballistic missile.'

Their high point was as part of the first British magazine team to be invited to the USSR. *Vogue*'s landmark trip began in Moscow and took them 7,000 miles through Tajikistan, Azerbaijan, Armenia and Turkmenistan. Locations included Red Square, a hydroelectric works and the Fire Temple at Baku. Parkinson also requested a fibreglass plinth inscribed with Cyrillic script – on one side, '*Vogue* 1975', and on the reverse, 'Jerry Hall'. Fashion magazines were not above Cold War surveillance. The authorities ordered the film to be developed in Moscow. Parkinson was convinced he'd never see it again. Jerry Hall agreed to smuggle a few rolls out just in case. As *Vogue* fashion editor Grace Coddington recalled. 'Clearly our plan had been overheard by the KGB. At the airport Jerry's stash was seized, until we convinced them that the film was unexposed. Back in London we compared print quality. Which was better? Moscow's, by far…'

Jerry survived her pioneering trips with Parkinson to become one of the most successful models of the 1970s, and one of the most recognisable names since then. All but unavoidable in fashion pages the world over – she was a regular, much-anticipated cover star in Britain, France and Italy – Hall received wider coverage as the mermaid on Roxy Music's LP *Siren* and in the video accompanying Bryan Ferry's single 'Let's Stick Together'. After a romance with Ferry, she left him for his friend Mick Jagger in the 1980s. Hall and Jagger's relationship was frequently disrupted, but in 1990 they married in a Balinese ceremony, not officially recognised back home in Richmond-upon-Thames. In 1999, Jerry filed for divorce.

She has also had a modest career as an actress, with parts in films such as *Batman* (as the girlfriend of Jack Nicholson's Joker) and on stage in *Bus Stop*, *The Graduate* (as Mrs Robinson) and the Cole Porter musical *High Society*. Along with her friend Iman, she is one of the few well-known faces of the 1970s who continues to work as a model today, though she is characteristically self-deprecating about it. 'It can be really awful,' she told *Vogue*, 'when all those girls are floating around looking marvellous and I come out looking like a squashed sausage…'

Jerry Hall (b. 1956, USA)

Left:
'Jamaica Love', May 1975, by Norman Parkinson. Fashion by Electric Fittings

Above:
'Jamaica: Blue and Beautiful', May 1975, by Norman Parkinson. Fashion by Wiki

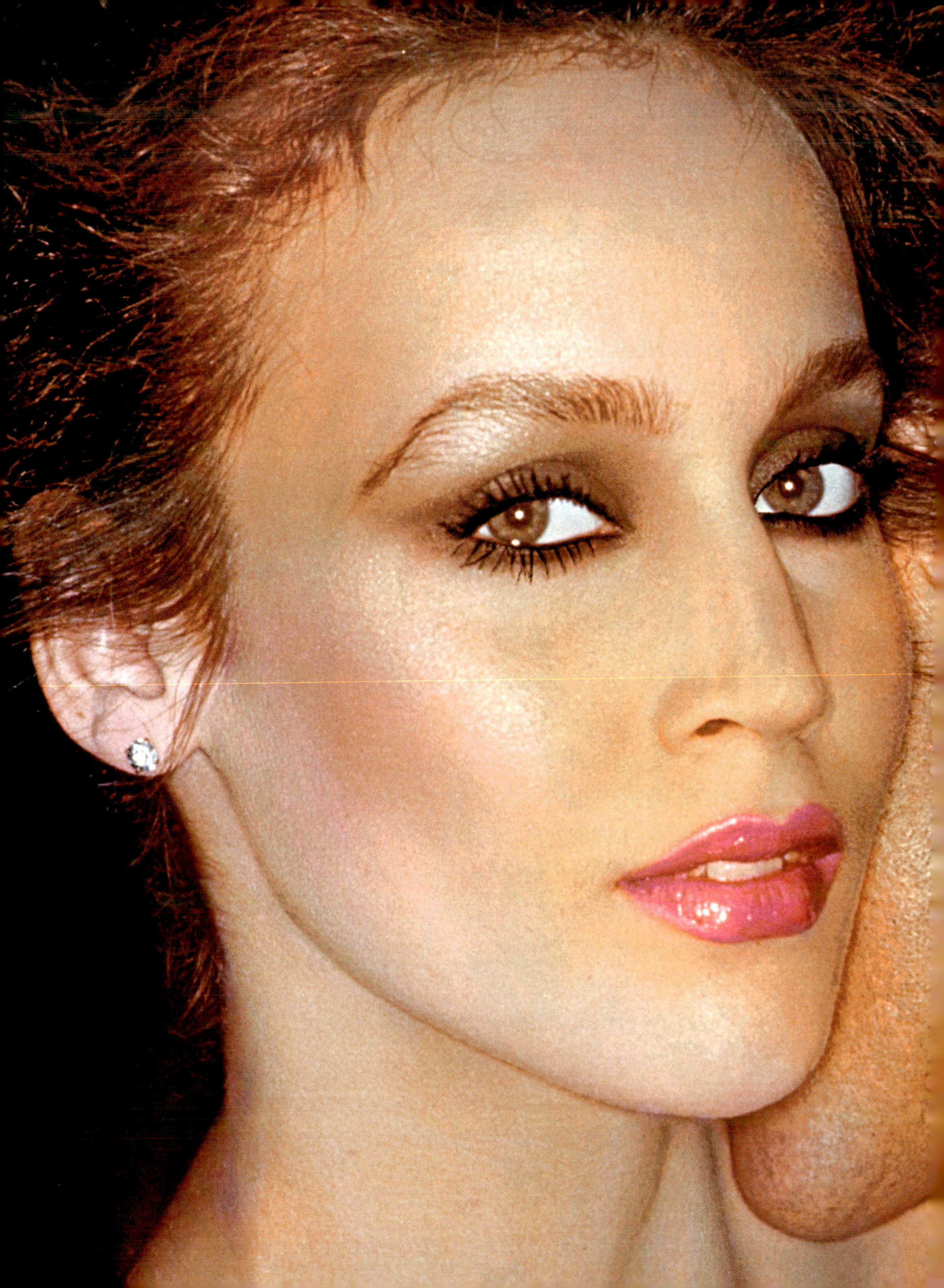

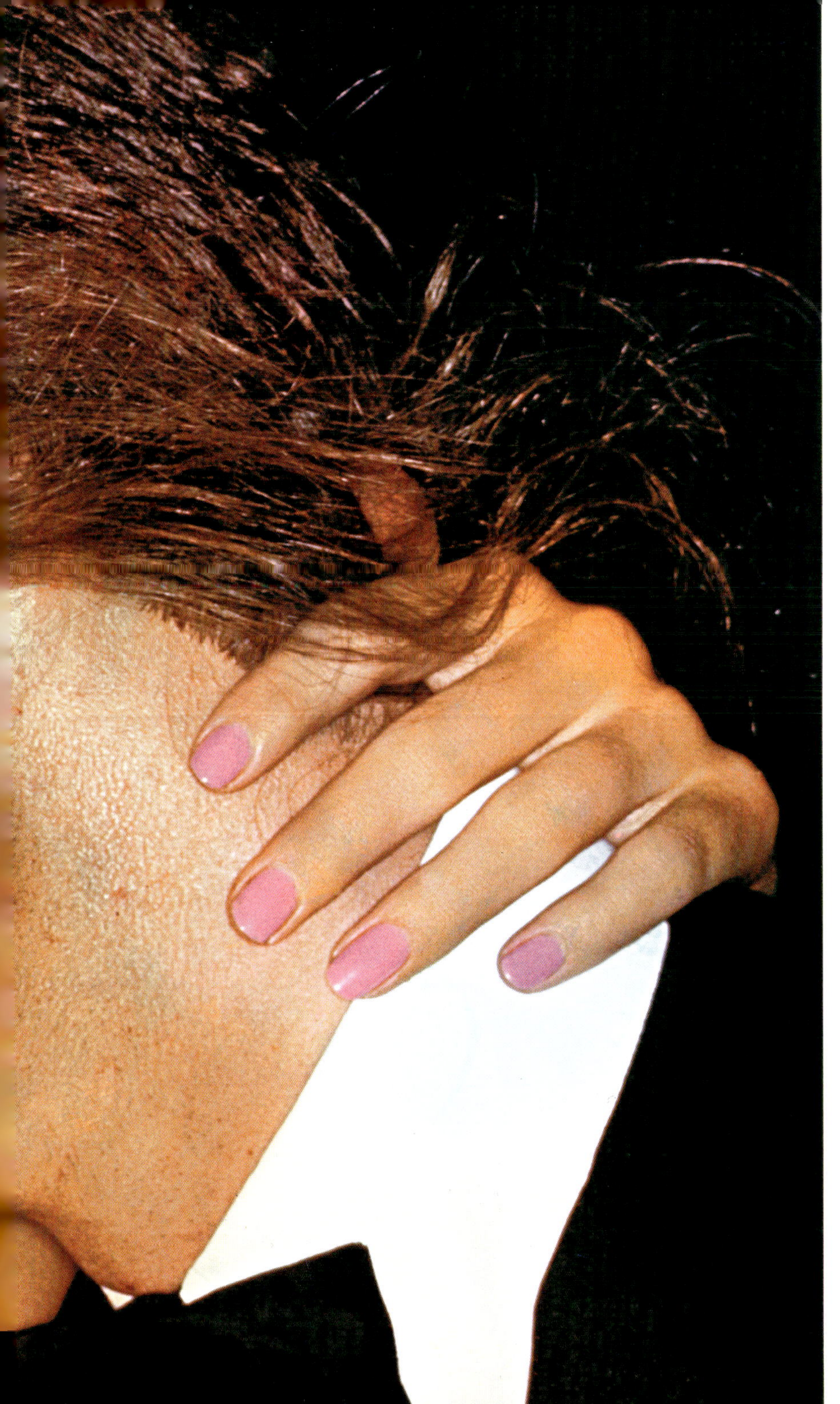

'Late at Night',
1976, by David Bailey

Jessica Stam

'Jessica Stam has always managed to bring a quiet femininity to her shoots,' says *Vogue* fashion director Kate Phelan. 'She is like a little cat who quietly pads around the studio.' Stam's doll-like face belies a steely determination and will to succeed. As the only sister of six brothers, she became as good as them at sport, and possibly smarter. Such an upbringing taught her 'to really understand the mind of the opposite sex', she says, though her innate sweetness camouflages it well. And this sweetness chimed with the times, as the prevailing trend for strongly etched personalities yielded to one for more delicately delineated faces.

Born in Kincardine, Ontario, on the edge of Lake Huron, modelling was not Stam's chosen career path – she had set her sights on dentistry. A chance encounter with a model scout in a coffee shop (she was on her way home from Canada's Wonderland amusement park) changed it, despite her hair being an awful shade of yellowy-orange. She then entered, and won, a Los Angeles-based modelling competition and the pace quickened.

It continued to do so, more rapidly still, when Steven Meisel caught a glimpse of her. 'Obscurity to model fame in one step…' *Vogue* noted. In fact, as she simply recalled it, 'he changed me'. This was not just a broad metaphysical comment on the course her life would take, but also a reference to an immediate physical transformation: he made her dye her hair, sometimes to a different new shade a week (quite possibly back to yellowy-orange at one point). This led to major advertising campaigns for Prada and Versace and, for a while, virtually every such assignment Meisel undertook. 'I guess,' she told an interviewer, 'I'm his muse. He brings out the best in me. He's inspired by works of art, old movies and paintings. If you work with him, you learn about the same things.' Of course this was not Meisel's first success from Ontario. The illustrious Linda Evangelista, from St Catherine's, was Stam's predecessor here.

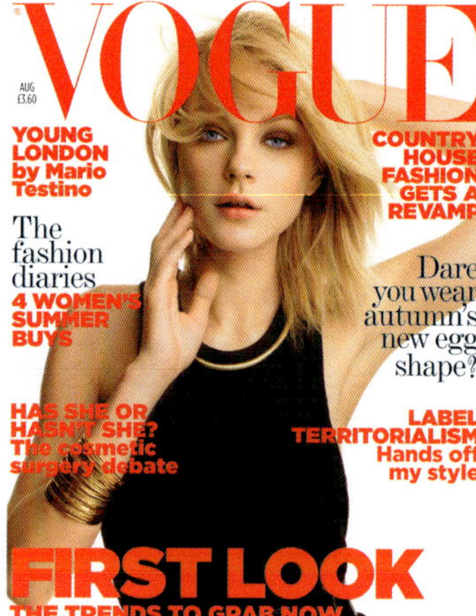

A strictly religious upbringing and common sense have led Stam to eschew the temptations and excesses of the fashion industry. Her wise head has also reassured her: 'with modelling, you are judged on your looks. It's easy to take that personally, but you have to realise that it's only your appearance that's being judged, not you as a whole. If you didn't, you'd be destroyed…'

If it all goes wrong, immortality is assured not just in the countless fashion pages of magazines the world over, but in the much-coveted, widely publicised it-accessory of 2005: the Stam bag from Marc Jacobs.

Jessica Stam (b. 1986, Canada)

Above:
'First Look', August 2006, by Patrick Demarchelier. Fashion by Yves Saint Laurent

Opposite:
'The Collections', February 2007, by Liz Collins. Fashion by Chloé

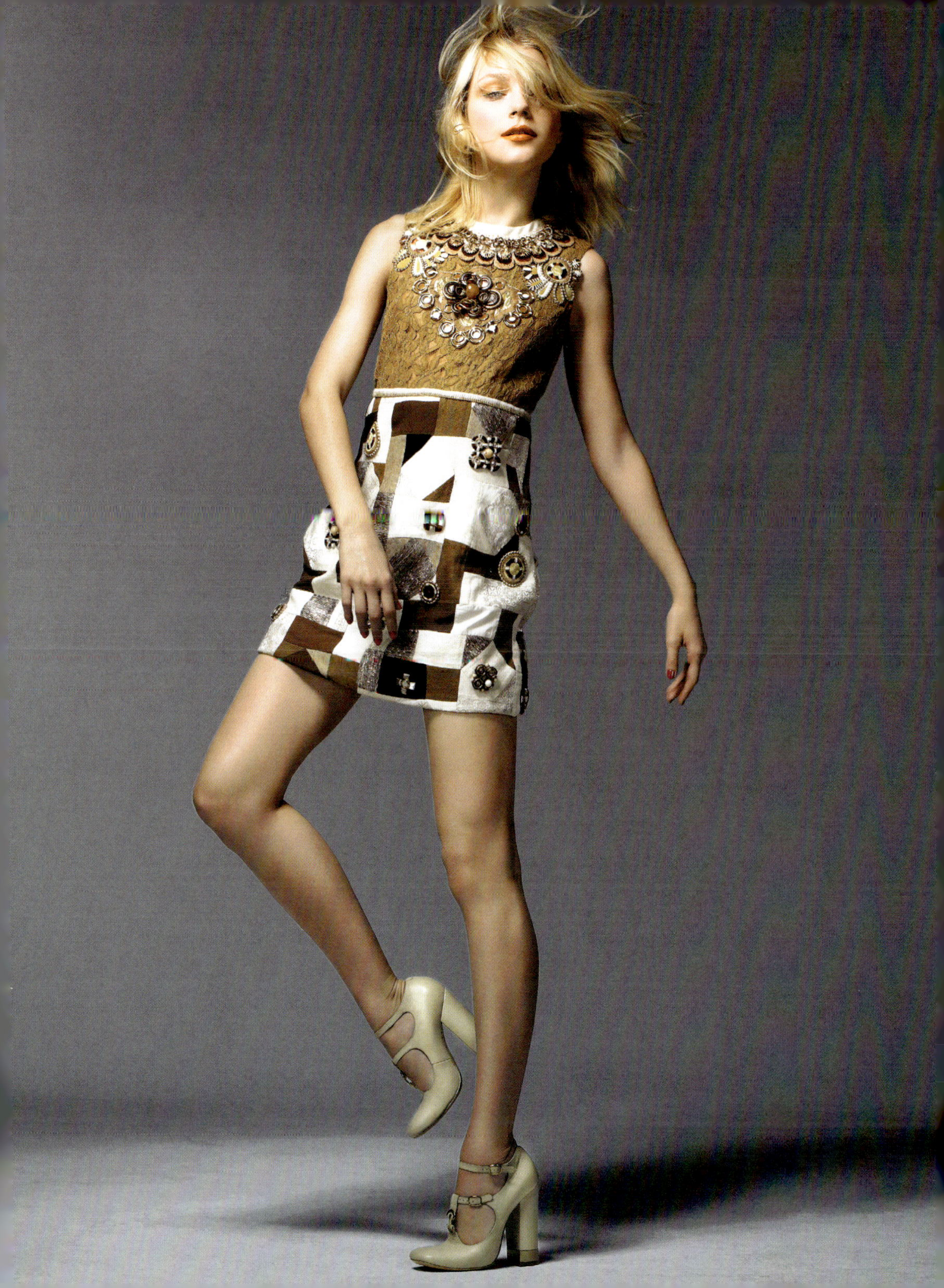

Jill Kennington

In 1967, Diana Vreeland issued a memorandum to the staff of American *Vogue*, one of her less absurd *pensées*. 'In my opinion,' it read, 'Jill Kennington is one of the best models around… She is not a beauty, but she has fresh air and dynamo… I sincerely suggest that when we are doing pictures we use her… She is usually in England… It has also come to my attention that she never did have a nervous breakdown and that was all a load of talk…' Run-of-the-mill in light of Vreeland's exhortations to rinse a blonde child's hair in dead champagne or to turn an old ermine coat into a bathrobe, it is nevertheless informative of the mystique surrounding a model who had begun to put distance between herself and the industry that had, in a short space of time, made her a star.

Kennington never had the global career of Jean Shrimpton, or her universal recognition, but she was for a time Shrimpton's only serious home-grown rival. They shared a rural background and a burgeoning middle-market appeal, but Kennington was cooler. 'I was known by teenagers, which struck me as odd,' she says. 'In the airport going to Cyprus with Terry Donovan, I got mobbed by a bunch of kids.'

Young and energetic and happiest *en plein air*, she was *Vogue*'s Face of '63, the Quintessence, and by 1964 could be found doing anything anywhere – modelling furs in the Arctic Circle or sarongs in the heat of the Arabian desert. By 1966 she had a role in Antonioni's film *Blow-Up*, an auteur's oblique survey of Swinging London, doing 'an awful lot of standing around in a graphic sort of way in front of a wind machine'. Simultaneously, her career at *Vogue* was ascending.

David Bailey had Jean Shrimpton and Terence Donovan had Celia Hammond. As fragile and alluring as either of them, Kennington wasn't anyone's in particular until she encountered John Cowan. In him she found a collaborator who allowed her an equal share of the creative process, at least at first. They were a dynamic, high-octane team. 'When I met him, I realised that I had come across a rare species, a magnetic, charismatic and powerful personality,' she told Cowan's biographer Philippe Garner. 'I felt my own power, personality and ability fully appreciated, which allowed me to be myself and stretched to the limit… He was never afraid of living dangerously and I matched him with guts and daring…'

Despite their rapport, she insisted on working with other photographers; increasingly, this disconcerted the possessive Cowan. She was the pliable star of the off-kilter photographs of two legends of fashion photography, Guy Bourdin and Bob Richardson – for Bourdin a Courrèges-clad space girl, for Richardson a heavy-lidded, faux-furred hooker. For a third, Helmut Newton, she posed languid to the point of torpor. For Cowan, meanwhile, she was anything she wanted to be: a sphinx, an ice maiden, a castaway on a balsa raft, a bareback rider, a daredevil parachutist…

Though it fizzed and glittered during its 60 or so months, Kennington's career was a short-lived one even by *Vogue*'s fastidious standards. Kennington, though, had other interests beyond fashion and walked away unscathed, for the most part. Despite inventing the scenario entirely, Bob Richardson's memoirs in note form give some idea of what fashion lost: 'Jill Kennington – a sensational beauty – love at first sight – she came to my studio with her boyfriend of the moment – he threatened me with a gun and fired two shots into the ceiling – I am still in love with her.'

Jill Kennington (b. 1943, UK)

Opposite:
'Newest Beauty Asset',
September 1966,
by Bob Richardson.
Fashion by Julian Robinson

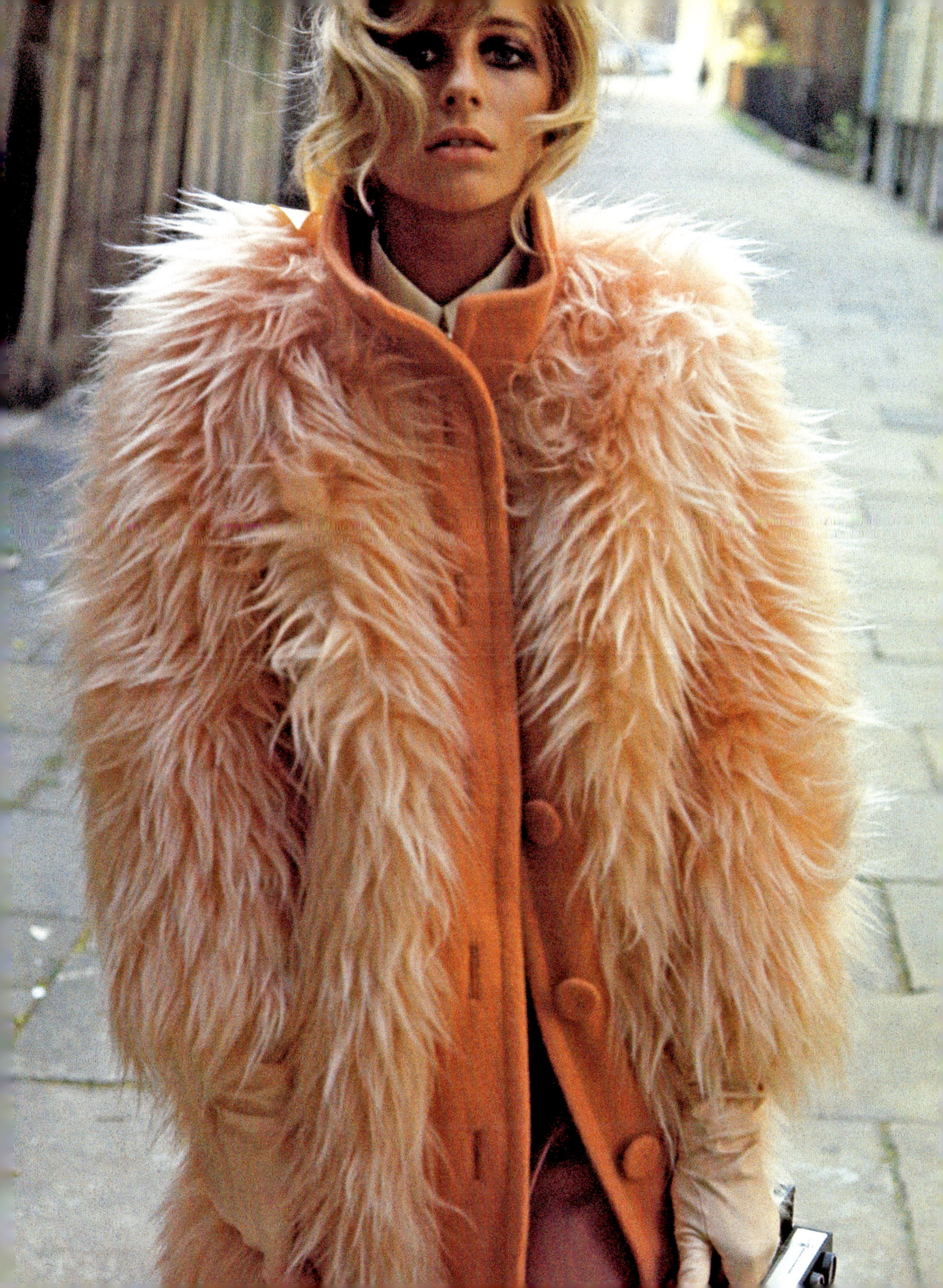

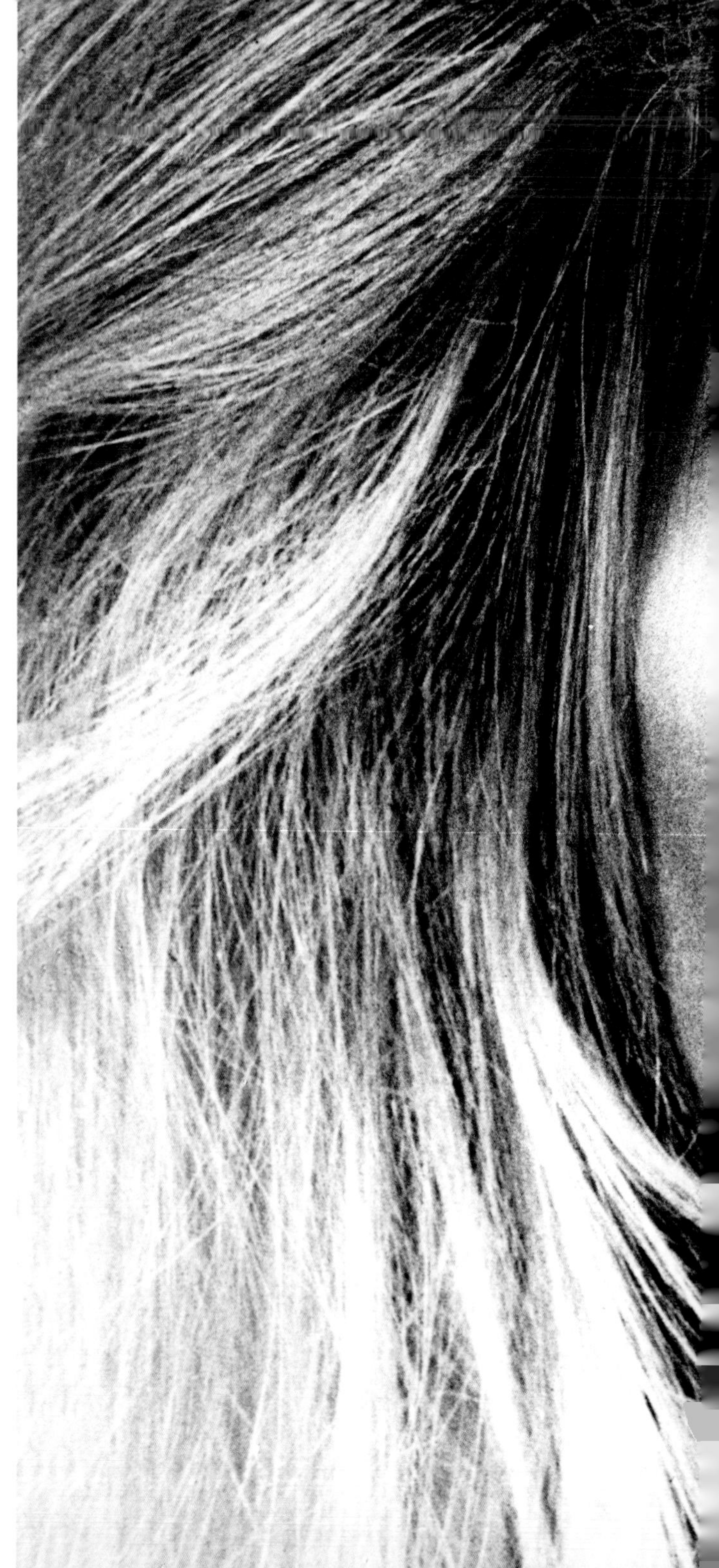

'The Face Makers',
September 1966,
by David Bailey

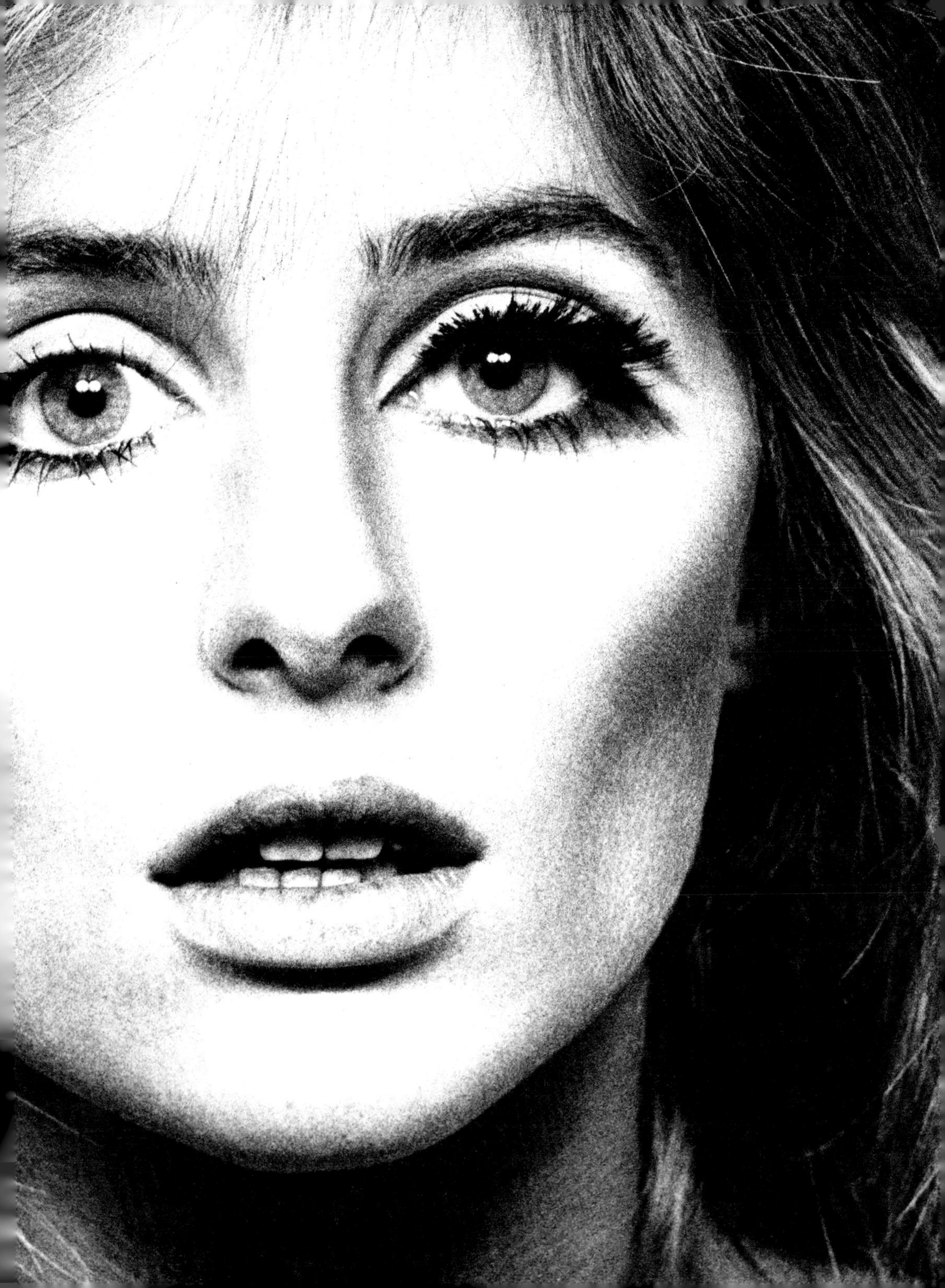

Karen Elson

She has, *Vogue* is always delighted to report, come a long way. Mistaken on starting out for a delivery girl by the top photographer who had booked her, she has in the intervening years become 'fashion royalty', as the magazine reminded readers, and more in demand than ever. She has put behind her comments, such as Karl Lagerfeld's – meant appreciatively – that she resembled someone from the Middle Ages *and* a 'mutant from another planet'.

It was photographer Steven Meisel who persuaded her to dye her hair a disturbingly violent shade of red, as well as suggesting she add to the quirk by shaving her eyebrows. 'And while there's been much talk,' said *Vogue* in 1998, 'about Karen being just another beautiful/weird British model, her increasing radiance suggests she'll last the course.' She has; no longer Le Freak, a funny-faced export for the overseas novelty market, she is a timeless beauty. 'You don't want to bite the hand that feeds you, because you're getting attention for being an individual,' she has said, 'but it was hard to be called the freak of fashion.'

Born and brought up in the north of England (specifically Oldham), Karen was a quiet and shy child, all the more so when teased at school for her unconventional appearance: alabaster skin and, as *Vogue* put it, 'long limbs then still knobbly from growth spurts'. Enrolled into a local modelling agency by her shrewd and sympathetic mother in order to help her gain confidence and self-esteem, she was (despite the opinions of others, and possibly herself) a success.

Meisel found her in 1997 and the quirkiness became an international phenomenon – and a lucrative one. 'It turned out to be one of the craziest and most amazing years a clueless, kooky 18-year-old could ever have,' she said. There was also an inevitability about it all. 'Just as Elson thought she'd discovered the place in which her looks were celebrated,' said *Vogue*, 'she found herself being called the same as at school, but on an international scale.'

Karen articulated her ethos to Tim Walker, with whom she has made memorable stories for *Vogue* (an alarming Brothers Grimm tin-soldier fairy tale, and a more prosaic road trip to Scotland with Erin O'Connor – 'what fun we had thawing out,' she recalled). 'Modelling is best dealt with by having an imagination about it. I have never believed I am a *model*, not in the conventional way. I find "acting" out a role for the camera more liberating than trying to stand in front of a white backdrop and pose. I get a story in my head and then I really believe in the story. That makes me feel free… I really feel the moment in a good picture. Even if it's a created moment, it's still a valuable moment.'

Elson has instituted a parallel career as a musician, kickstarted by her marriage to Jack White of the White Stripes. She has also been a member of quasi-eco-political cabaret troupe the Citizen's Band; its membership revolves (it has included, among others, Maggie Gyllenhaal and Zooey Deschanel), but a constant is Karen's arresting vocals. 'It's a way,' she told *Vogue*, 'of making people politically conscious without hectoring them.'

Whatever she turns her hand to, *Vogue* opined, 'she's the one you can't keep your eyes off.'

Karen Elson (b. 1979, UK)

Opposite: 'Sculpture Class', October 2008, by Nick Knight. Fashion by Stephen Jones Millinery

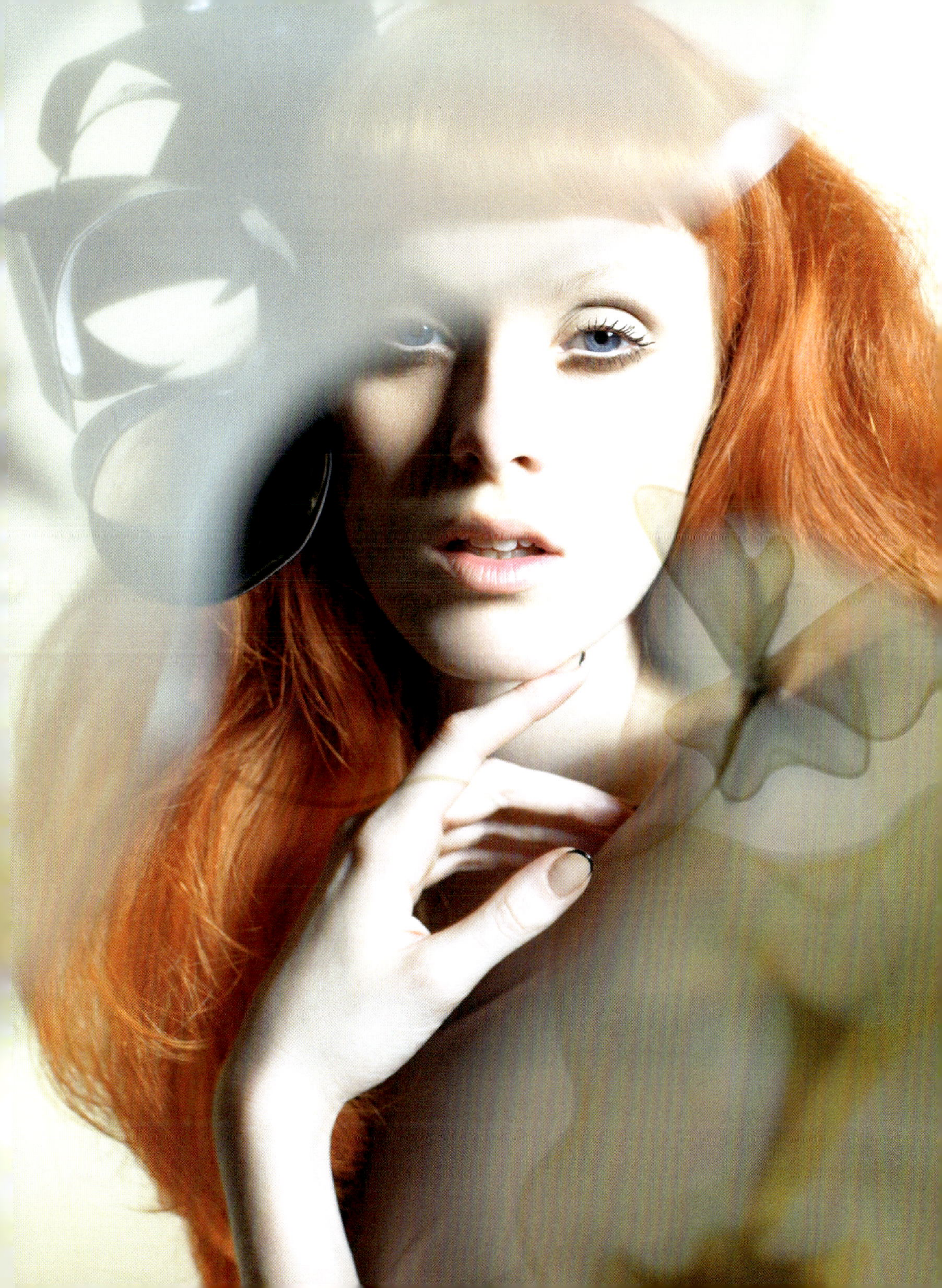

Karen Mulder

'Remote confections of cultured image and cherished dreams, they had come to epitomise modern beauty and grace,' Michael Gross has written of the supermodels. 'They seemed to be in charge of their lives and their careers.' This was certainly true for the majority and it was, for the most part, true for the bewitching Karen Mulder, before illness led her to withdraw from the modelling industry before her time.

Raised in the Hague, Mulder had her feet firmly on the ground and, on the face of it, a strong sense of proportion. 'The Dutch hate to encourage vanity or conceit, and that's why I feel so at home in Britain,' she explained to *Vogue*. 'The British have exactly the same sense of humour and cynicism about success. They may be proud of you, but they don't say it in case it goes to your head.' Perhaps, with hindsight, someone should have said it sooner, and often.

The genes that produced captivating feline eyes and a just-shy-of-6ft frame, with almost cartoonishly long legs, also spawned an overbearing sense of unworthiness and guilt that was both charming and worrying. 'I want to give something back,' Mulder told *Vogue*, 'because I can find no justification for supermodels earning so much' – and with that she set up a foundation to provide holidays for underprivileged children in a French château she had bought for the purpose. Such kindness was typical of her disposition, but she might have exorcised further demons had she followed through with an idea formulated with her boyfriend Jean-Yves Le Fur – a documentary about the lives of the supermodels. It came, however, to nothing. 'Sometimes it's a plus to be insecure,' she told Arthur Elgort. 'It makes you try harder.'

Mulder was always driven and would always be punctilious, whatever the demands of her schedule. Her back-story started when she spotted a notice inviting applicants to the 1986 Elite Look of the Year contest – she was the runner-up, but it was a given that she'd be trained up by Elite and handed a contract. There was no gradual limbering up for the top slot, no paying dues in forgettable catalogues; it all happened quickly.

Within a year Mulder was a star, within two a supermodel. She was a 'rare commodity', as one observer put it, 'a mannequin who can turn a rigorously plain dress into one as alluring as a satin negligée'. Her walk earned her legendary status, and she took to the catwalk for Valentino, Yves Saint Laurent, Versace and Armani and others. 'At Calvin Klein's presentation,' wrote the *New York Times*, 'Mulder's voluptuous outline and undulating walk transformed an understated grey tunic into a seductive showpiece…' An entire edition of Italian *Vogue* was given over to just pictures of her. Le Fur, by 1995 Mulder's fiancé and manager, made the most of her considerable earning power. There were Karen Mulder dolls and beauty and exercise videos. Then, around 1999, she gave up modelling.

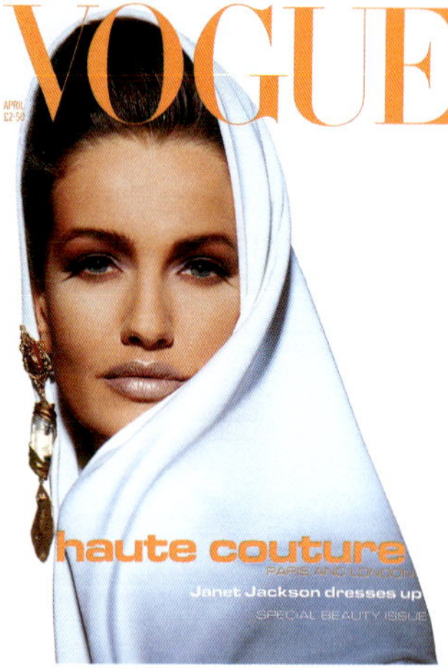

She hated being photographed, she said, and not knowing who she really was. She was also anxious to try other avenues. The first was acting, which foundered after one outing, *Un Vol, La Nuit* (2001), a French romantic comedy in which she played a famous model slightly the worse for alcohol. She also made a foray into music.

For several years Mulder received treatment for acute depression. She reappeared again in 2004, releasing a CD of self-penned songs. A return to the catwalk came in 2007, and her appearance was warmly applauded. However, two years later there were reports that she had been arrested for abusing a Paris-based cosmetic surgeon. The career of one of the fashion world's startling beauties seemed to be over. Her heyday – when her agent bragged 'she could sell a paper bag', and when she confided 'what could be better than to be young and beautiful and make a lot of money?' – suddenly seemed very long ago.

Karen Mulder (b. 1968, Netherlands)

Above:
'Haute Couture', April 1991, by Tyen. Fashion by Bianchini

Opposite:
'The Wanted Man', May 1991, by Peter Lindbergh. Fashion by Strenesse

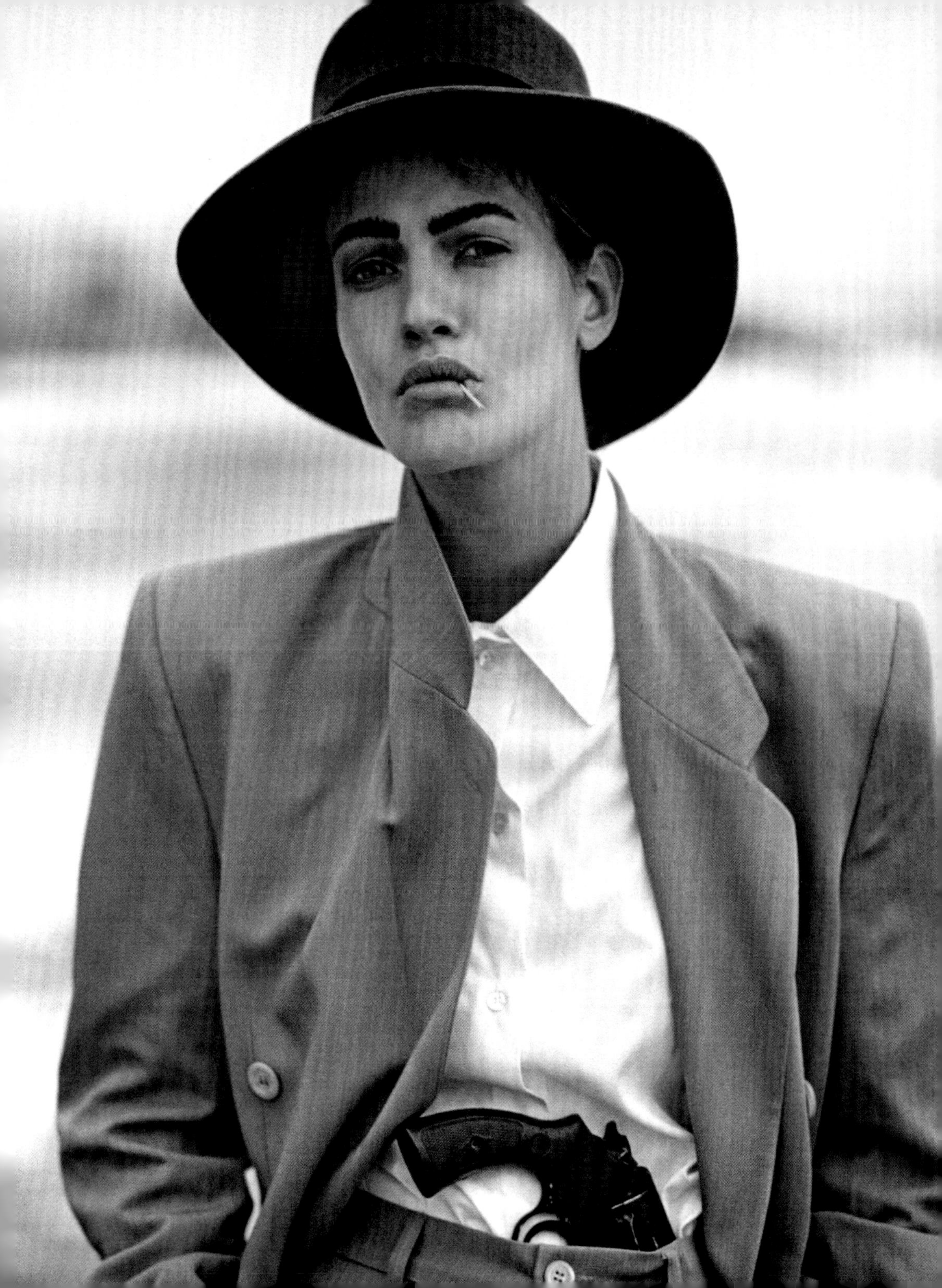

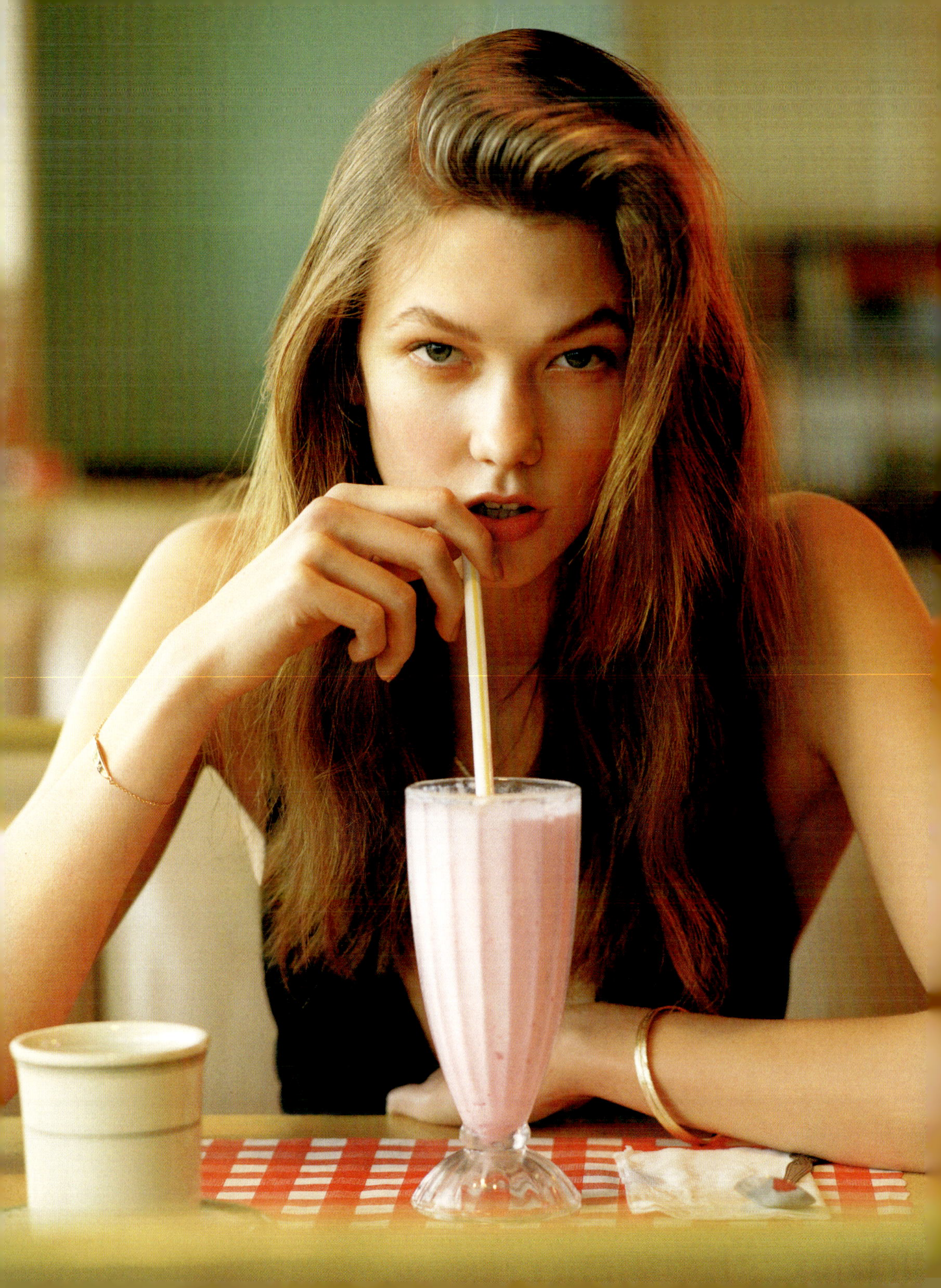

Karlie Kloss

Sometimes, like Pallas Athena springing from the head of Zeus, models appear fully formed as if from nowhere, hurling high-wattage thunderbolts of charisma before them. Karlie Kloss, of the mesmeric, much-parodied catwalk 'death stare', is one such. (*New York* magazine tells us that she 'moves in slow motion, swaying her head from side to side in such a way that if laser beams were to suddenly shoot out of her eyes – and we suspect they might any minute now – she would obliterate everyone in the first two rows.')

This goddess, 6ft tall with impossibly long legs, sprang from St Louis by way of Chicago and was discovered in her early teens at a charity fashion show. 'I just got incredibly tall – I just grew six inches,' she told American *Vogue*. She signed up with the Elite agency but was subsequently the subject of an unseemly tug-of-love with a rival agency. Before modelling claimed her, she was fulfilled by a nascent ballet career, having studied at Caston's Ballet Academie in 2002 and danced with the main Caston Chamber Ballet in 2007. She is currently its most prized alumna.

'I'm the stick that stands out above everyone in St Louis – and all my co ordination went out the door.' Well, not quite. Karlie is an imposing and ornamental addition to catwalks the world over; the ballet deportment and the Caston performances have left her with self-possession and an ability to move with grace in public and to remain unconcerned in the glare of the spotlight. Steven Meisel, the acknowledged authority on models *de nos jours*, his studio an unofficial finishing school for fashion fledglings, says: 'She's an amazing model. She knows clothes. She has tons of energy. She will add things to the shoot that I would never have thought of.' Perfect for the face of Pringle Scotland, one of their most recent collaborations.

Compared to a young Christy Turlington by Arthur Elgort and accorded 'the Evangelista factor' by American *Vogue* – much to live up to there – the St Louis supernova is poised to go further into the stratosphere. Bringing her safely back down to earth will be her three sisters, her easygoing nature and her baking skills (cookies, predominantly).

Karlie Kloss (b. 1992, USA)

Opposite:
'Born in the USA', May 2010,
by Alasdair McLellan.
Fashion by Louis Vuitton

Kate Moss

It can be bluntly put: Kate Moss, the travel agent's daughter from Croydon, is the most celebrated beauty of her era, and after the Queen the most recognisable living British woman. Possibly more so, as there are few corners of any foreign field untouched by fashion magazines, Calvin Klein advertising, Chanel perfume marketing strategies, paparazzi and tabloid-style newspapers. Like the Queen, her likeness has been painted by Lucian Freud and, like the Queen, she refuses to speak publicly on a host of issues. In fact, for the most part, she – Kate – refuses to speak publicly at all.

She came to prominence in the early 1990s, the personification of the 'waif', almost anti-fashion in appearance, or at least against the then-prevailing type (amazonian, high maintenance, impossibly dignified). At 5ft 6½in tall, Kate was demonstrably petite for a top model and slight in build. As her star rose, the slightness was wrongly perceived as first-stage anorexia or heroin-induced skinniness. Despite the woeful connotations, it made her name known.

Kate was brought to *Vogue*'s attention by way of youth-culture magazines, specifically *The Face*, for which she was photographed in 1989 by Corinne Day, who would herself have a distinguished *Vogue* career. Editor Alexandra Shulman and fashion director Lucinda Chambers were instrumental in providing Kate with an arena, the former remarking of Corinne Day's photographs: 'The way she looks at women is the way a girl appreciates a girl's looks; not the way women judge other women. There is a warmth and intimacy there.' *Vogue* heralded a new spirit in fashion, which some labelled 'grunge'. But it really meant a relaxing of rules and of stereotypes, so that a south London teenager could wear a homemade T-shirt and tattered leggings, a pale pink and ice-blue tweed bustier by Chanel or a grubby eiderdown and look like the germ of a fashion icon.

These early photos were defiantly unglamorous, like pale and eerie stills from a gritty documentary or freeze-frames from someone's home movie. Whatever they were, they weren't fashion photographs as were then expected. They were raw and natural, completely without 'style' – in the sense that there was nothing artificial in their conception, as there always seemed to be in every other fashion story. Moss's hair was ungroomed, her make-up minimal and the clothes all but incidental. It's the stuff of future fashion theses that far from presiding over the death of the cult of the model she ended up coaxing model stardom to even greater heights. Everyone who follows her is compared to her, and in truth no-one has got whatever it is she has.

'She was just this cocky kid from Croydon,' recalled Corinne Day, pinpointing what made it work, 'she wasn't like a model... but I knew she was going to be famous.' Nearly two decades since her first *Vogue* pictures, Kate has changed the perception of beauty and fashion across the globe, without appearing to expend any effort. 'There wasn't any teaching and that was quite good,' she said, 'because that's why I was a natural. I was a normal teenager.'

As Day predicted, Kate became famous quickly and she remains so. And mostly for her fashion and modelling career. There have been well-documented extra-curricular activities and 'issues', but more important are the covers, the clothing lines, the appearances in best-dressed lists, the smouldering sensibility that makes even the most quotidian accessory look way beyond the reach of anyone else. 'Her incredible personal style,' wrote Sarah Mower in American *Vogue*, 'is what put Kate Moss up there on the Olympus of supermodeldom, inhabiting that special peak of fame reserved for the few who have crossed over to pop-cultural goddess.'

Now, in her thirties, Kate Moss remains unsinkable and untouchable. She is a cipher for her times, an inscrutable sphinx of a woman, who never explains and never apologises, and if she possesses a riddle, has not yet made the mistake of letting us know what it is.

Kate Moss (b. 1974, UK)

Opposite:
'In Her Own Style',
January 1997,
by Craig McDean

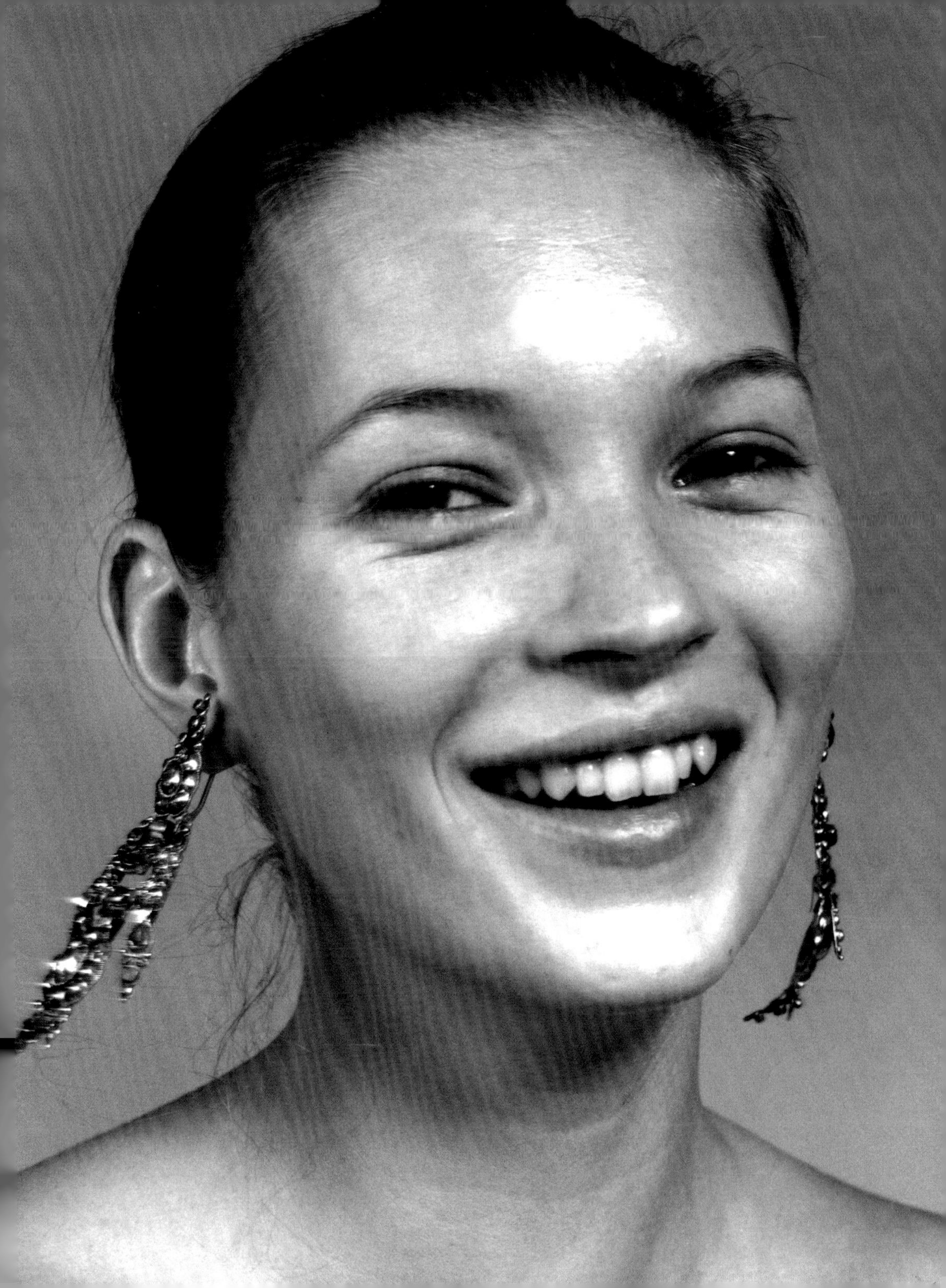

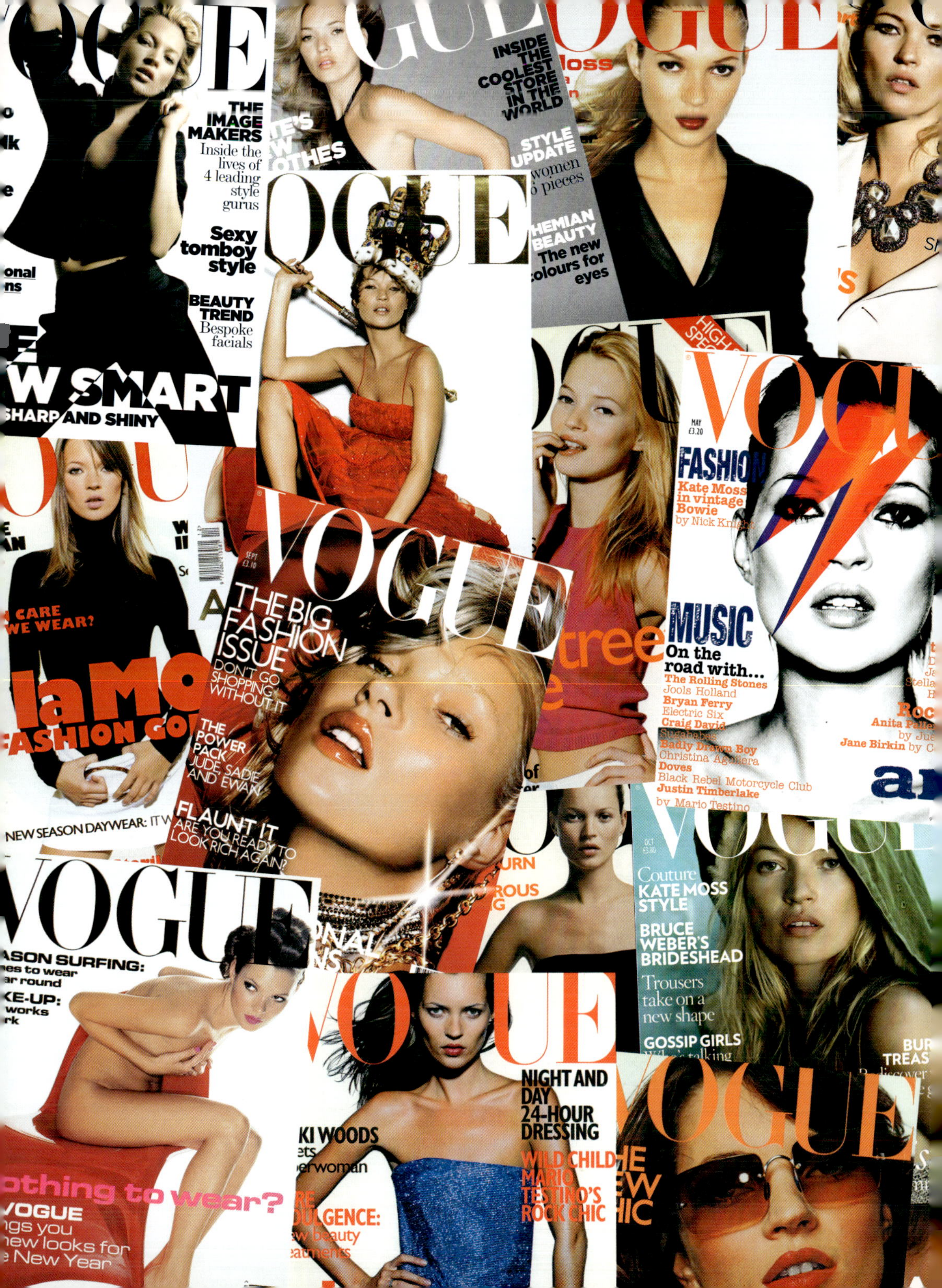
VOGUE
THE IMAGE MAKERS
Inside the lives of 4 leading style gurus
Sexy tomboy style
BEAUTY TREND
Bespoke facials
SMART
AND SHINY
INSIDE THE COOLEST STORE IN THE WORLD
STYLE UPDATE
The new colours for eyes
VOGUE
VOGUE
MAY
£3.20
FASHION
Kate Moss in vintage Bowie
by Nick Knight
MUSIC
On the road with...
The Rolling Stones
Jools Holland
Bryan Ferry
Electric Six
Craig David
Sugababes
Badly Drawn Boy
Christina Aguilera
Doves
Black Rebel Motorcycle Club
Justin Timberlake
by Mario Testino
Anita Pallenberg
Jane Birkin
VOGUE
SEPT
£3.10
THE BIG FASHION ISSUE
DON'T GO SHOPPING WITHOUT IT
THE POWER PACK
JUDE, SADIE AND EWAN
FLAUNT IT
ARE YOU READY TO LOOK RICH AGAIN?
NEW SEASON DAYWEAR:
tree
VOGUE
OCT
£3.80
Couture
KATE MOSS STYLE
BRUCE WEBER'S BRIDESHEAD
Trousers take on a new shape
GOSSIP GIRLS
VOGUE
SURFING:
VOGUE
NIGHT AND DAY
24-HOUR DRESSING
WILD CHILD
MARIO TESTINO'S ROCK CHIC
KI WOODS
VOGUE
to wear?
VOGUE
New Year

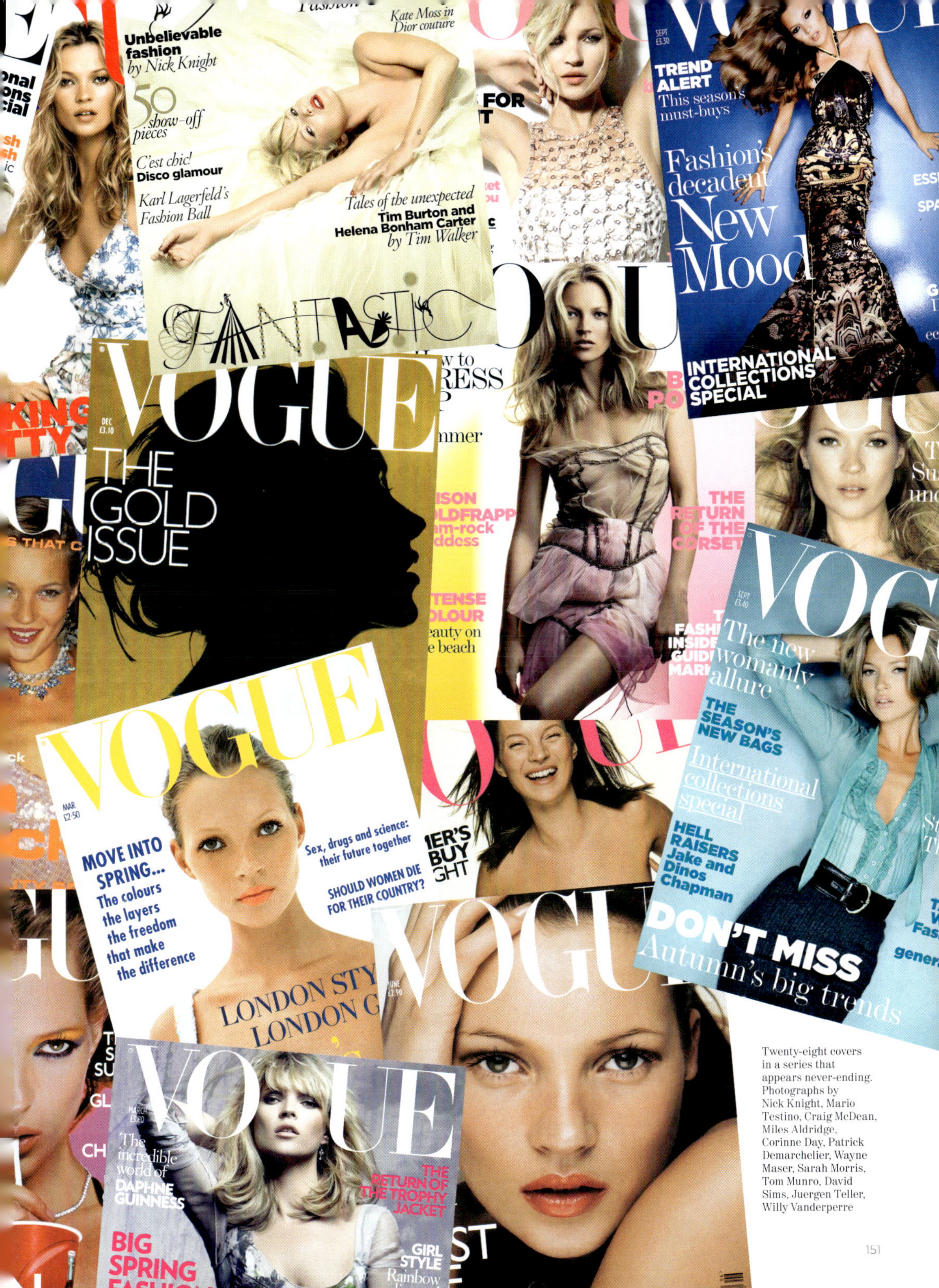

Twenty-eight covers in a series that appears never-ending. Photographs by Nick Knight, Mario Testino, Craig McDean, Miles Aldridge, Corinne Day, Patrick Demarchelier, Wayne Maser, Sarah Morris, Tom Munro, David Sims, Juergen Teller, Willy Vanderperre

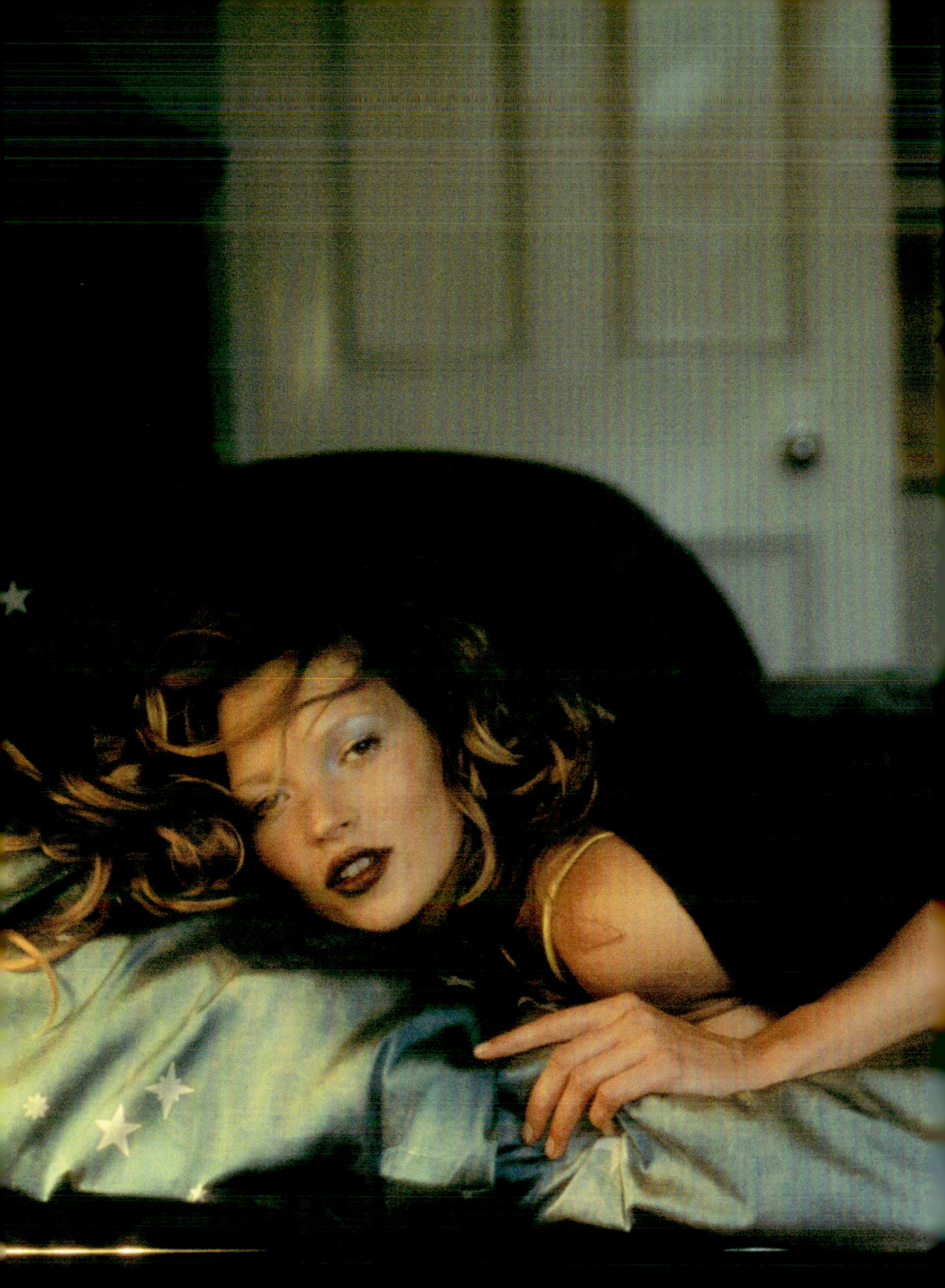

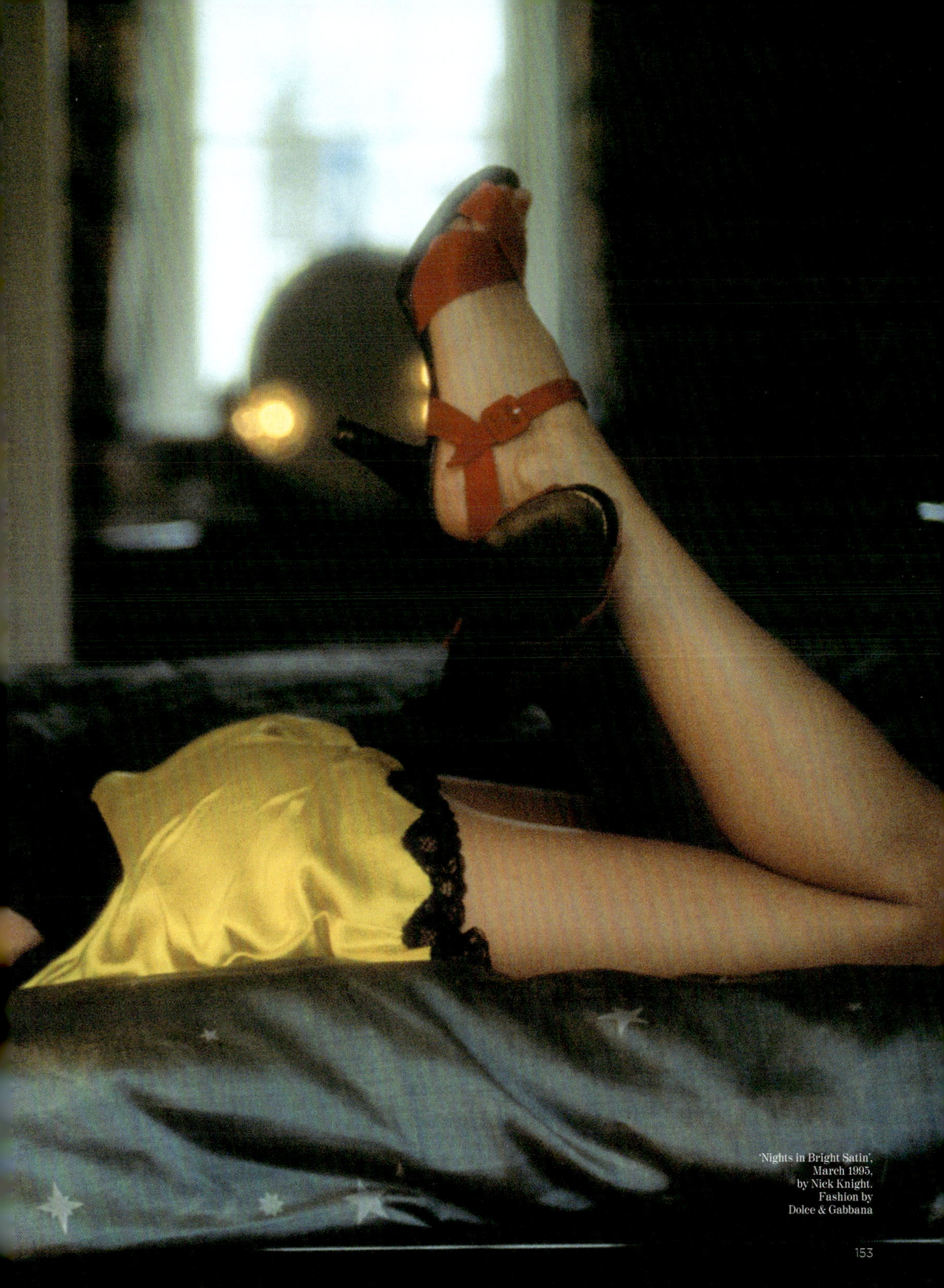

'Nights in Bright Satin', March 1995, by Nick Knight. Fashion by Dolce & Gabbana

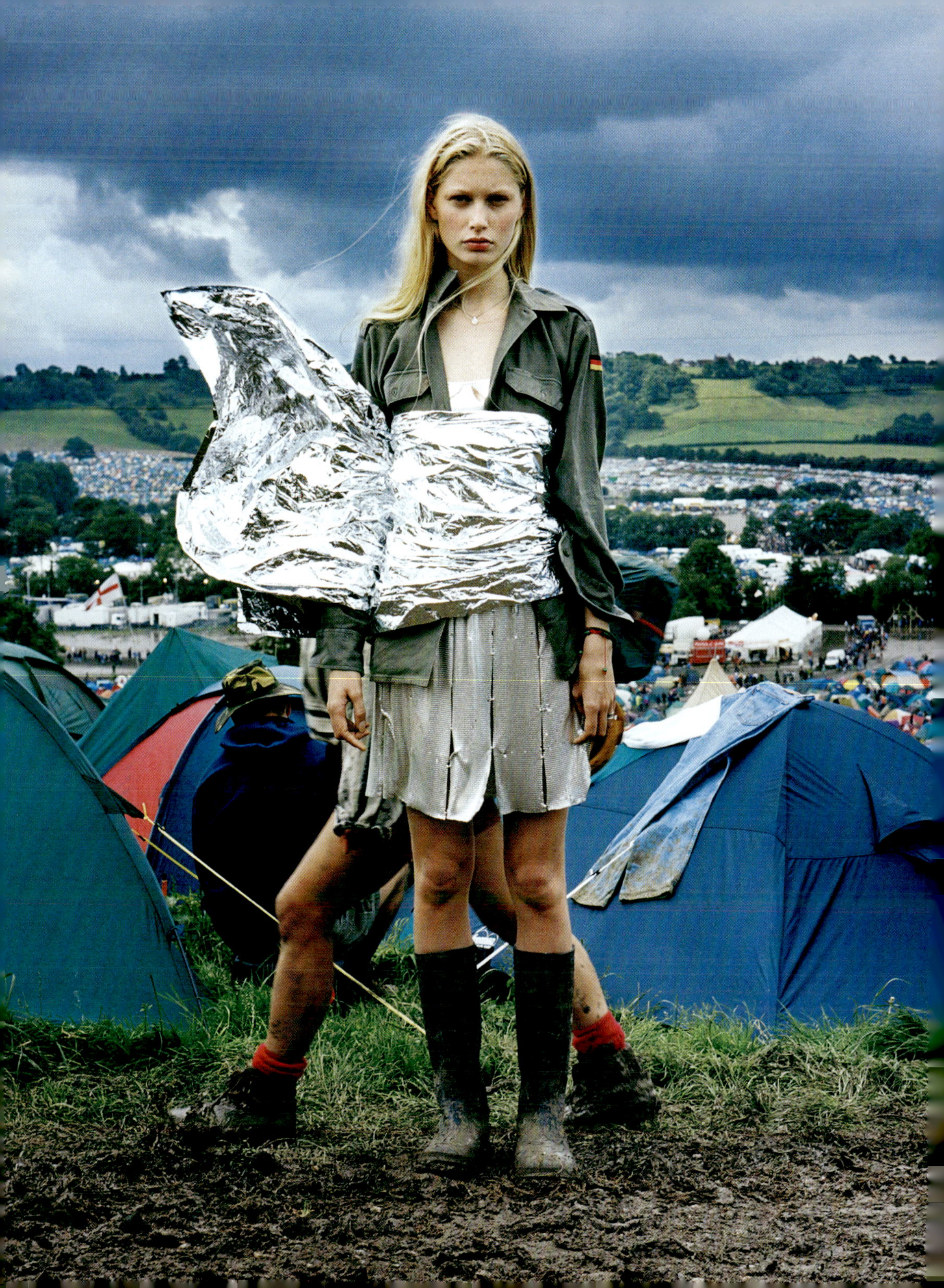

Kirsty Hume

Kirsty Hume's name was for a while intertwined with that of her handsome, epicene husband, Donovan Leitch Jr, son of 1960s folk balladeer Donovan. Arthur Elgort's shoot 'Seasoned Simplicity' for American *Vogue* showed both parties in an easygoing homage to the 1960s against the idiosyncrasies of the British landscape, while Steven Meisel photographed their wedding for the magazine (her dress was gothic in inspiration). Kirsty herself had something of the Summer of Love about her: lean, at just under 6ft tall, with considerably past-the-shoulder-length sunlight-coloured hair and a vulnerability that spoke of simpler times. She further possessed an unassuming nature, which *Vogue* found refreshing. 'It's true that I'm on the list of top models,' she said in 1996, 'but I don't think I've done anything with my life yet that I deserve to be called a "star"…' *Vogue* was also touched by her frantic efforts in running around her New York apartment to capture two sick kittens, which needed their medicine dispensed by eyedropper.

Fame had crept up on 20-year-old Kirsty Hume from Ayr to catch her unawares: 'It's hard to adapt from being a little girl in Scotland with no responsibilities to living in a big city,' she told *Vogue*'s Charles Gandee, 'earning money and travelling all over the place and having phone bills to pay and an apartment to clean and all the rest of it. When I left Scotland I didn't even have a credit card.'

A one-day modelling class taken for fun at 13 gave Kirsty a grounding in poise and deportment. At 16 she was snapped up by a modest Glasgow modelling agency, and within a couple of years was in Paris trying her luck. She was encouraged by Patrick Demarchelier to take it seriously, which she did – and rose stratospherically – before withdrawing from view slightly to study art. 'I'd rather be remembered as a famous painter than a famous model,' she once said, 'so I'd better start the ball rolling now.' Modelling, she admitted, was a means to an end. She wanted to earn enough money to retire and 'live a tranquil life', which she accomplished quickly and with her husband moved to upstate New York, near Woodstock.

The whippy, trippy, carefree 1960s feeling continued further in *Vogue*'s approving account of her off-duty uniform: 'part hippy with pagan tattoos, part boho de luxe.' She and Donovan Jr were the perfect models (along with Trish Goff and her husband, Aaron) to star in the magazine's 'Earth Girls' festival shoot with Tim Walker. It was photographed at Glastonbury in the British summertime, so naturally it rained. Kirsty was dressed in a Versace diffusion-line camisole, a chainmail miniskirt and a silvered thermal blanket, and recalled: 'We'd have to put on waterproof trousers and jackets over our clothes. For some shots we'd simply push the waterproofs down to our knees and stand there, while Tim shot from the knees up.'

Kirsty Hume (b. 1976, UK)

Opposite:
'Earth Girls',
December 1998,
by Tim Walker.
Fashion by Versus

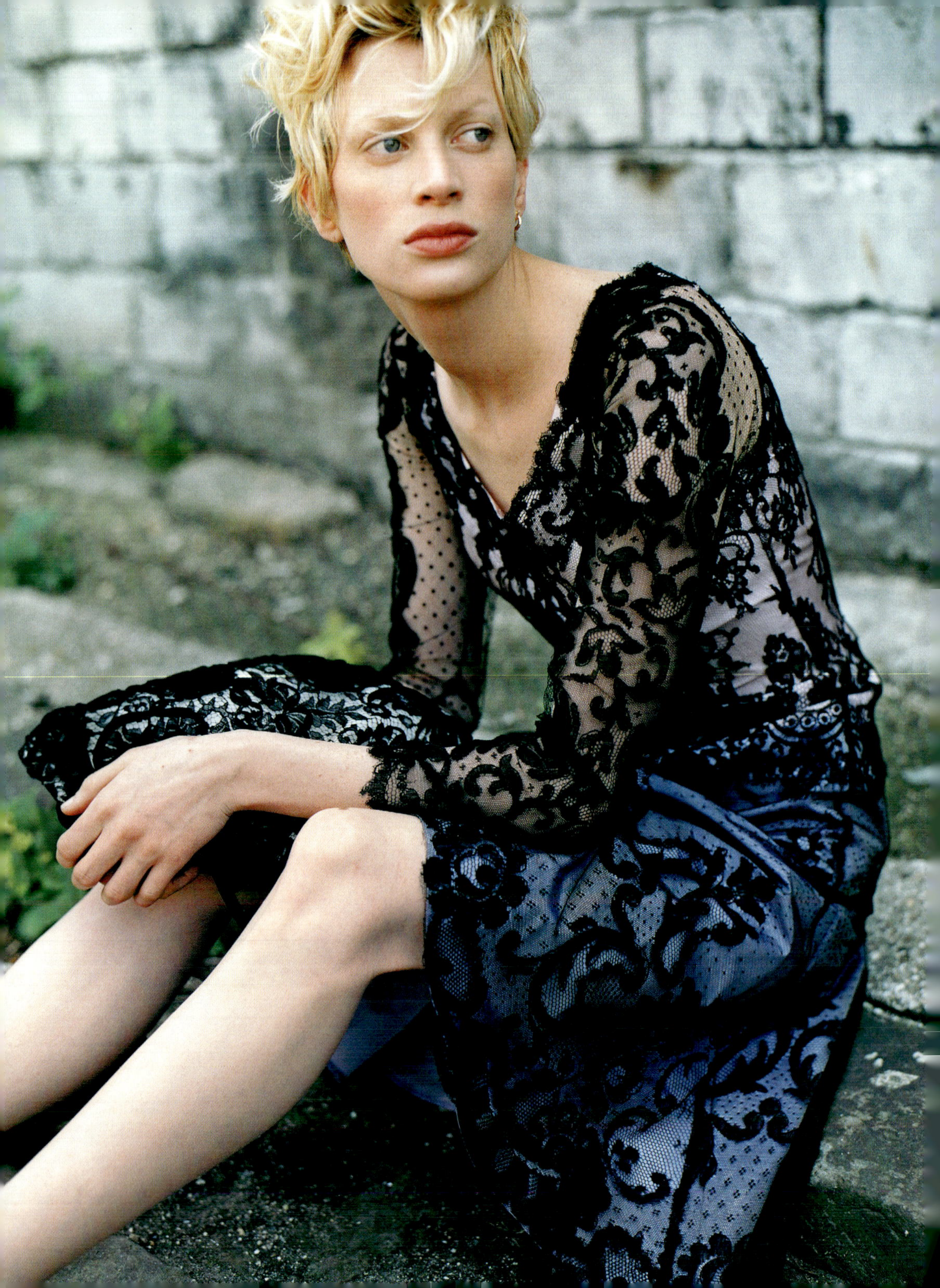

Kristen McMenamy

On paper, it shouldn't have worked – stick-thin angularity, barely discernible eyebrows above drooping eyelids, small breasts, large hands, an androgynous schoolboy crop and a wide mouth (which admittedly lit up the room when she smiled, although for a considerable time she rarely smiled in print). But it did work. Sensationally.

It helped only a little that Kristen McMenamy sprung out of nowhere at just the time photographers and magazines decided to veer off into uncharted territory – anti-fashion. That is to say, not biting the hand that fed them, but just deciding that beauty could be found in unpromising and improbable places and in those who might never consider they had anything much to offer at all. They called it unlikely beauty, then extreme beauty, just occasionally weird beauty and squint or skewed glamour. American *Vogue* put it politely. In McMenamy they had found 'the model-with-a-difference extraordinaire'.

The most extraordinaire bit was that McMenamy was, of course, absolutely beautiful, no matter what you put her in nor what you asked her to do: to pile on the neon-blue lipgloss, vinyl and metal body sculpture, pumpkin-hued stretch mini-shorts, or just to stand there backstage, naked and exhausted like a bruised pugilist. So beautiful, in fact, that Karl Lagerfeld appropriated her as a muse. He also took the first pictures of her for British *Vogue* (and gave her away at her wedding to fashion photographer Miles Aldridge in 1997). 'She is like a piece of paper. Whatever I cut on her works. Above everything else, she is always herself. She *is* modern fashion, which is not to be obsessed with beauty but with life, personality, versatility.' Touchingly, she was entirely unaware of her impact and considerable personal magnetism, quitting a Richard Avedon shoot for Versace in tears, saying 'the [Versace] woman thing is so major! Well, I felt like a eunuch…' (They implored her to return; she did; the pictures remain magnificent.)

Born in 1966 in Easton, Pennsylvania, McMenamy – nicknamed Skeleton at school – was an avaricious reader of fashion magazines and in due course sent in her pictures to a *Cosmopolitan* model contest. The winner was a suntanned blonde from California. Undaunted, she attended modelling school, and, armed with a local photographer's slightly out-of-focus snapshots, made the rounds in New York with a friend in tow for support. The friend was useful, as agency after agency discouraged her. The last ignored her, but thought her friend might just have what it took.

However, the fuzzy pictures worked and somewhere along the line another smaller agency took her on, sending her to Paris, where notions of contemporary beauty have always been less rigorous and less humdrum. Still there were the dispiriting rounds of go-sees for yoghurt commercials before the German photographer Peter Lindbergh spotted her. Channelling Weimar-era androgyny and Fritz Lang's Expressionist films, McMenamy was perfect for Lindbergh's atmospheric *mise-en-scène*. 'You can put her nowhere,' he explained to the *New Yorker*, 'and say, "Do something", and you get the most incredible pictures.' She went back to New York a star, albeit one slightly out of kilter with the prevailing mood (still suntanned Californian blondes).

On the catwalk she was a star, her long, pale limbs turning into the spotlight like flowers bending towards the sun. The *New Yorker* found her backstage at a Comme des Garçons show, looking at her colleagues being frantically shoehorned into ballgowns. '"Oh why couldn't I have a ballgown?" she wails, to no-one in particular. "Well, I do have a ballgown at Yohji Yamamoto." She pauses, still thinking, looking not quite consoled. "It's wood," she explains.'

Esoteric and ethereal, her beauty may not be of the classic kind, but she challenged notions of what it might be and in so doing revealed herself as an endlessly beguiling siren. The more you fixed yourself on her gaze, the more beautiful she became – but you felt she didn't quite believe she was beautiful at all, and that, tragically, she might *never* believe it. She has kept little from those years to hand down to her children. But there is a happy ending. 'Fashion,' she said recently, 'actually gives me a sense of self-worth.'

Kristen McMenamy (b. 1966, USA)

Opposite:
'Sheer Heaven', November 1995, by Mario Testino. Fashion by Christian Lacroix

Lara Stone

'At this moment,' American *Vogue* trumpeted in 2010, 'the face of beauty is Dutch'. By Dutch, the magazine meant Mirte Maas, Doutzen Kroes, Anna de Rijk and Kim Noorda, but mostly it meant the least Dutch sounding of all, Lara Stone. As it turns out, she is only half-Dutch (the other half is British), but she counts all the same, having been born and raised in the Low Countries, in Geldrop-Mierlo. Photographer Mario Testino, who knows these things from Rotterdam to Rio, called her 'the embodiment of beauty today', adding, in admiration: 'We went through an anorexic phase, but now we have Lara.' This is an incontrovertible, approving reference to her looks, from which you cannot unlock your gaze – she is curvaceous (with 32D breasts), gap-toothed, full of figure and undeniably of real life.

In fact, conjectured *Vogue*, not since Kate Moss appeared fresh out of south London in 1990 have a model's face and body been the subject of so much in-depth scrutiny. Both caught the fashion industry unawares: 'the sheer originality and wrongness of her beauty and the sexy voluptuousness of her figure'.

She was discovered some time ago on the Paris Metro, aged 12 – this is the second bite of the cherry for Lara Stone. It didn't work initially; the skinny, odd-eyebrowed ingénue needed time to coalesce into the harmonious hourglass-figured woman. 'Everyone at school said I looked funny, weird,' she told *Vogue*. She entered – and failed to win – the Dutch Elite modelling competition, but the agency took her on anyway. Years of struggle followed until she made it in 2008, after an absence and a change of agents, and opened the season's Prada show.

'She literally bounced down the catwalk,' recalled *Vogue* editor Alexandra Shulman. The bouncing may have been due to her slightly smaller than average feet, which tend to fit uncomfortably in the standard runway shoe. The Prada show led to a busy period. 'I fly to New York every week,' she told *Vogue*, 'sometimes twice a week.' She travels to Paris, too, several times per month.

Lara is seen as something different, she says with candour, because she is fat (which is not strictly true): 'If I had the discipline to be super-skinny, I would be.' But then her sex appeal would not shimmer enough to be Karl Lagerfeld's 'perfect girl of the moment' or, for that matter, *Vogue*'s 'icon the fashion world never admitted it was waiting for…' Forward into the Stone Age.

Lara Stone (b. 1983, Netherlands)

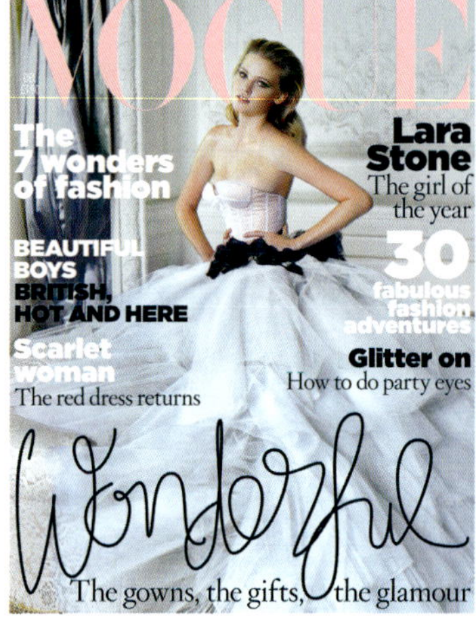

Above:
'Wonderful', December 2009, by Mario Testino. Fashion by Dior

Opposite:
'Go Figure', April 2010, by Alasdair McLellan. Fashion by Michael Kors

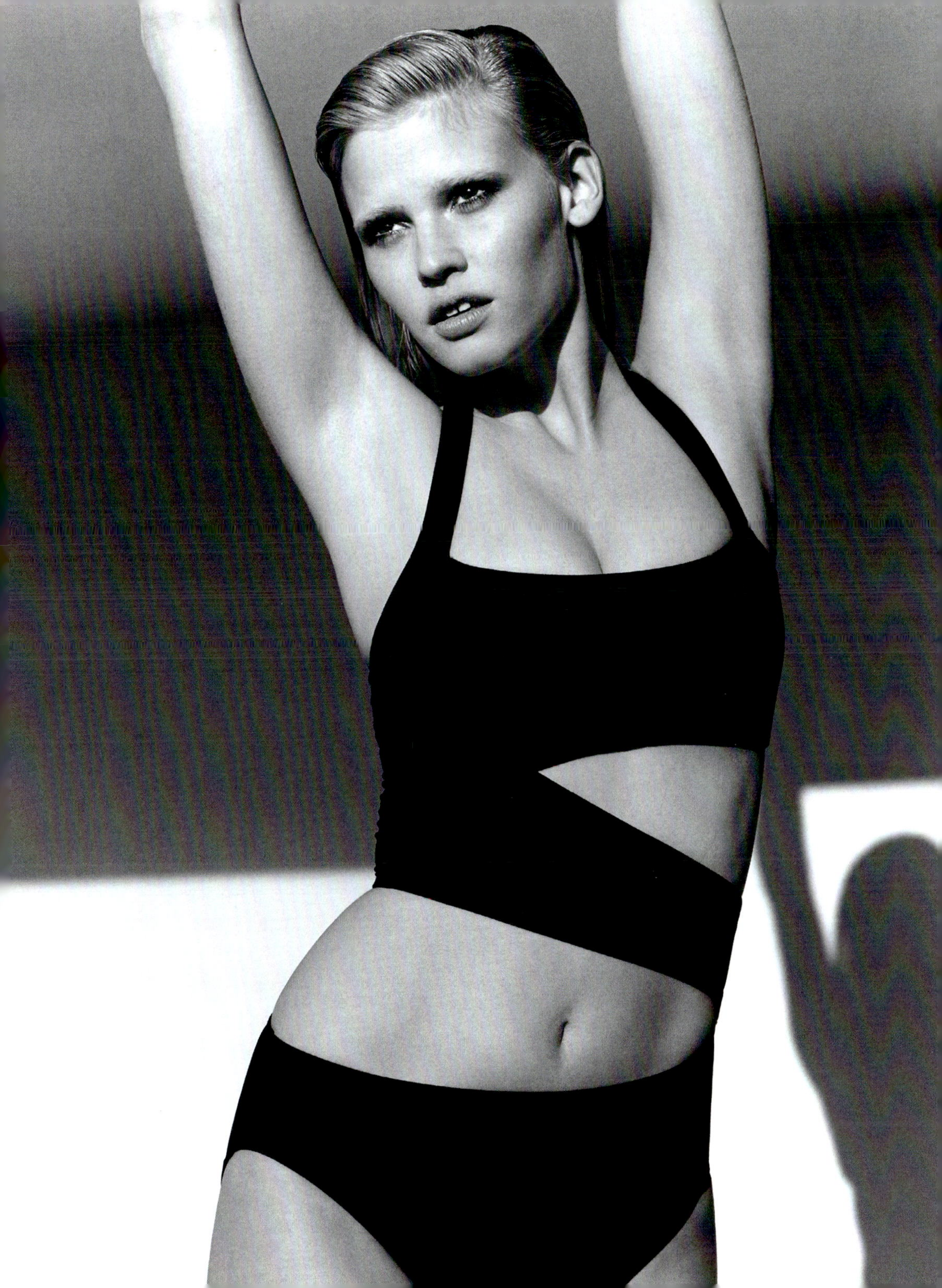

Lauren Hutton

In the mid-1970s, *Vogue* was agog at the new commercialism: 'Girls next door not only look like a million dollars, they sometimes make it, too.' By 1974 a gap-toothed, banana-nosed swamp skunk (her own words) from South Carolina was the world's highest-paid model. Thirty years old, Lauren Hutton earned a quarter of a million dollars a year alone as the face of Revlon's Ultima – and she kept that going for a number of years. In so doing, she almost single-handedly raised the pay scale and expectations of thousands of young model girls around the world. She was also a rising Hollywood star, acting when modelling assignments allowed. She had succeeded at both, not despite her 'flaws' but because of them.

Hutton came to New York in 1964, aged 21, with $200 and a determination to get to Africa somehow. In time she was turned down by every modelling agent except Eileen Ford, who agreed to take her on if she had her nose fixed and teeth sorted. It was a condition she agreed to, but never found the time to honour. 'I promised I would, once I had the money,' she told *Vogue*, 'but inside I figured it would take me a long, long time to get around to it.'

Her first job was as a house model for Dior at $50 a week. 'I would sit there all day, and when a buyer came in I'd do my thing. It was incredibly dull, but it was a guaranteed job.' At 5ft 5in and 124lb, she was known in the showroom as the Baby Elephant. She lost the weight that she felt she ought to, and became a catwalk model. 'In those days,' she continued to *Vogue*, 'photography models wouldn't be seen dead on the runway. But, hey, it was $50 a runway. And I did some bra-and-pantie stuff because it paid $300 an hour *and* it was less revealing than my bikini…'

An antipathy to the highly made-up and lacquered look of the era – Peggy Moffitt being the *ne plus ultra* – meant that Hutton's scrubbed-clean, girl-next-door ordinariness was a novelty. Somehow she bleeped on *Vogue* editor-in-chief Diana Vreeland's radar ('You! You have quite a presence'), and that was it. Hutton was off on a go-see to Richard Avedon. She protested to Vreeland that she had seen him already and the maestro had refused to photograph her. 'Tomorrow,' the editor twinkled back at her, 'tomorrow he will.'

After the pictures came out, she recalled she was 'basically triple-booked every hour for the next 10 years'. In time – and it took a long time – the modelling career faltered, to be replaced by Hollywood and movie-making. During the 1980s Hutton was making around five movies a year. For every *American Gigolo* there was, however, a *From Here to Maternity*. 'I was the Grade-B Cheese Queen,' she told *Vogue*. 'I modelled my way through movies.'

By 1988 (the year of four guest-starring episodes of *Falcon Crest* and the not overly well-received *Timestalkers*), a call came through from 'some Steven Meisel guy', and at 45 Hutton was back on the cover of Italian *Vogue*, the new face of respectable early middle age. 'With Steven taking the pictures and Laura Mercier doing my make-up, I was alright,' she explained. 'With anyone else I was in trouble. I looked like a madam from a bordello. It was just tragic.' Fortunately Meisel was on hand slightly later to photograph the nearly 50-year-old face of Revlon's Eterna 27. 'One of the nicest things about Steven is the way he encouraged me to be my age,' Hutton told *Vogue*. 'He didn't want me to look pert or this and that… he wanted me to look as I felt at this time, which means I can feel 15 one day and 150 another – and, of course, look it!'

Naturally she does not act her age, which helps, too: she is a dogsledder, scuba diver, strong swimmer (preferably with sharks), indefatigable traveller and motorcyclist. The last enthusiasm nearly killed her. On a trip outside Las Vegas with easy-riding celebrity friends, including Dennis Hopper, Laurence Fishburne and Jeremy Irons, she crashed at 100mph, flew 20ft in the air and crash-landed to break her sternum and ribs, and pulverise part of the tibia in her right leg. Even in a semi-comatose state she had to be tied down to her hospital bed, as she was trying to get up and walk gracefully away from the trauma. A lifetime in modelling had left her body lithe, given her endless reserves of patience and the strength of spirit to keep moving on. Quite possibly it saved her life.

Lauren Hutton (b. Mary Laurence Hutton, 1943, USA)

Opposite:
'The Million-Dollar Girls Next Door', December 1974 (unpublished), by Eva Sereny

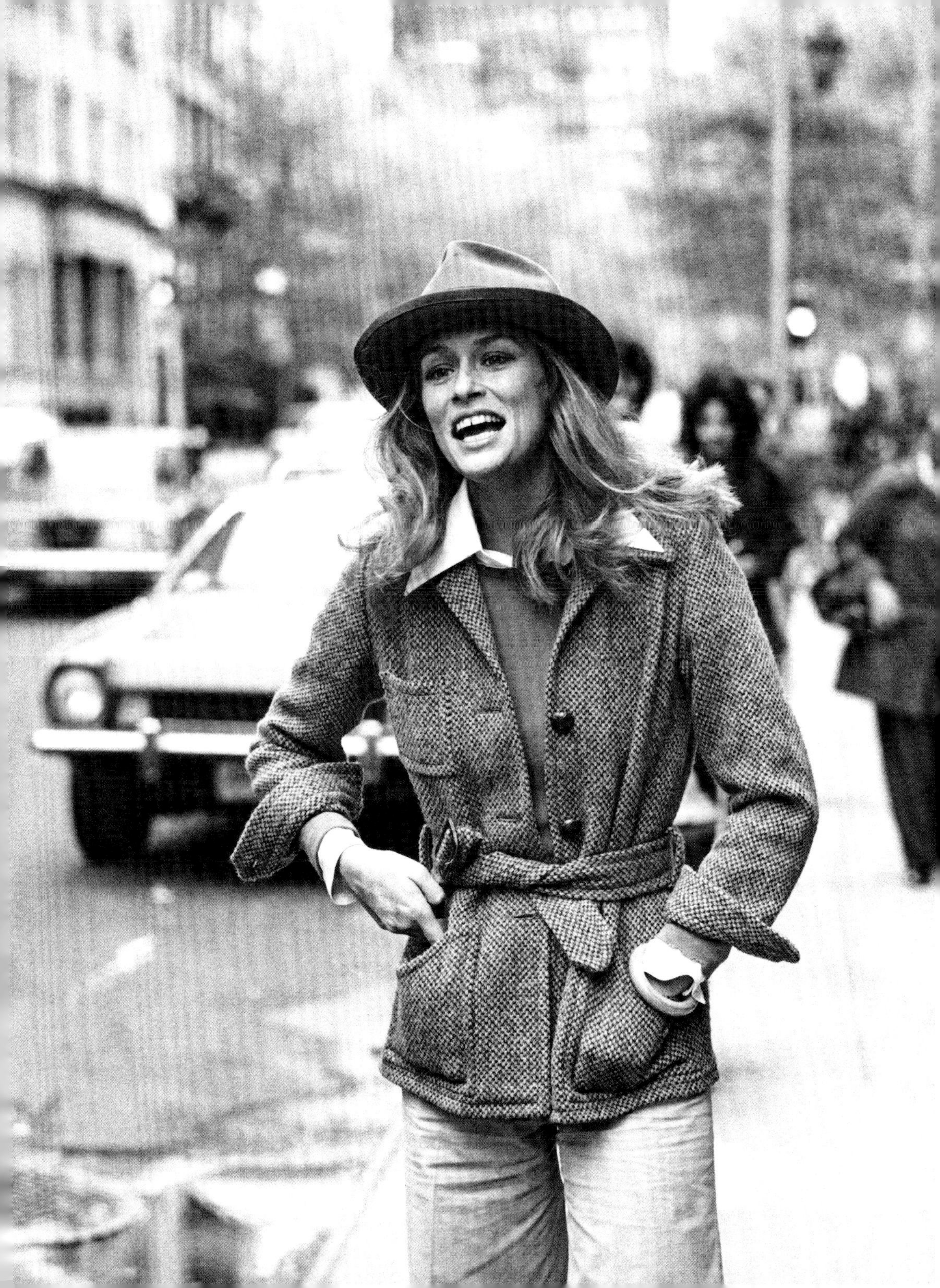

Lee Miller

Manhattan, 1926. An 18-year-old girl, fresh from Poughkeepsie, New York, walked off the sidewalk into the path of an oncoming car. A fellow pedestrian caught her elbow at the last minute. The girl was Lee Miller; her saviour, the redoubtable Condé Nast, king of American magazine publishing – and owner of *Vogue*, in front of whose offices the catastrophe was averted. The businessman took her up to his office and offered her work as a fashion model for *Vogue*. This was not as hackneyed as it might sound. Nast had guided *Vogue* from being a substanceless society weekly into the glossiest publication of its time precisely because he knew what faces sold it at the newsstand.

The progress of Lee Miller appears scarcely credible: from small-town girl to fashion model, to sophisticated expatriate in Paris, to fashion photographer, to photo-essayist, to confidante of Picasso. She remains one of *Vogue*'s heroines – and, for a time, one of its most beautiful models. When her modelling career was over (it was a brief one) her association with the magazine continued. She had previously picked up a camera and tutored herself in the studio of Man Ray, and her life with *Vogue* lasted well over a quarter of a century. Far from the hothouse atmosphere of the studio, it was her war photography, unexpected and astonishing, that made her name. It also propelled Nast's *Vogue* into the modern era. Lee's war reportage – in words as well as pictures – gives the magazine's history real substance, so that its pages, viewed years later, do not shimmer only with images of beautifully attired women.

She was, though, one of those herself; a favourite of Arnold Genthe, Edward Steichen, George Hoyningen-Huene and briefly Horst. Cecil Beaton was mostly resistant to her charms, calling her 'a sun-kissed goat-boy from the Appian Way', though conceding that 'only sculpture could approximate the beauty of her curling lips… languid, pale eyes and column neck'.

Barely 10 years after the last of her fashion appearances, the neatly coiffed model-turned-photographer witnessed the Thousand Year Reich's *Götterdämmerung* as a dirty, battle-hardened war correspondent in combat fatigues, and confronted the full depth of the Holocaust first-hand, entering Dachau and Buchenwald shortly after liberation. Not for nothing was the first compilation of her work, found at *Vogue* and locked away in her attic, titled *The Lives of Lee Miller*. Awful as it is to see, the war turned out to be the making of her and she was lost when it was all over. She tried to spin it out after peace was declared and reported Europe's attempts to rebuild itself. Cabled 'Go home' by *Vogue*'s editor she did, at length; but nothing would be the same again. She strung out her career there until 1953.

Lee was never comfortable modelling, as her subsequent career path suggested. Horst found that out early on, discovering on one shoot that she eschewed direction and did precisely what she wanted. 'With strong-willed girls,' he ruefully concluded, 'you let them do it, you don't suggest.' Hoyningen-Huene's fashion pictures of Lee reflected the new type of modern woman – stylish, relaxed and independent – that Condé Nast sought to invigorate his dynamic magazine still further.

Lee Miller (b. 1907, USA; d. 1977)

Opposite:
'Coiffure by Callon',
1930 (unpublished),
by George Hoyningen-Huene

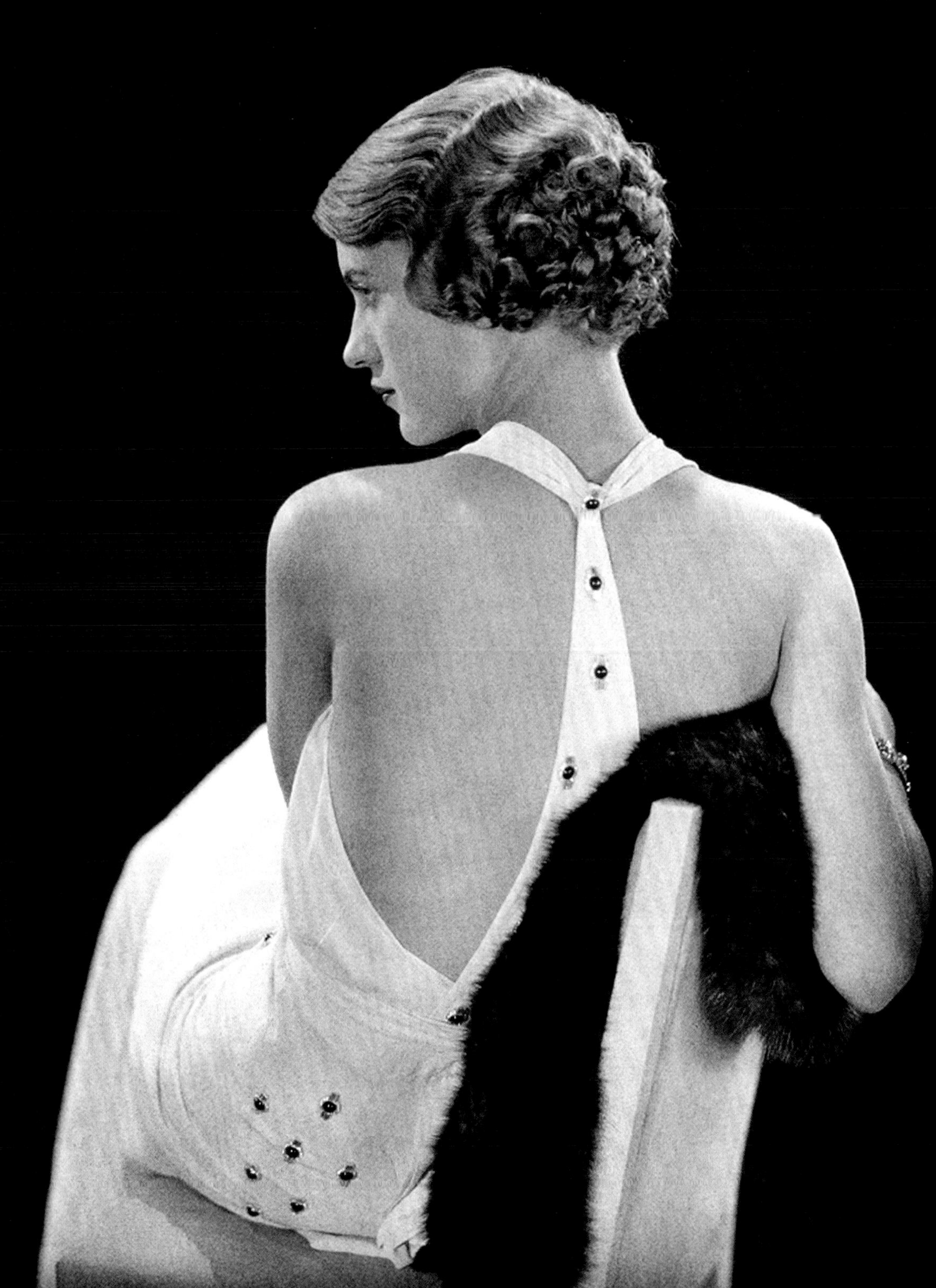

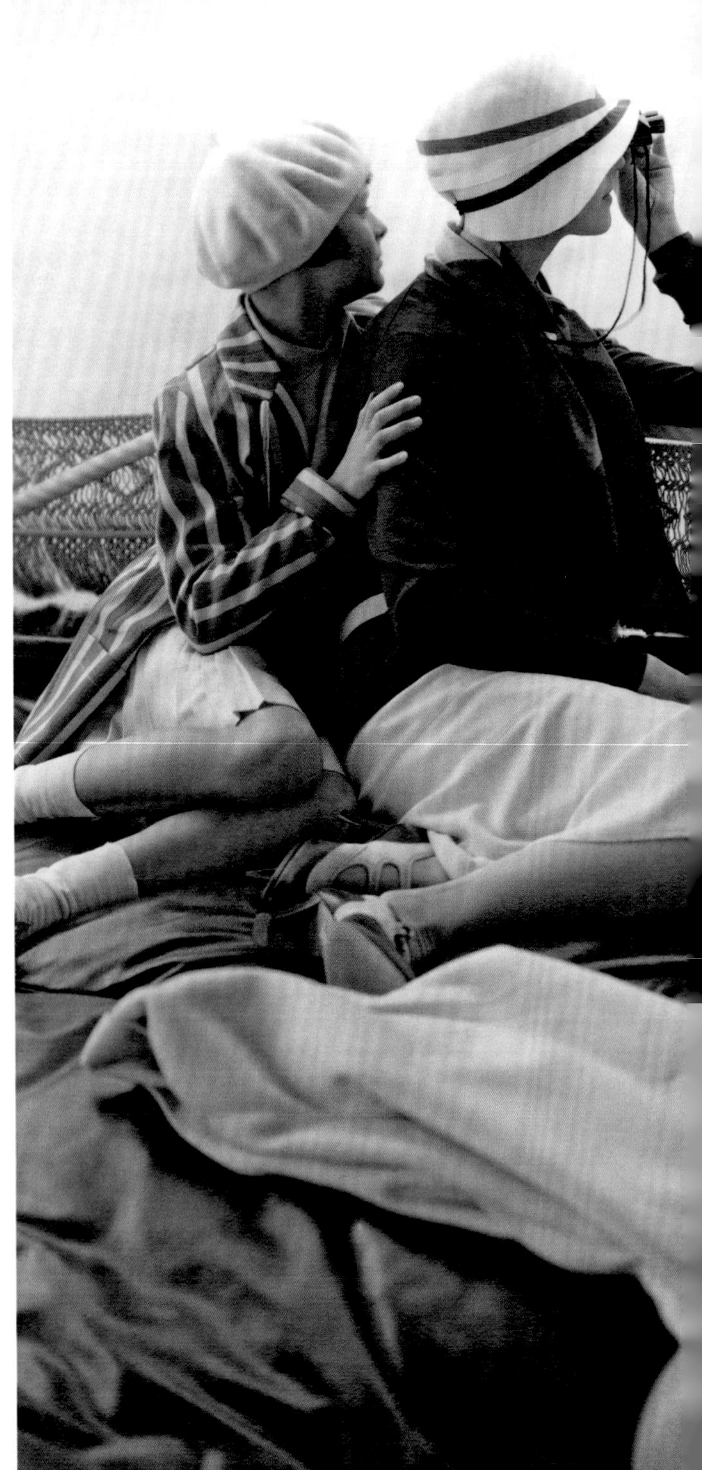

'The Mode Puts Out to Sea',
July 1928,
by Edward Steichen.
Fashion by Saks

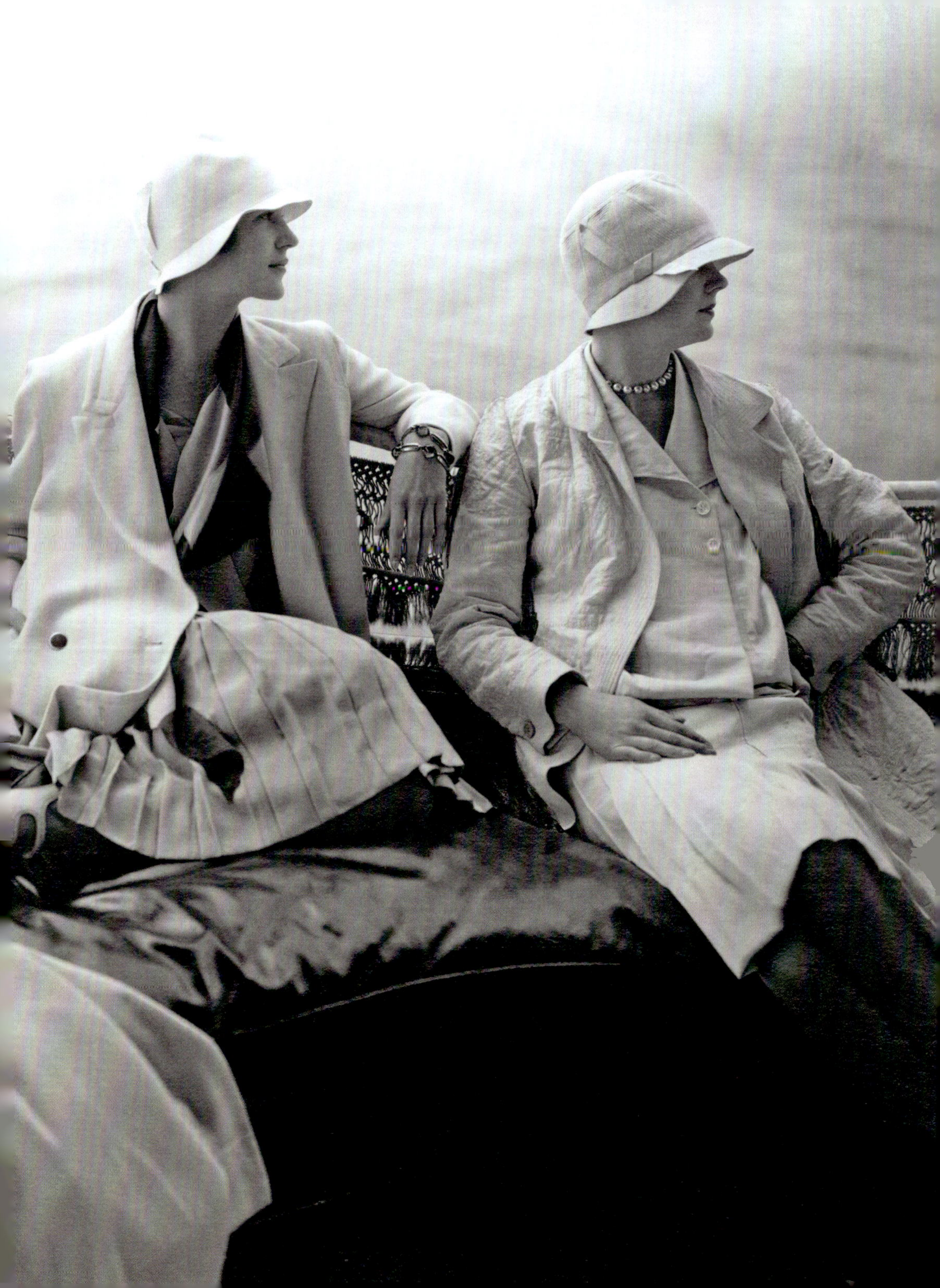

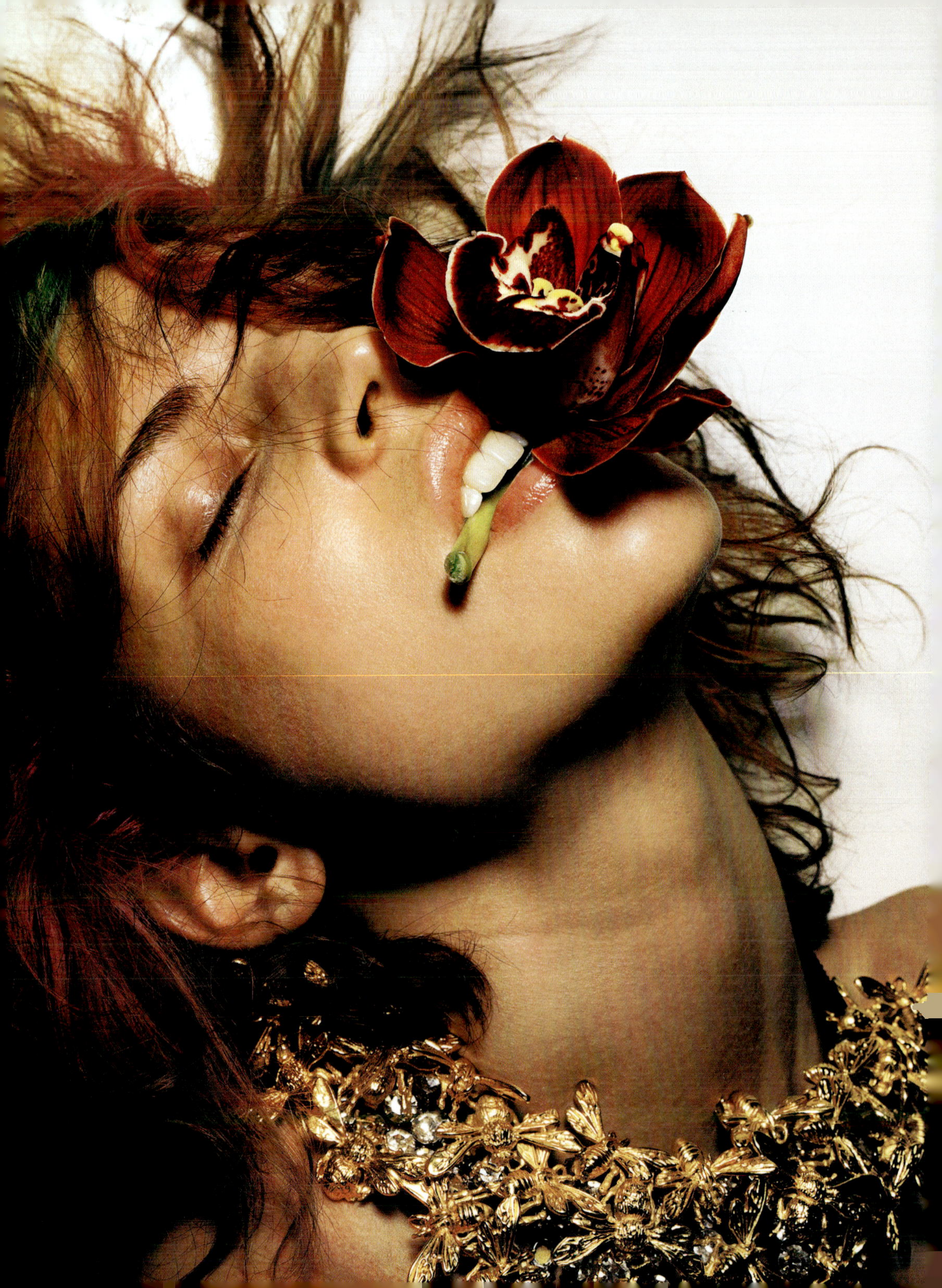

Liberty Ross

One of the high points of Liberty Ross's *Vogue* career was her 'guest editorship' of the magazine's fashion pages in 2002. In collaboration with photographer Nick Knight, she imagined, as the magazine billed it, 'a powerful vision, a daring artistry and an understanding of beauty's inherent decadence'. It involved long-dead and desiccating Valentine's Day roses and heaps of sundry flowers. She intended for there to be hundreds of live insects but settled instead on some bee-inspired jewellery. There was, however, fruit in all stages of over-ripeness and decay, from which the insects might just have crawled. Liberty summed up the theme as 'violent nature, beautiful, fertile, powerful, and decaying'. The results made an impactful statement: 'Next to [Knight's] close-ups of fruit, ripped open and spilling its seed, and flowers, dry and shrivelled, or oozing decay,' *Vogue* reported from the hothouse of a set, 'Liberty appears supine and sexy, with the blood-coloured juice of pomegranates dripping down her skin.'

As much as her suite of pictures was unexpected and avant-garde, Liberty Ross's upbringing was enviably unconventional. Her father, Ian Ross, co-founded Flipper's, the legendary but short-lived roller disco on Santa Monica Boulevard. His partner was Denny Cordell, the record-industry mini-mogul. Ross himself had impeccable music-biz credentials as one of the founders of the pirate station Radio Caroline. Flipper's was closed by the LAPD after a riot, so Ross, with six children to feed (Liberty is the second youngest), took a position as butler to a wealthy American family. In time the family relocated to Britain and Liberty started her career in fashion as a child model. (*Vogue*'s archives contain a charming and neat handwritten thank you to Norman Parkinson, who once took her picture.) She did not capitalise on this early launching pad and only modelled seriously in the mid-1990s, often for Mario Testino. In time she would become a catwalk regular, though she did not altogether enjoy the experience. 'I have very small feet,' she said, 'so shows were always torture, as the shoes were too large…'

Fashion aside, she was often a fixture in the social pages of magazines and was perennially on lists of best-dressed women. She was also *Vogue*'s guest motoring correspondent, reviewing four of the latest sports cars. It was an assignment that delighted her: 'I'd wanted a sports car ever since I was told the story of my parents' first date. My dad had driven my mum back to his Chelsea pad with every intention of luring her in – but while unlocking the front door, she attempted to hijack his convertible MGB…'

Liberty's own marriage (to film director Rupert Sanders), and the birth of her first child, did not slow down an enviable productivity rate. She did, however, stop to bring up their second. She has recently returned to modelling from her home in the Hollywood Hills, not so far from the site of Flipper's. Out there on a visit, *Vogue* was delighted to find that, just as her new family house was a collection of beautifully proportioned elements, so too was Liberty's face, familiar to *Vogue* readers from the end of the last millennium: 'saccharine cuteness undercut by jet-black hair, a strong Roman nose and exceptionally large, oval eyes'.

Liberty Ross (b. 1978, UK)

Opposite:
'Forbidden Fruit', July 2002, by Nick Knight.
Jewellery by Johnny Rocket

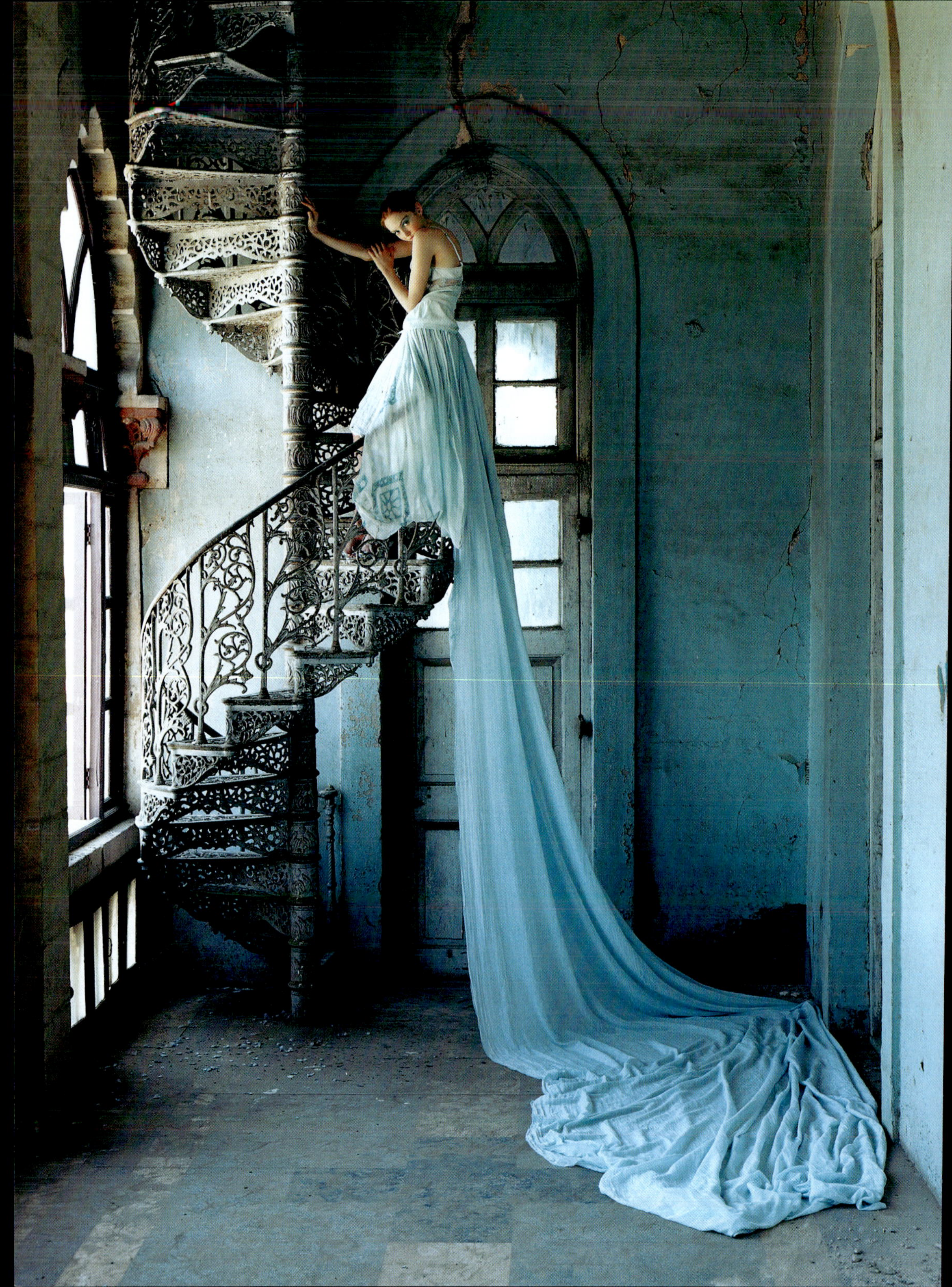

Lily Cole

By the end of 2005, Lily Cole – puckish despite her commanding height (she is 5ft 10in) – was surely accustomed to the grand *Vogue* gesture. The summer's portfolio of pictures showed her in opulent if dusty Rajasthani palaces and bouncing balloons in their equally luxuriant grounds. Previously, she had assumed a starring role in photographer Tim Walker's Christmas extravaganza, a [illegible]-page 'Vogue Pantomime', quite possibly the most expensive *en plein air* shoot the magazine has yet commissioned. She had also started at the top: her first appearance in *Vogue* was on its cover (in April 2004), sharing the limelight with Gemma Ward – the youngest models yet to appear there. For Walker, Lily is something of talisman as well as a muse: 'Some models,' he says in admiration, 'know how to stitch and weave themselves into a picture. Lily knows instinctively how to be a part of it.' Walker was among the first to photograph her. He recalled the 15-year-old Lily coming to see him in her school uniform. 'She was a little bit stiff. I wondered if we'd picked the peach a little too early…'

Lily must be accustomed to fairy tales; her path to modelling stardom started unexpectedly, as all good fairy stories do. This one has a hint of the quotidian and unglamorous, but it's good nonetheless: she was discovered, aged 14, by a talent scout eating an oversized hamburger in a café in London's West End. (Lily was eating, not the talent scout.) She fled his advances, but thought it over and came back. Her alabaster skin and red hair (she was recently voted fourth sexiest redhead of all time, a place behind Prince H[illegible]) and, as *Vogue* put it, 'her otherworldly looks' attracted the attention of fashion's Fairy Godfather and off she went, quite quickly, to a shoot with Steven Meisel for Italian *Vogue*.

Her sweet-natured, Dresden-shepherdess looks mask a steely determination to succeed. In tandem with her successful modelling career (and to date she has made around 200 catwalk appearances), Lily has not resisted the call of academe, reading history of art at King's College, Cambridge.

She is shrewd enough to know that modelling careers, unlike diamonds, are not forever and a foray into acting has been, on the whole, well received. It started quietly, though popularly, with a part in the 2007 revival of the *St Trinian's* films. It became memorable with a part in Terry Gilliam's *The Imaginarium of Doctor Parnassus*; the film was fraught with its own particular difficulties, but Lily triumphed in a lead role. The gothick theme (and long titles) continued with *Phantasmagoria: The Visions of Lewis Carroll*, directed by the occasionally controversial musician Marilyn Manson. The decision to appear in it, and perhaps as the cover model of French *Playboy* in white socks and clutching a teddy bear, may have been prompted by her avowed intention to provoke discourse. 'How boring,' she said, 'to always conform.'

Lily Cole (b. 1988, UK)

Opposite:
'Lily Takes a Trip',
July 2005,
by Tim Walker.
Fashion by Stella McCartney

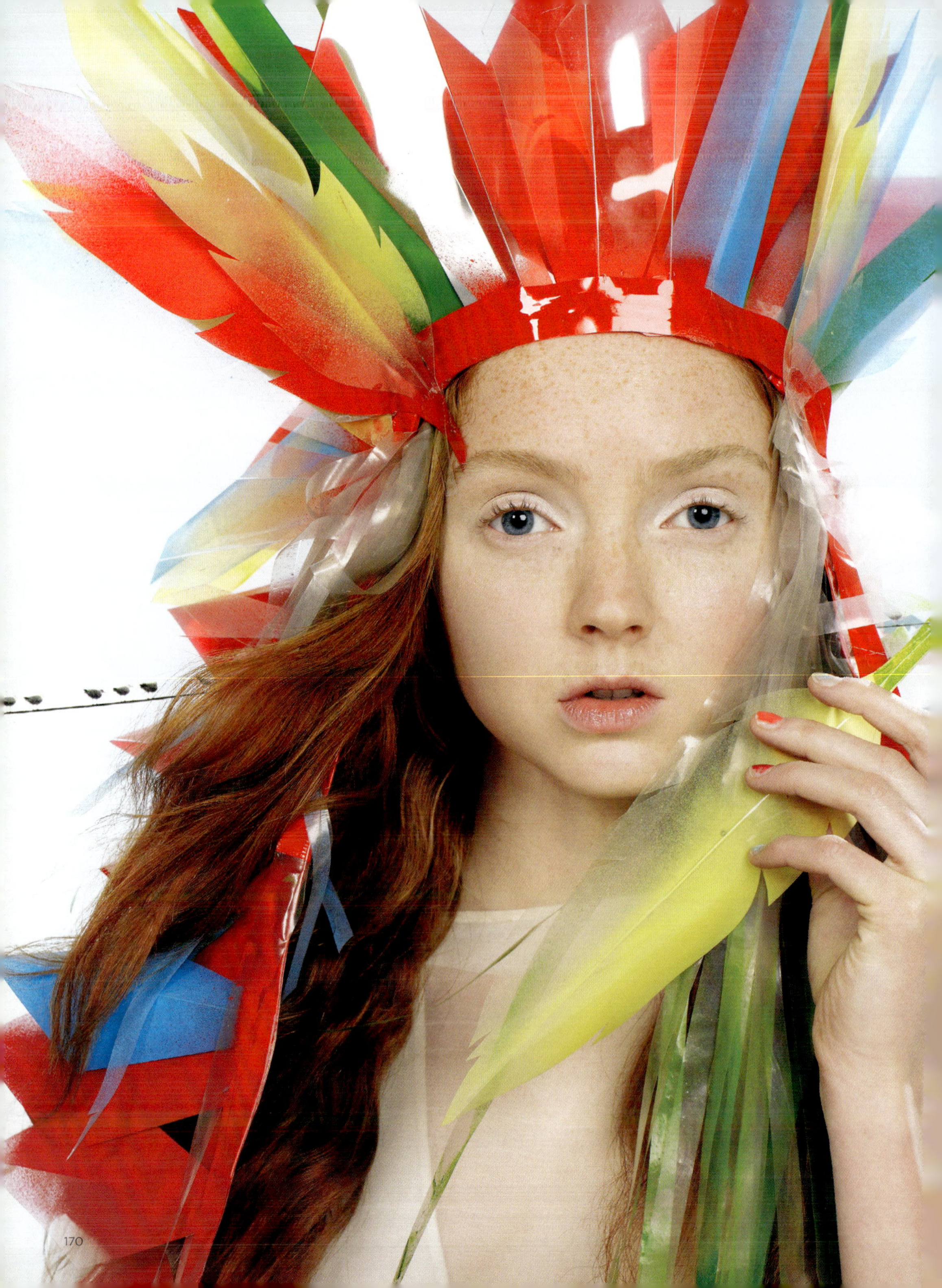

This page:
'Rumpelstiltskin',
December 2004,
by Tim Walker.
Fashion by Gucci

Opposite:
'Plastic Fantastic',
May 2007,
by Nick Knight.
Fashion by Calvin Klein

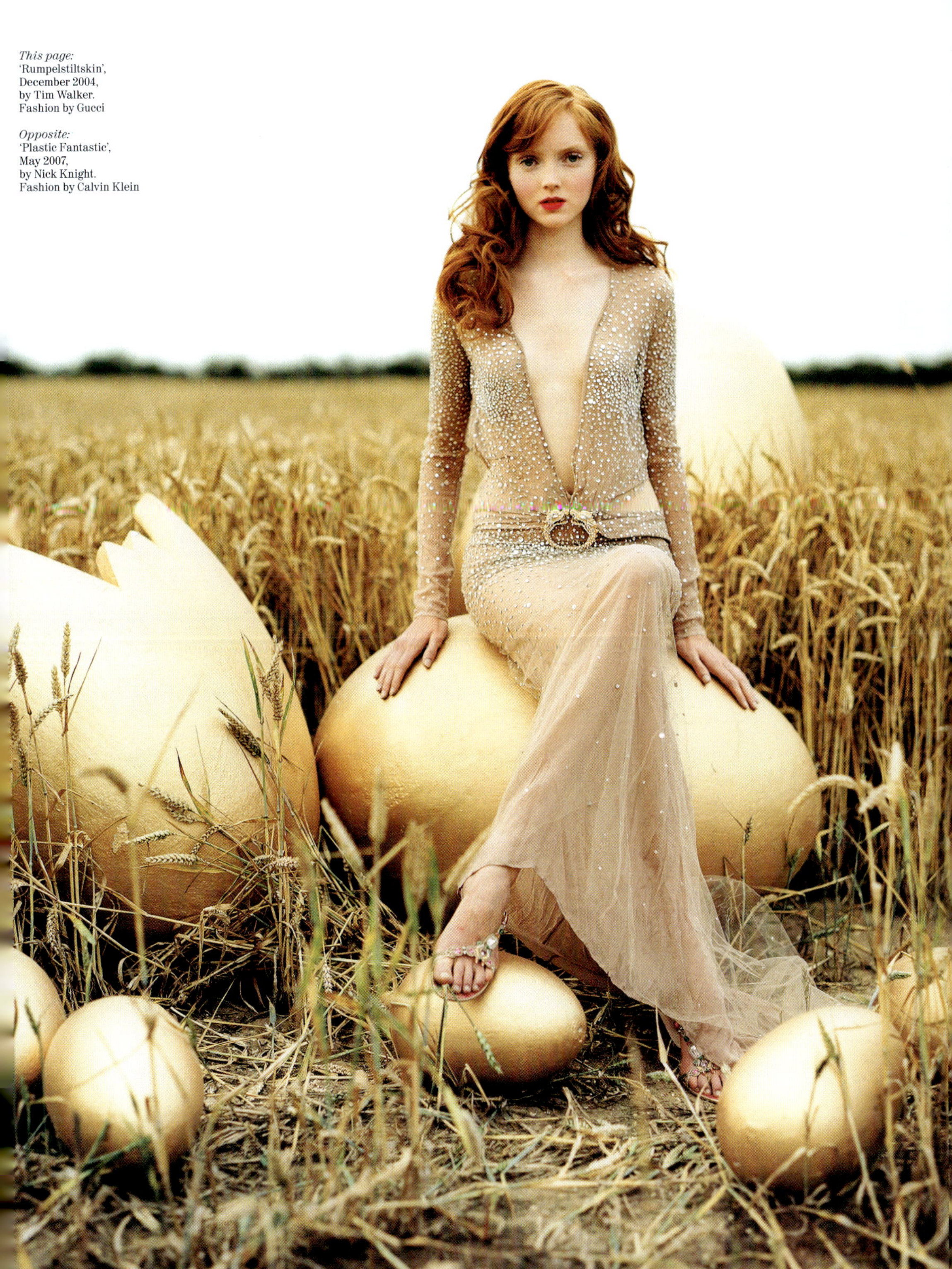

Lily Donaldson

Though it was for Italian *Vogue*, the most enviable launchpad for any neophyte model, Lily Donaldson's first shoot had a slight air of the inauspicious. She was made up to resemble an injection-moulded showroom dummy and placed in a shop window to fool passers-by. She succeeded, and her dexterity won her admiration – 'the consummate chameleon,' said one observer.

This may not have been the *Vogue* entrée dreams are made of, but her British *Vogue* debut was, by contrast, in at the top: a 20-page fashion extravaganza in October 2004 photographed by Mario Testino to celebrate Englishness. She was 17, a sophisticated English rose who still felt, she said, 'like a kid inside'. Her notes, relayed to the magazine from the shoot's location, betray her easy-going charm: 'I threw a few things in my bag for overnight but still managed to forget my coat and it's freezing! (I always manage to forget something – usually it's my toothbrush or pyjamas.)... From what I understand, my "character" is pretty batty and eccentric – she probably lives in some attic somewhere!'

Known back then to few outside the industry, Lily became recognisable in a season that brought her significance thrice over: large-scale campaigns for Burberry, Dolce & Gabbana and Dior. A few years later it was easier, said the *Sunday Times*, to detail the fashion houses that had not taken up this option. 'Amazingly, she achieved all this without looking like most of the alien waifs who drag their feeble carcasses up and down the catwalks...'

One gets the impression that the leap to fame was not too difficult to manage for the daughter of photographer Matthew Donaldson (himself no stranger to the pages of *Vogue*); her mother is an artist and jewellery designer. It is not a rags-to-riches, plucked-from-nowhere, small-town story, nor is it one of excessive privilege, but it is one that clearly allows Lily to be consistently – and charmingly – underwhelmed by it all. Perhaps, suggested *Vogue*, having spent her early life among artists she is able to collaborate on making great pictures.

Lily was discovered, aged 16, while shopping in north London, and began modelling part-time while she studied for her exams. (She was a pupil at Camden School for Girls, where, one interviewer put it, if you look like Lily 'and hang around the school gates long enough, getting discovered is a bit of a cert'.) She intended to go to art school, but it didn't pan out that way because her ascent was rapid. In succession, she was a staple in Italian *Vogue*, a cover girl on American *Vogue*, prolific in British *Vogue* and the star of a Pirelli calendar. The modelling world has few accolades left to bestow.

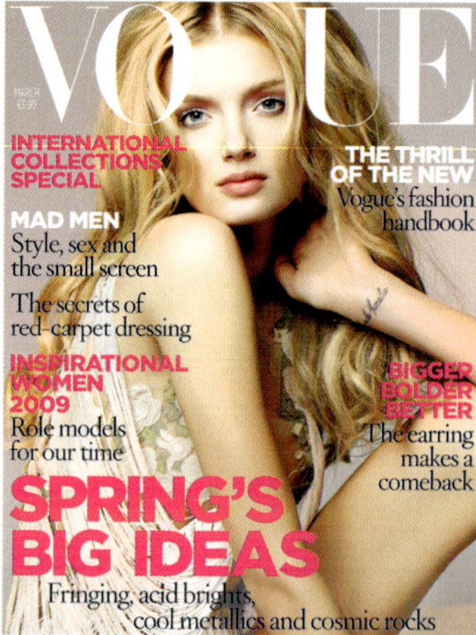

Lily stands out for her height (5ft 10in) and her implausibly slight, willowy frame – which, *Vogue* hazarded, does not exactly make her a *rara avis* of the modelling world. What was unusual was that 'her looks make sense, as she is classically beautiful, which marks her out from many of her wonderful but slightly strange-looking colleagues'.

Becoming a household name will, one gets the impression, discomfort her only briefly and then she'll shrug her shoulders and get on with it. So far Lily has eschewed, by luck or clever design, the kind of close scrutiny impossibly beautiful English models tend to attract. 'I don't know whether it's because I don't find it interesting, or maybe it's because I'm not very interesting...'

Lily Donaldson (b. 1987, UK)

Above: 'Spring's Big Ideas', March 2009, by Nick Knight. Fashion by Alexander McQueen

Opposite: 'Brilliantly British', October 2009, by Mario Testino. Fashion by Jasper Conran

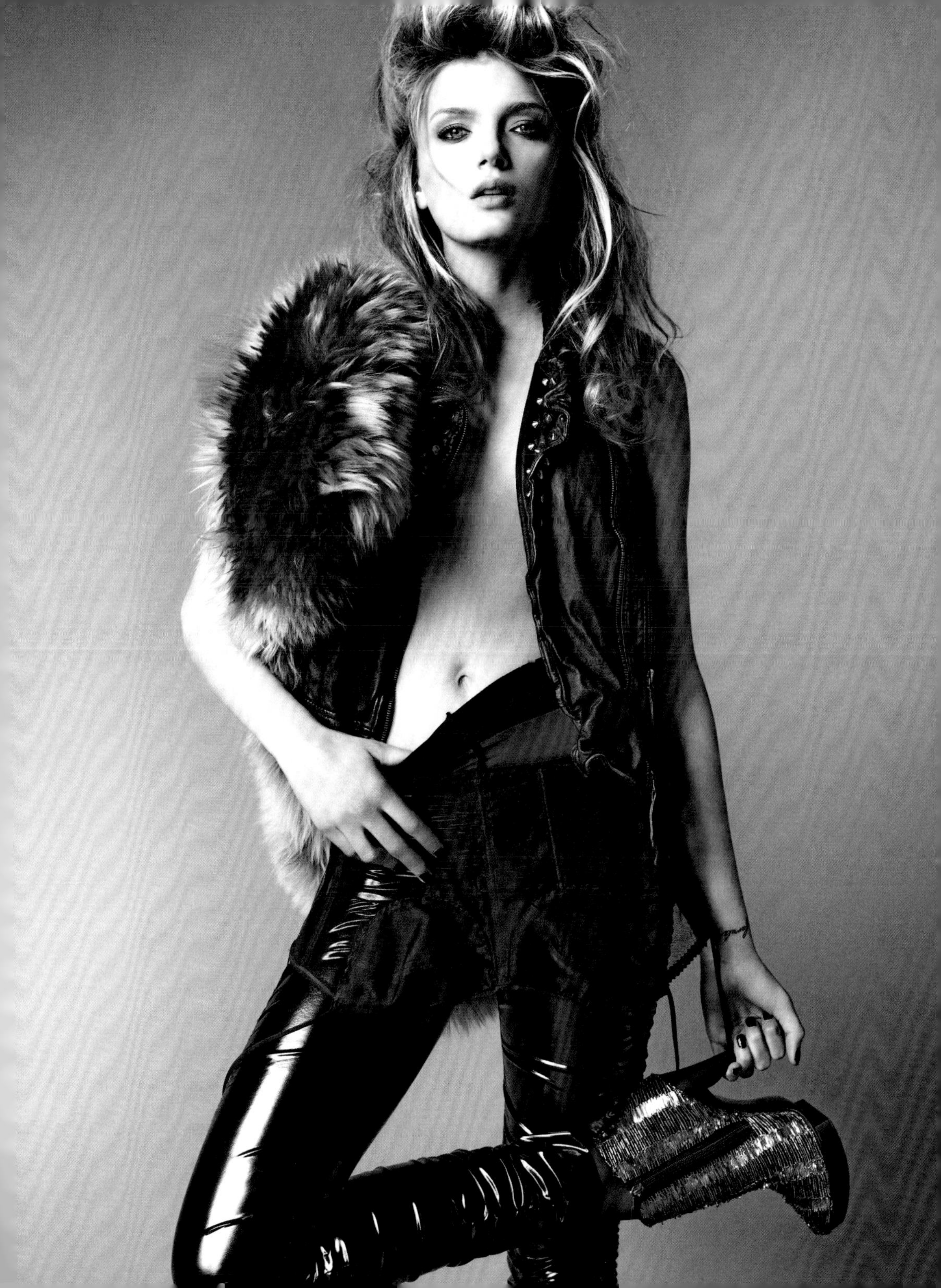

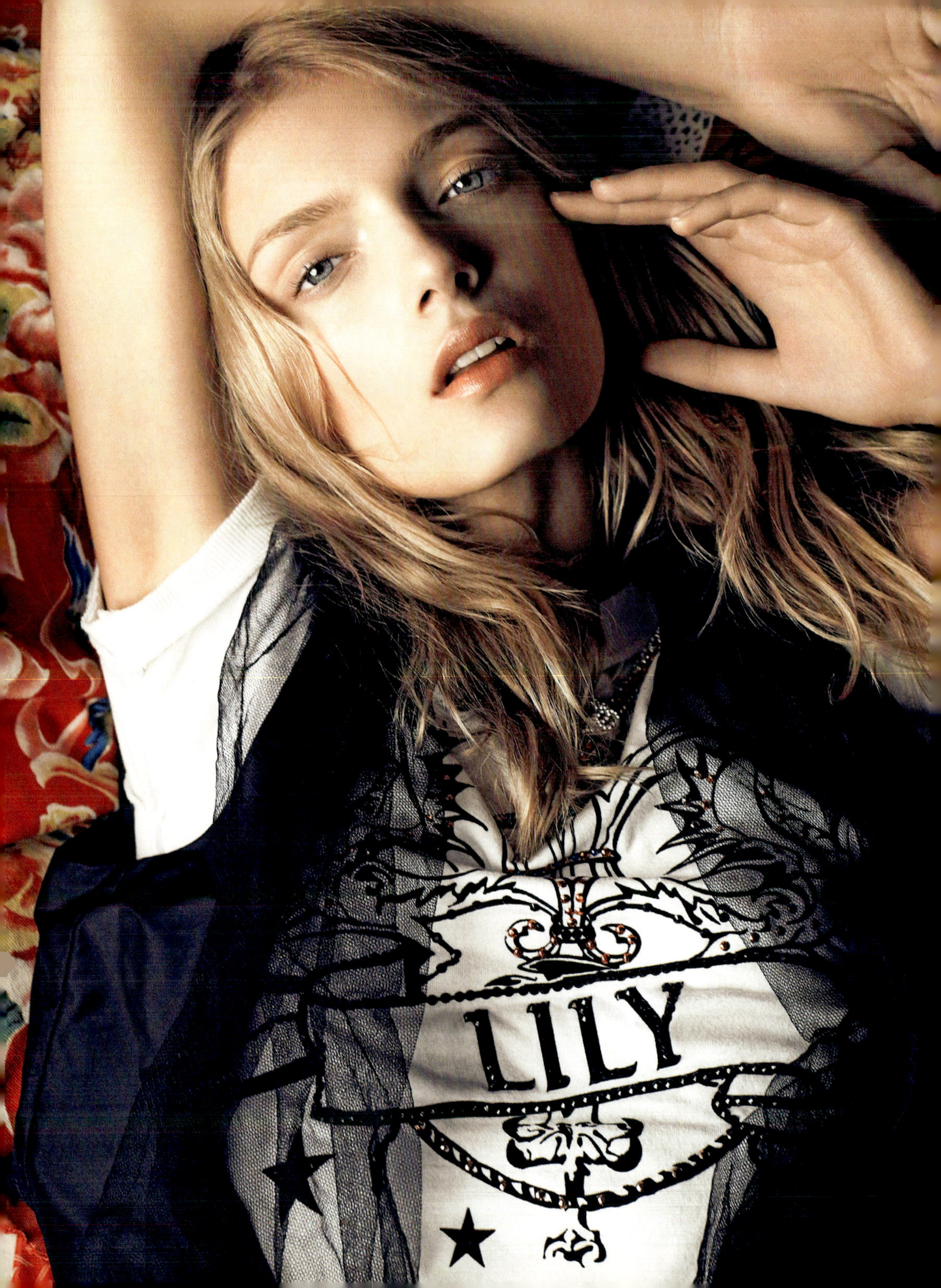
LILY

Opposite:
'Camden Cool',
January 2008,
by Lachlan Bailey.
Fashion by Simon
Parchment

This page:
'Fringe Festival',
March 2009,
by Nick Knight.
Fashion by Alberta Ferretti

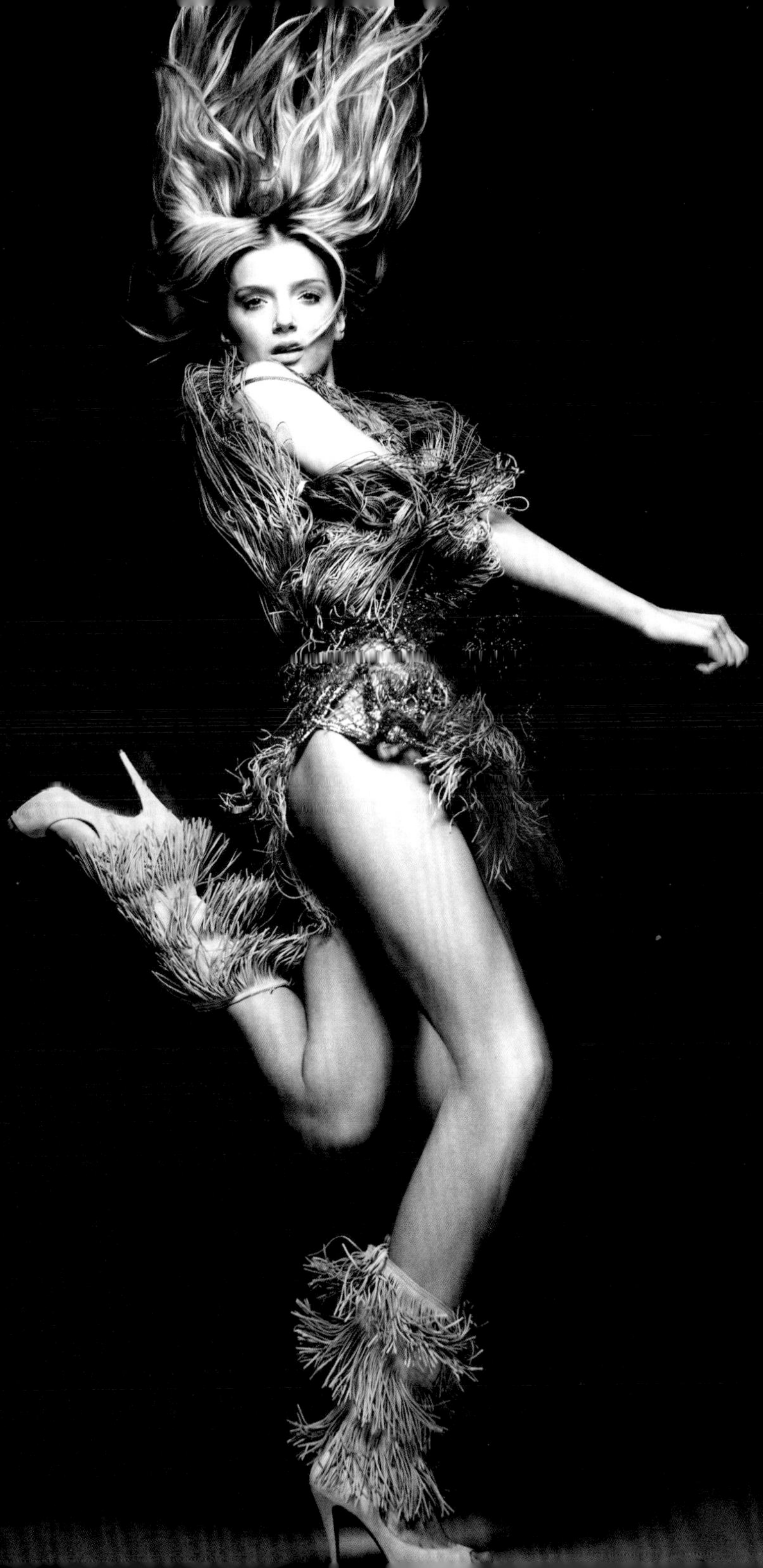

Linda Evangelista

'From Christy Turlington's stupendous pout to Tatjana Patitz's feline eyes, Linda Evangelista's boyish crop to Cindy Crawford's much-debated beauty spot or Naomi Campbell's puckish grin, they're all emphatically individual,' noted *Vogue*. They were also emphatically among the highest-earning young women of their generation, a generation marked out against a backdrop of conspicuous consumption. The supermodels seared themselves in the public consciousness as living exponents of the multi-billion-dollar power of the fashion business, their otherworldly glamour a marketing tool for a ruthless industry of conglomerates, franchises, licensed entities, bought out and kick-started couture lines. As the 1980s drew to a close, *Vogue* surmised that should you wish to book the three main supermodels for, say, a single day's advertising work, it might set you back around $100,000. None of their predecessors ever commanded those sorts of fees, no matter how much you ratchet up historical monetary equivalents, and few had a resonance, like them, way beyond the fashion pages of magazines.

'We don't wake up for less than $10,000 a day.' Hubris came no more excessive and no less warranted than that era-defining line. 'I feel like these words,' says Linda Evangelista, 'are going to be engraved on my tombstone.' She also famously maintained that 'no-one is born with perfect eyebrows'. Both these Marie Antoinette-isms belied a fierce intelligence, a keen sense of self-mockery and an extraordinary capacity for sheer hard work. Of all the supermodels, Linda was, they say, the one that turned up first, 'gave' the most, stayed till the lights went out. Her job was – and remains – to make the best pictures possible, to help the product on its long marketing journey and perhaps, along the way, to justify the fees and the fuss. And it does not come without a little self-doubt: 'I definitely do not see perfection in the mirror,' she told *Vogue*. 'I see a crooked face. I see burned hair. I see the truth… I'm a supermodel, not a superhuman.'

Linda retired from modelling in the mid-1990s but returned triumphantly in 2001 with 28 pages in American *Vogue*, photographed by Steven Meisel, who had championed her from the beginning. When Linda reappeared, the designer Michael Kors told *Vogue*: 'People say "Oh we hate supermodels", but the reality is, it's just like a fabulous box-office actress. Julia Roberts opens a film and people are waiting in line around the block. With Linda it's the same thing. She brings the whole thing to life so much quicker and with a lot less effort.'

The whole thing – longevity and staying power in particular – was in fact a bit of an effort, but one worn lightly. No supermodel kept the appellation for long without an almost seasonal change in haircut or hair colour, an acute sense of photographic trends and a readiness to embrace them full-on. But modelling was all Linda Evangelista ever wanted to do. The Catholic girl from St Catherine's in Ontario had something of an epiphany in 1978, aged 13 – 'I started perming,' she told *Vogue*. 'Mistake.' At which point her mother enrolled her into a quasi-finishing school, which taught her how to set a table, walk through a door satisfactorily and how to descend a staircase with grace, charm and ease. Much of this proved useful. A modelling course followed the self-improvement one. A wildcard entry to a Miss Teen Niagara pageant got her noticed by insiders and the slow rise to public attention began. And it was remarkably slow for so astounding a personality. It all changed, though – at least as fashion folklore has it – when hairstylist Julien d'Ys cut her long hair a bit shorter into a bob.

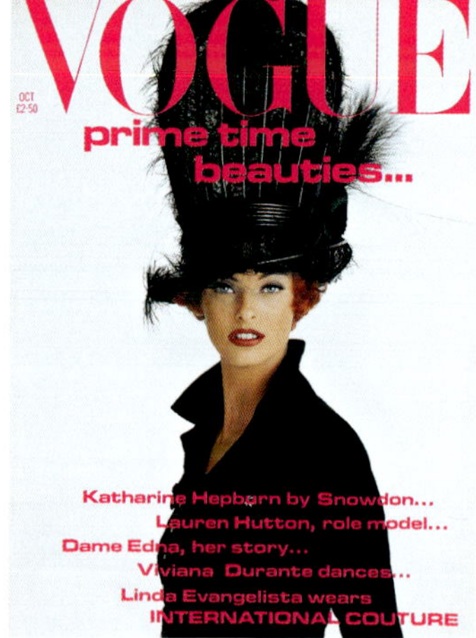

She once claimed she wanted to model for the rest of her life: 'I really love going to work. I've never slagged the business. But I know what the reality is. I know that it'll end one day. Or maybe not.' At 43, Linda Evangelista was the autumn/winter '08 face of Prada. She shows no signs of giving up, nor does the industry appear to have any intention of letting her do so.

Linda Evangelista (b. 1955, Canada)

Above: 'Prime Time Beauties', October 1991, by Patrick Demarchelier. Fashion by Chanel

Opposite: 'Send in the Gowns', October 1991, by Patrick Demarchelier. Fashion by Gianni Versace

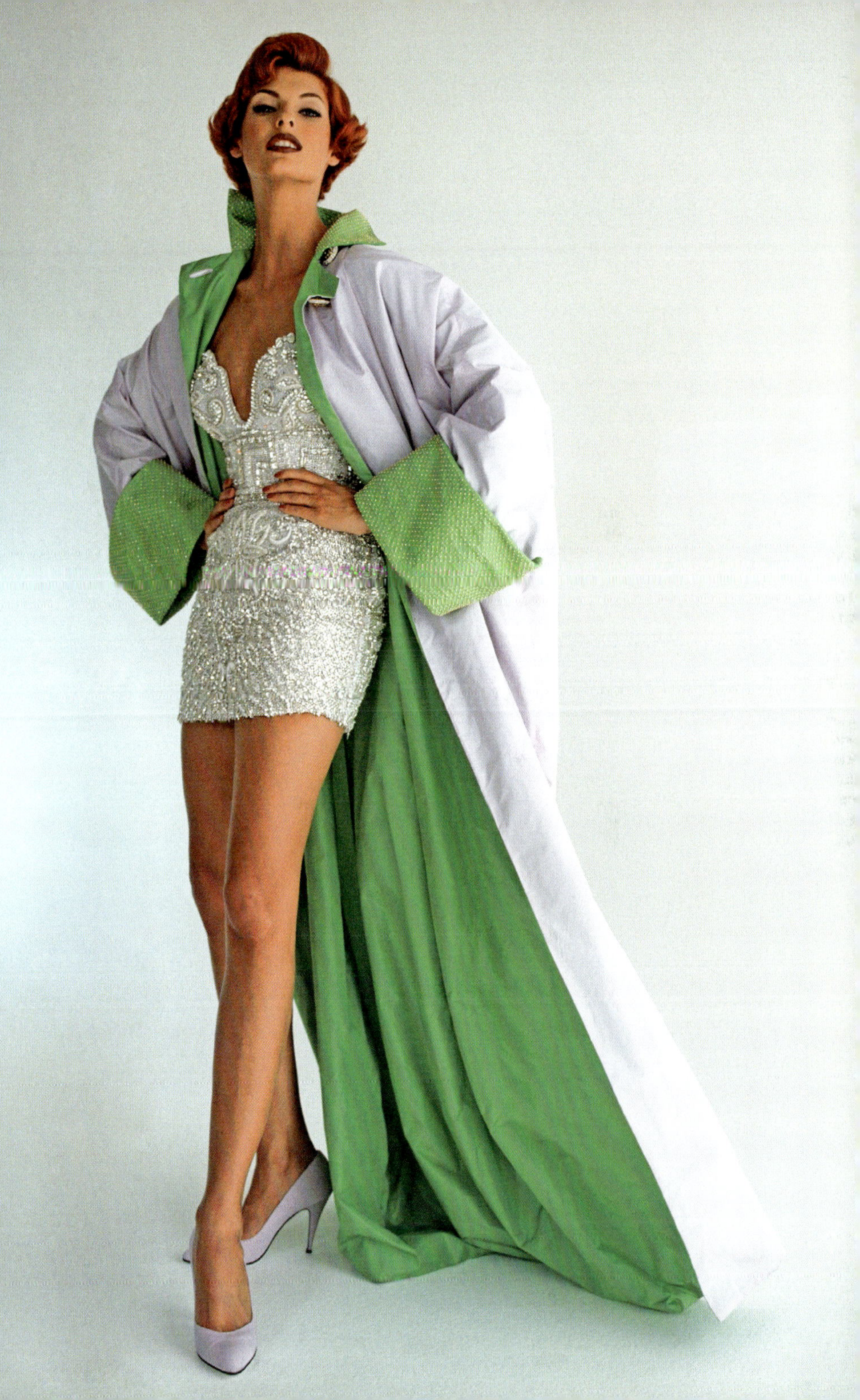

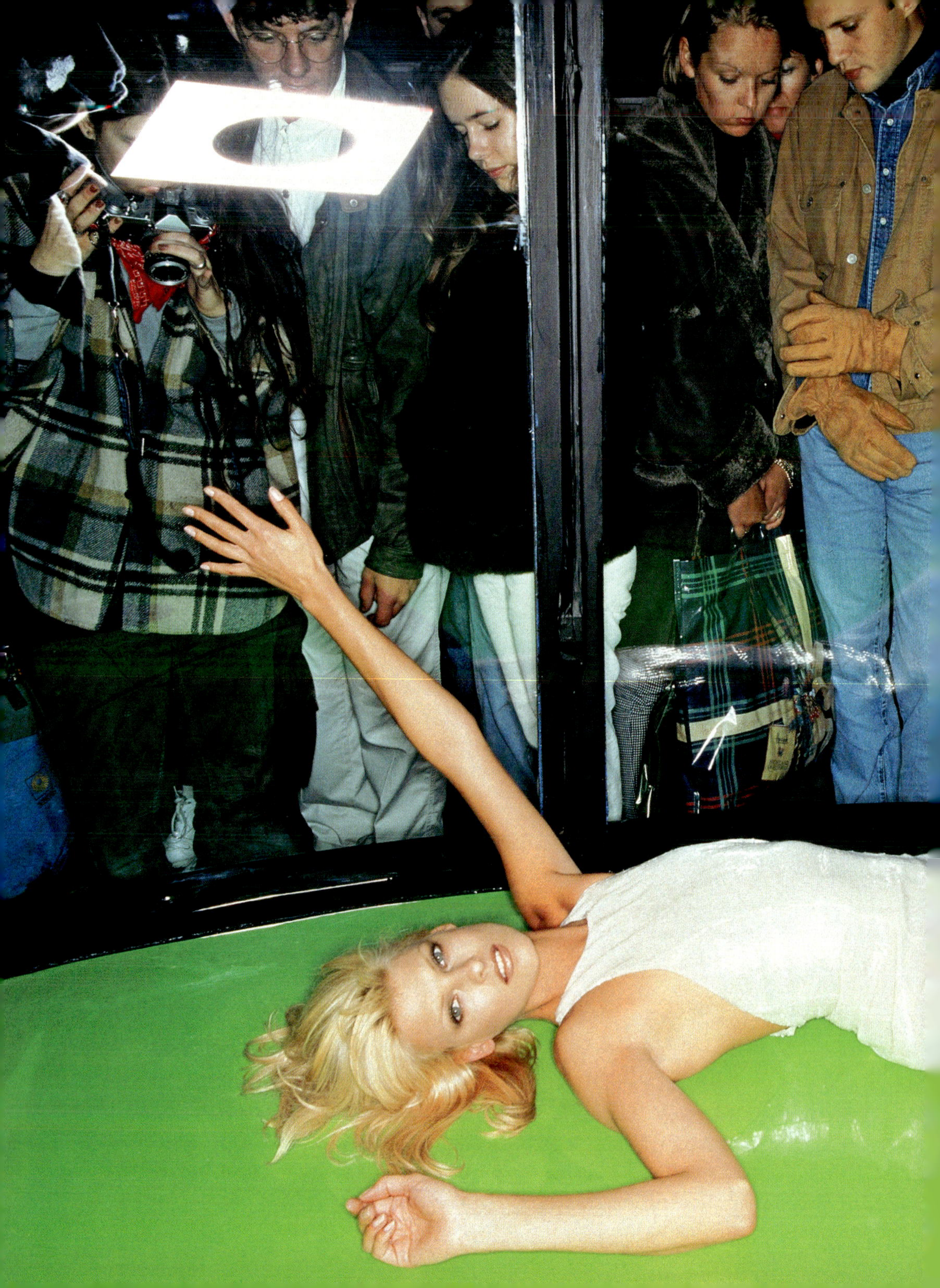

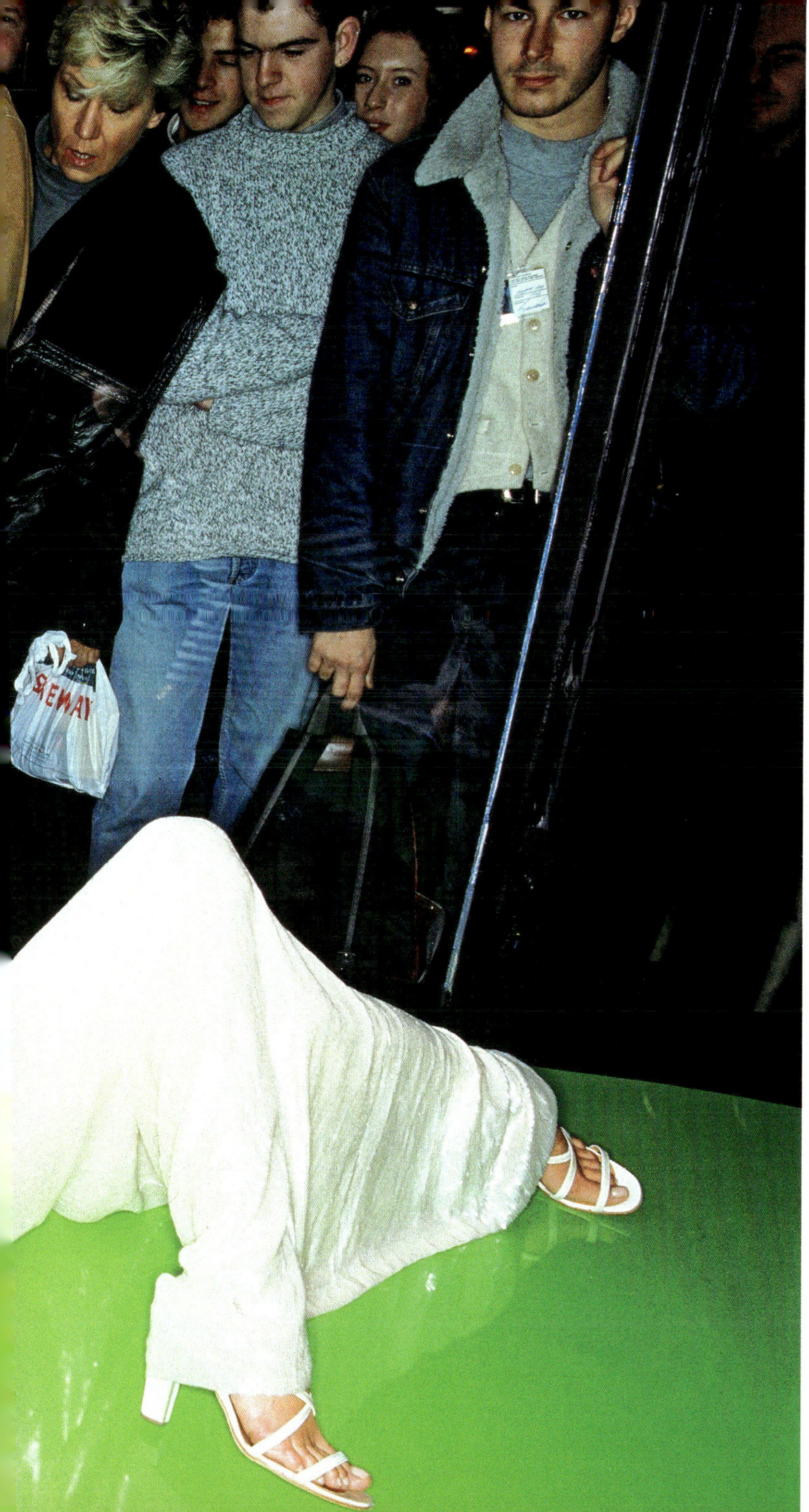

'Dress to Dazzle',
March 1995,
by Nick Knight.
Fashion by
Polo Ralph Lauren

Lisa Fonssagrives

Lisa Fonssagrives was the most successful professional model of her time and, in the days before models opened restaurants or took acting lessons, she was, by dint only of public recognition, the first 'supermodel'. The term does her no immediate favours, as she loathed the limelight. She modestly referred to herself as 'just a clothes hanger' – though, as one of the most well-known faces of the 1930s and 1940s outside Hollywood, she was constantly under scrutiny. *Time* magazine put her on its cover above the tagline 'Do illusions also sell refrigerators?', noting the sackloads of fan mail she received and her unsought popularity as a forces pin-up. Her *soi-disant* reserve and air of unapproachable hauteur covered up an intense shyness. One fashion editor compared her to a kitten 'in her quiet, clinging affection'. She was also, from 1950, Mrs Irving Penn, collaborating with him on some of the 20th century's masterpieces of fashion photography.

Born in 1911 in Sweden, she had trained as a dancer but turned to modelling when work fell off. She travelled to Paris in 1933 to participate in a dance competition, a ballet with a score by Gershwin. She did not win but fell in love with the city, she recalled later, and decided to stay. She studied art at the Sorbonne, modelling on her days off, and married the photographer Fernand Fonssagrives, whose name she kept after their divorce.

Thereafter, Fonssagrives was so prolific in the fashion pages of *Vogue* and *Harper's Bazaar* that her face, it was said, was as recognisable as the *Mona Lisa* to three decades of magazine readers. She parachuted over Paris for Jean Moral, leaned precariously from the iron struts of the Eiffel Tower for Erwin Blumenfeld, and disrobed for Louise Dahl-Wolfe. She was Horst's favourite model a decade before she became that of Penn. They both started out together. Horst remembered her 'trembling with fear' but he recognised her potential straight away. 'On the day of my first test with Horst, I was terrified,' she recalled years later. 'I knew nothing about fashion and had never even looked at a fashion magazine. I had no idea what was expected of me. I didn't know what to do with my hands or how to pose. Horst was very kind to me but was nearly as inexperienced as I was.'

Penn fell in love with Lisa the minute he set eyes on her. They married at Chelsea Register Office, 'sandwiched between sittings of TS Eliot and a fishmonger,' in Penn's words. The two had also recently shot a remarkable series on the Paris collections for *Vogue*: simple compositions against seamless grey paper in a daylight studio. These remain a pivotal moment in the history of the discipline, for many years the yardstick by which studio fashion photographs were measured. Penn brought the same spirit of wonderment to chronicling Lisa in haute couture as he would bring to documenting rediscovered tribespeople – an ethnographic interest he found time to pursue, and *Vogue* found space to display.

When Fonssagrives died in 1992, *Vogue* paid tribute to 'one of those rare women who become legends. Through the unsentimental camera she sent out a clear conception, maybe a revolutionary one, of the modern woman.' Of the 85 platinum/palladium prints Penn gave to the National Gallery of Art in Washington in 2005, he chose only photographs of Lisa to encapsulate the peak of his *Vogue* fashion years.

Lisa Fonssagrives (b. Lisa Bernstone, 1911, Sweden; d. 1992)

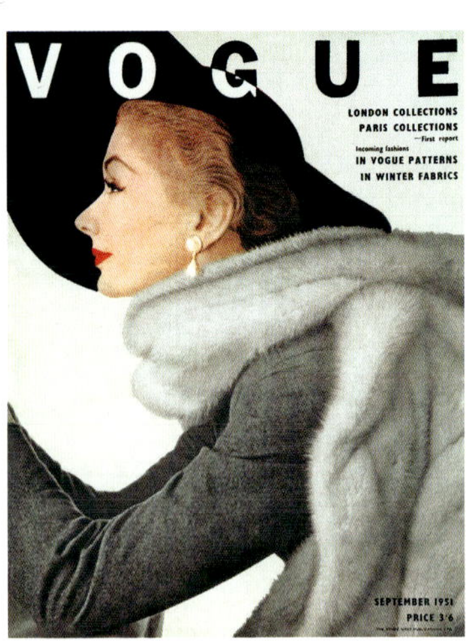

Above:
'In Winter Fabrics',
September 1951,
by Irving Penn.
Fashion by Maximilian

Right:
'The Black and White Idea',
April 1950, by Irving Penn.
Fashion by Jerry Parnis

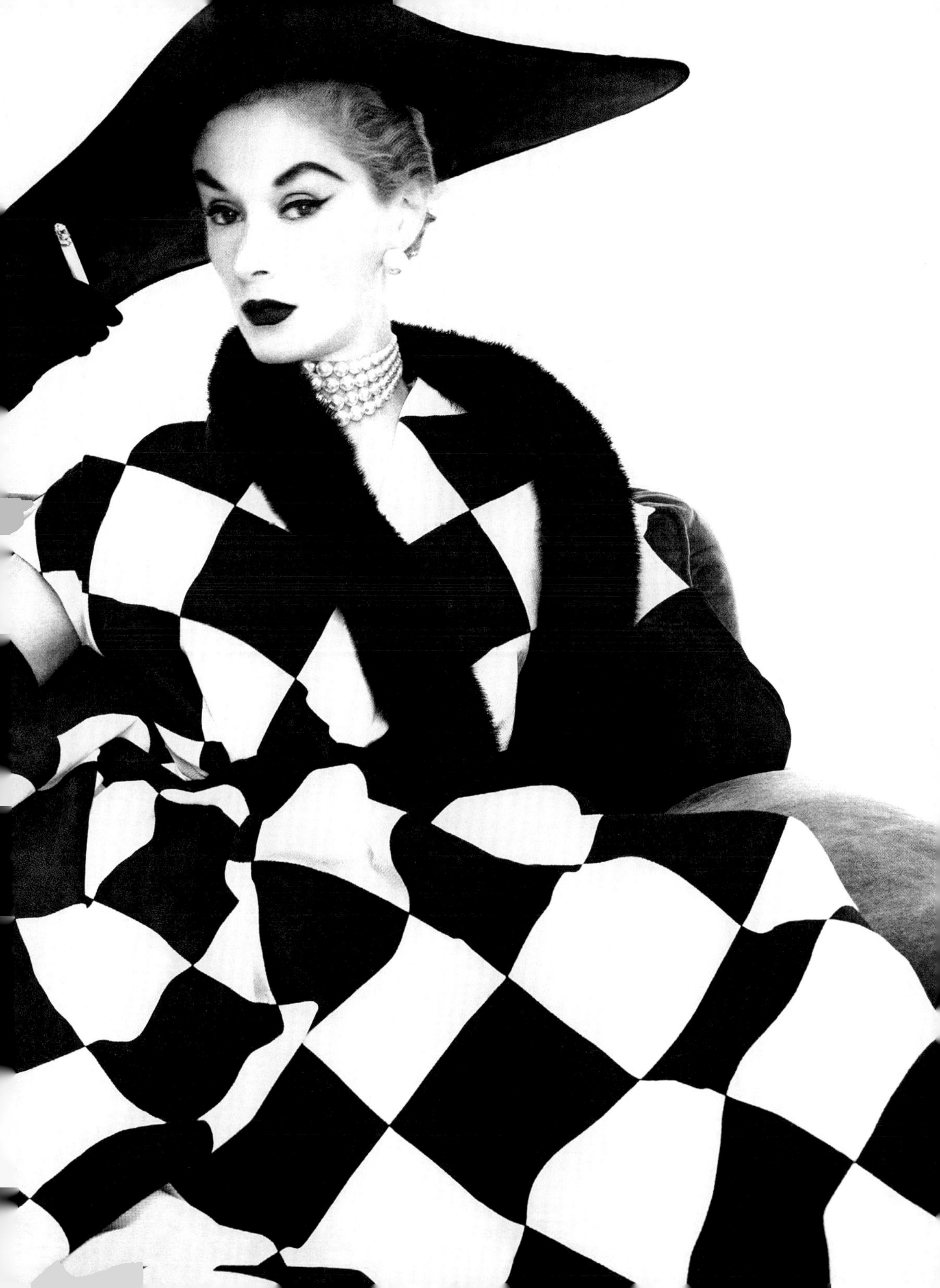

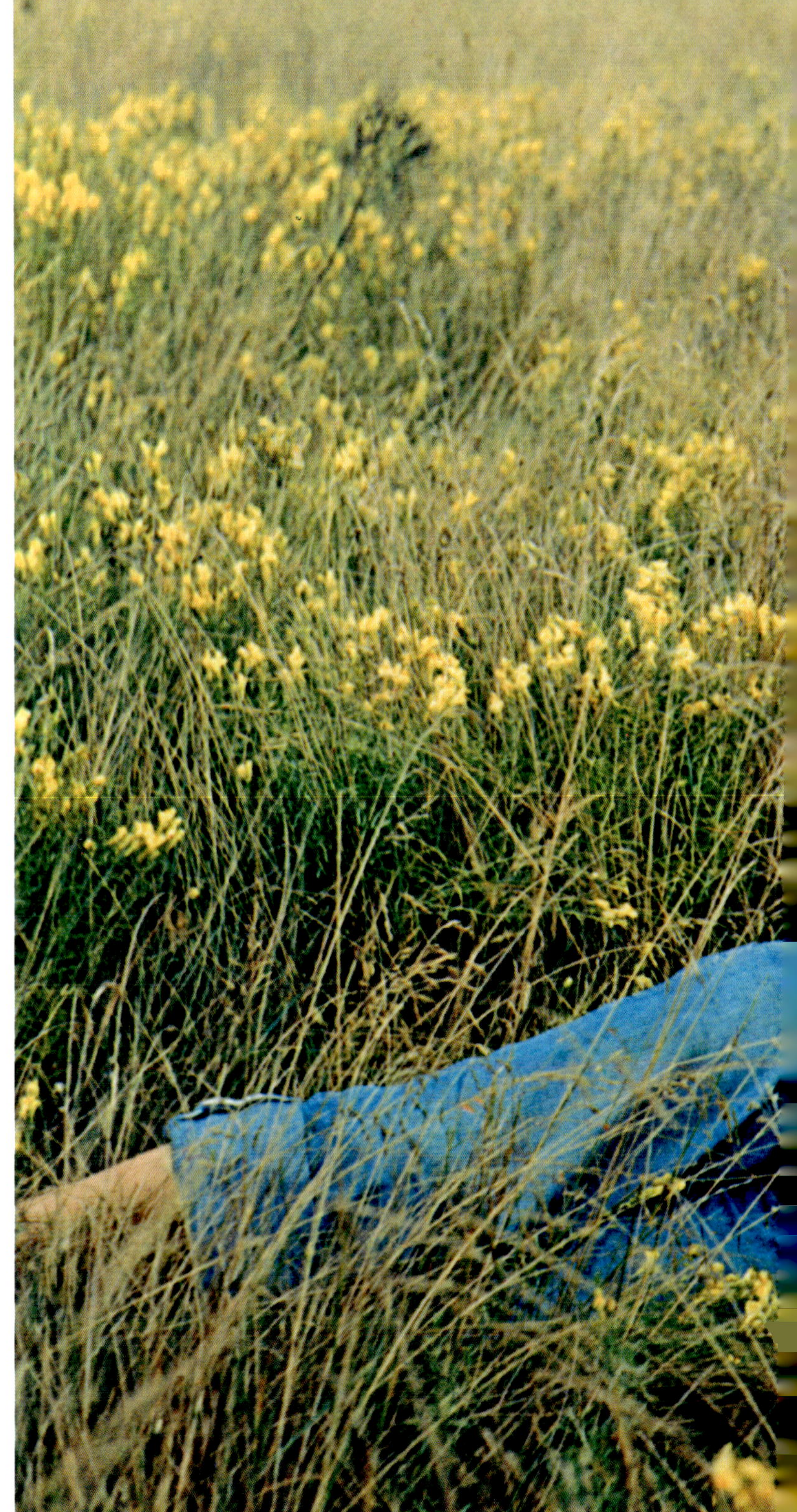

'Summer Reader',
July 1952,
by Irving Penn

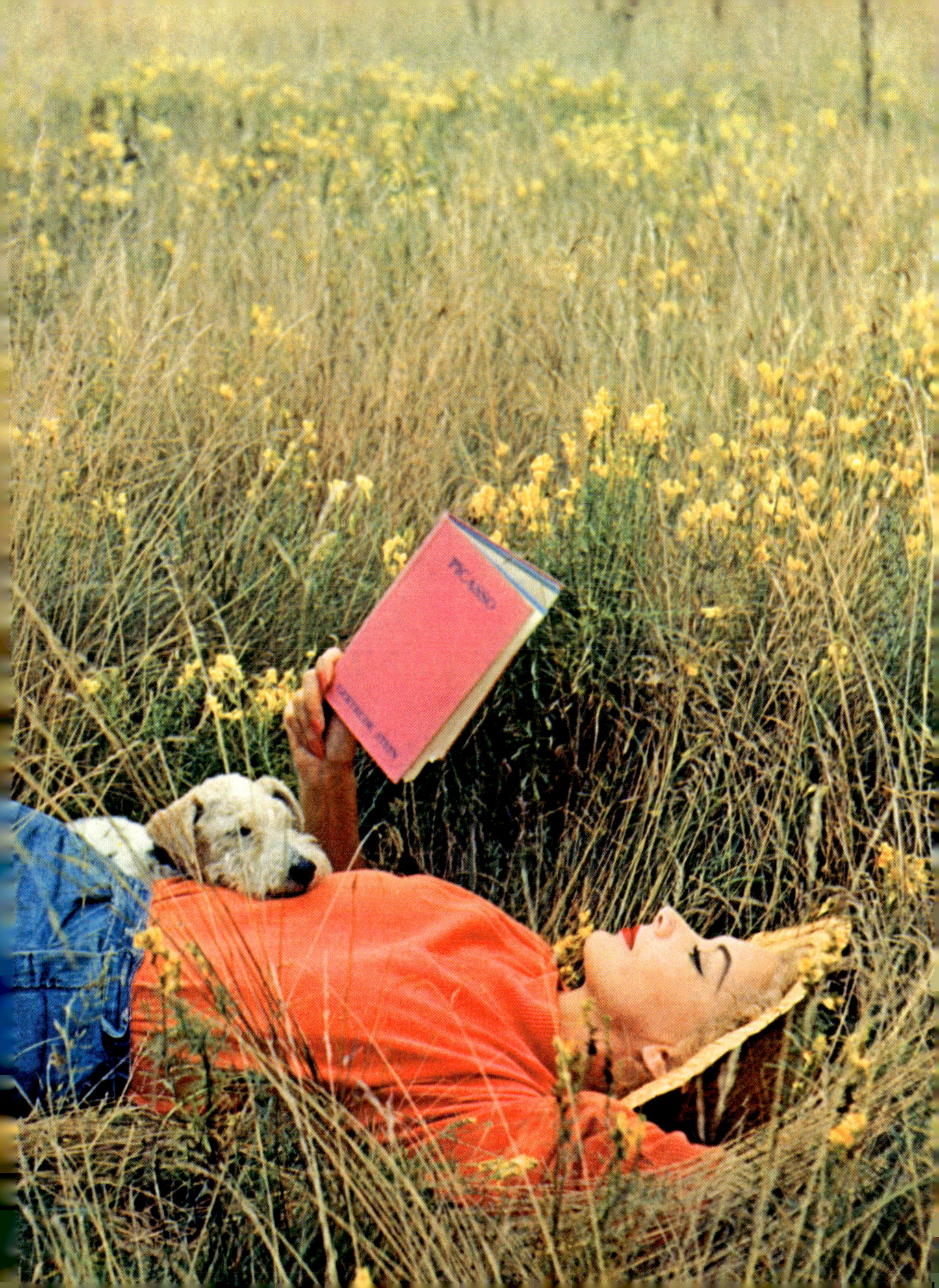
PICASSO

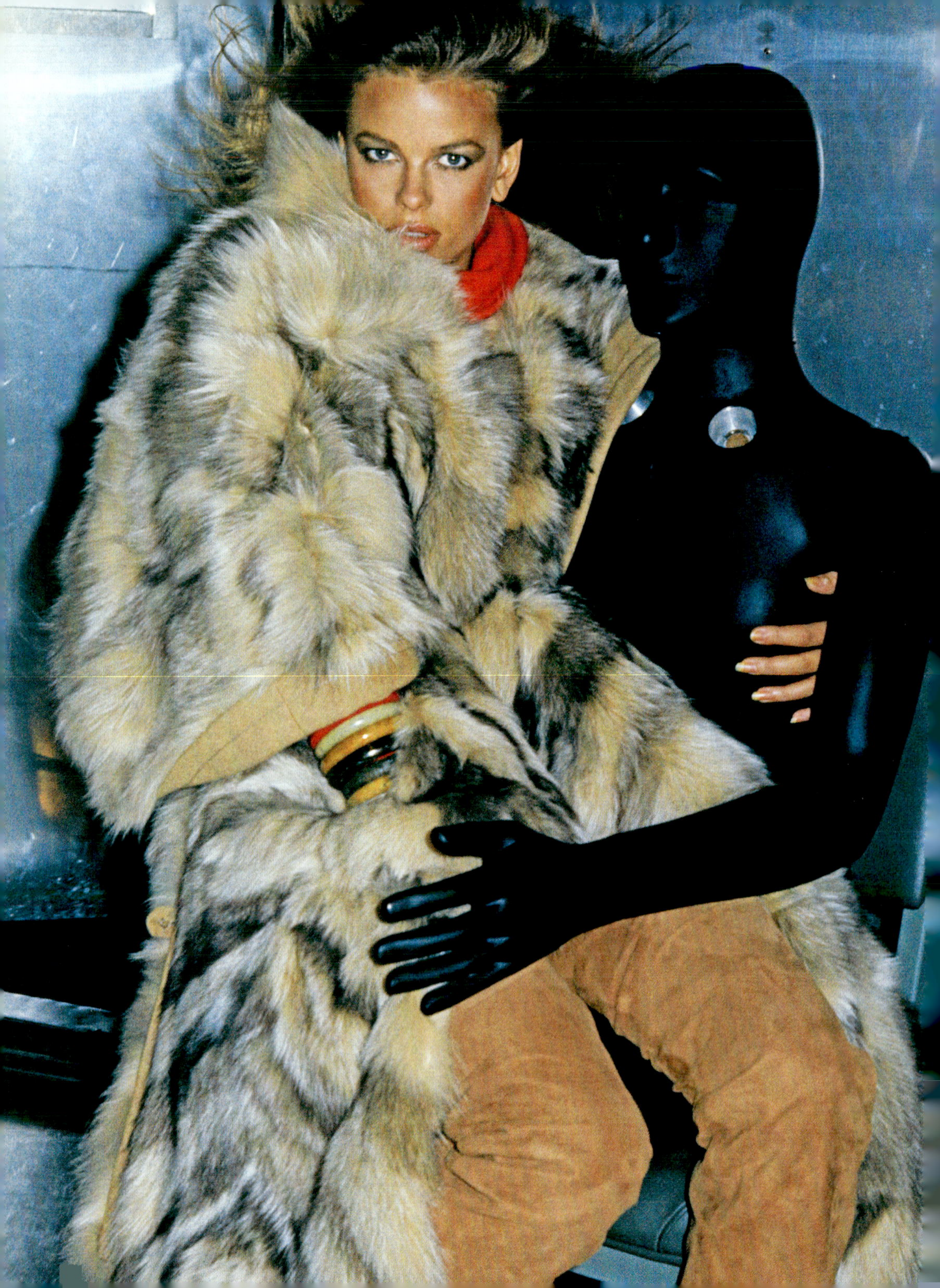

Lisa Taylor

Lisa Taylor was one of the most photographed models of the 1970s, though she rarely made it into British magazines, at least in the years of stardom. 'When I first met Lisa Taylor,' Arthur Elgort recalled, 'she looked like a sporty rich kid.' Despite that, Elgort made her name with some of the decade's most enduring and inspirational fashion photographs. She summed up, for him and many others (not least American *Vogue*), precisely the woman to whom they strove to appeal. 'The modern woman who has something on her mind – and going places fast,' said Elgort, putting Lisa into a Mercedes 450SL and getting her to drive, windswept, across the George Washington Bridge.

She *was*, as it happened, a sporty rich kid (from Oyster Bay, Long Island, the daughter of a textiles company executive). She was sporty enough to turn that enthusiasm to dance and, around 1971, modelling was a part-time way of financing her classes. 'It was so easy,' she told the writer Michael Gross. 'I went in and started working.' She landed a cover for *Mademoiselle* very quickly and her career was launched.

Lisa admitted that she found the life stultifyingly dull – 'modelling isn't the most inspiring, intellectual thing to do'. Nothing, however, would halt her early trajectory. She was the girl whose wrist, dripping in diamonds, was clamped between the jaws of a snarling Doberman in Chris von Wangenheim's Dior shock ads. 'Fetching is your Dior,' ran the strapline.

'That picture of Lisa Taylor sitting down in the dress with her legs very casual with those very cheap little sandals,' said former *Vogue* fashion editor Candy Pratts Price of a 1975 Helmut Newton shoot, 'that inspired me. I've got to have that attitude as a woman. It wasn't the clothes. That girl looked like she was in command of herself. It was a way of living.' Female empowerment was also something of a novelty for mainstream fashion magazines – the shoot was the 'Story of Ohhhhhh!', a tongue-in-cheek reference to the erotic novel *The Story of O* (1954), which had recently been republished. For Newton's lens, Lisa lay sprawled on a chair, her legs apart, eyeing men who passed her by – as, traditionally, they would have been eyeing her. It caused a full *Vogue* mailbox and a flurry of cancelled subscriptions. The writer Polly Devlin believed that 'it was perhaps her [Lisa's] total connection with reality that was so provoking'. The age of 'porn-chic' had truly begun.

Lisa Taylor gave up modelling before it all became too much – but she had a renaissance in the early 1990s, when Calvin Klein chose her as a model for a clothing range. Even those who were not *au fait* with the history of high glossy magazines could see, some two decades after it had all begun, quite what the fuss was all about.

Lisa Taylor (b. 1951, USA)

Opposite:
'Test Your Cool',
December 1976,
by Chris von Wangenheim.
Fashion by Maximilian

Lud

In the dressing room of the *Vogue* studio in between-the-wars Paris, where temperament ran high, Russian-born Lud was a class apart. It wasn't merely her high Slavic cheekbones or her eyes that appeared (as one commentator put it) 'the blue of ice one moment, the blue of warm bright gemstones the next', but her capriciousness and disdain. As *Vogue*'s Bettina Ballard recalled: 'Lud would look over the dresses, choosing what she wanted to wear and leaving the rest for the other girls. There was no point in trying to put her in anything that she didn't like – she would throw away the picture by posing badly.' She was, as Ballard explained, utterly ruthless with herself as much as anyone else. In order to enhance her figure, she had undergone cosmetic surgery, which was botched. 'We could never put too low a dress on her because her nipples pointed upwards.'

Lud smiled sparingly, and usually only for Horst, with whom she was probably a little in love. Horst responded in the only way he could – she became his favourite model. In one of his best-known photographs, she stands sinuously between two columns wearing a dress by Alix, whose hallmark was draping material in a Graeco-Roman style. This appealed to Horst's love of the classical civilisations and was, as he readily admitted, influenced by Edward Steichen's portrait of Isadora Duncan at the Parthenon. He said of his muse: 'I spotted her when she was working as a messenger. She was delivering a package at the *Vogue* studio and I immediately wanted to use her as a model... She revolutionised the look of the model. She was not at all remote or cold, not at all like a sleepwalker; she was sensual and catlike. When I met her she was poor, but no amount of money could get her to pose in a dress she did not like.'

When war broke out and Horst left Paris for the US army, he heard she had married a lion tamer, the two of them travelling the world with the circus. At length she returned to fashion, but not to Horst. 'One night at a party given by Molyneux,' the photographer recalled, 'Schiaparelli came up to me. "You can't have Lud. No, no, no! She is mine now."' And what Elsa Schiaparelli desired, Gabrielle Chanel wanted the more. Lud was pulled between the two great rivals like a rag doll (if a rag doll might ever have been described as 'a lethally beautiful Medea').

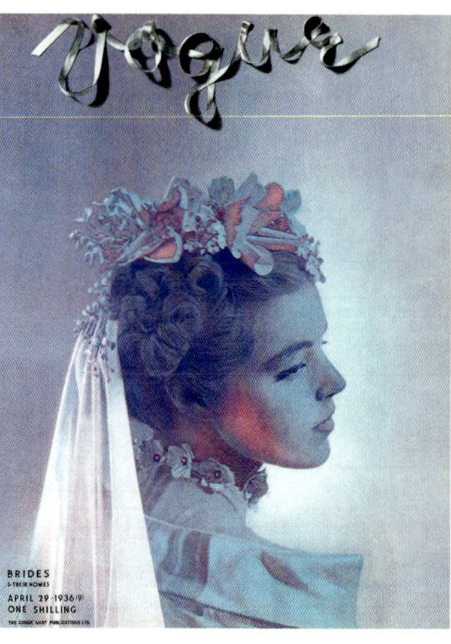

Her marriages (to the lion tamer, a marquis and a naval engineer) failed, and she tried to make it in films, without much luck. Ballard was unsparing: 'After the war, I found her thickened and saddened... with her husband in trouble on a black-market charge.' By the early 1950s she was working for the couturier Balenciaga and helping out in the chorus of the Paris Opera. In turn, as her career in fashion diminished and her savings dwindled, she ended up in Le Touquet as an airline clerk and later as a caretaker at an old people's home. In 1982 she married again, happily, to a childhood friend, and moved to the French Alps, where she died in 1990.

Lud (b. Ludmila Feodoseyevna, c. 1913, Russia; d. 1990)

Above:
'Brides and Their Homes', April 1936, by Cecil Beaton. Headdress by Beaton

Opposite:
'Not All Skirts Are Mile-Wide', March 1938, by Horst. Fashion by Alix

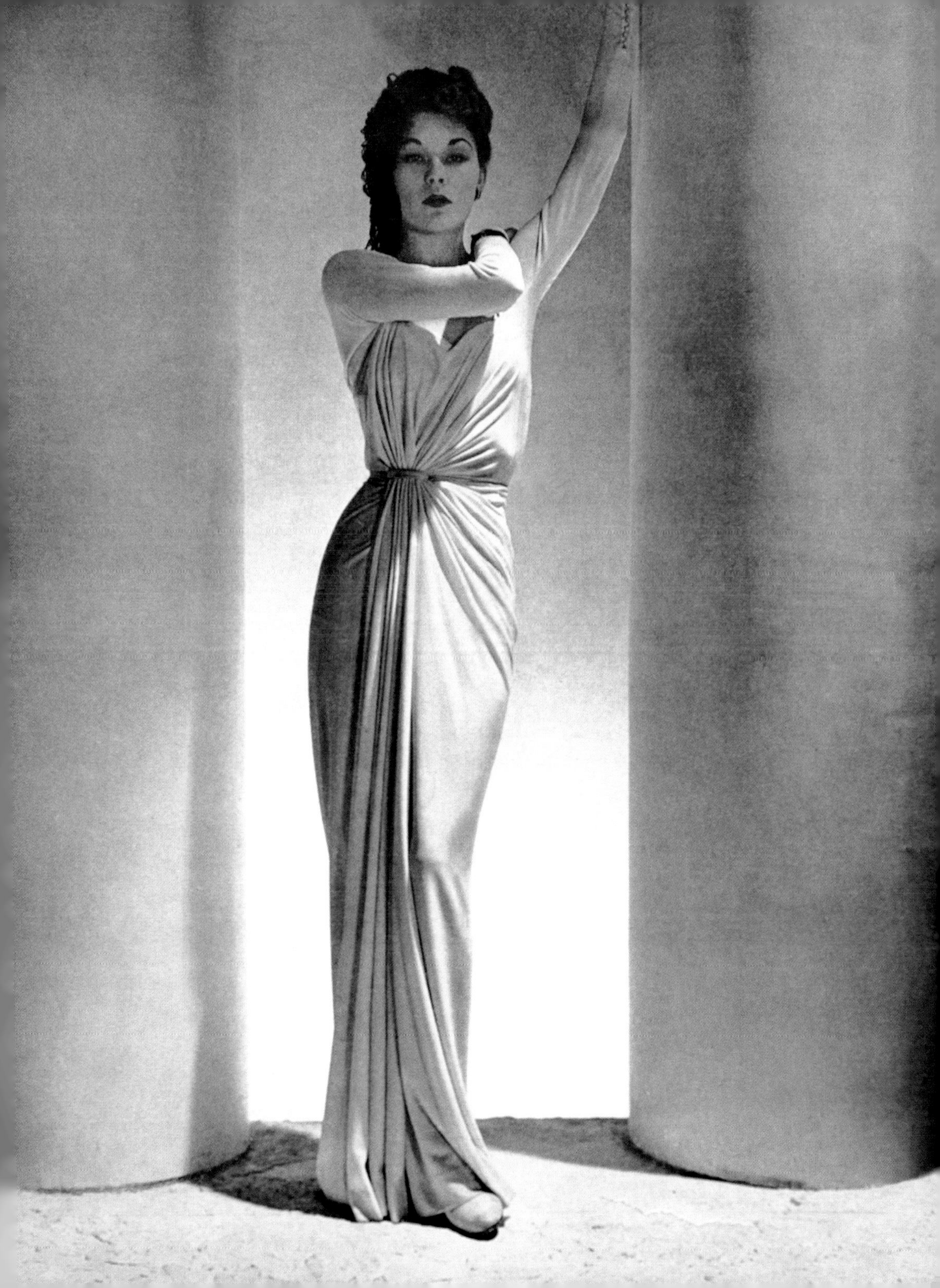

Maggie Rizer

'She is a model,' ran one early profile of the strawberry-blonde, fresh-faced Maggie Rizer, 'who likes what she does but is unusual in that she really doesn't seem as if she would be devastated if it all ended tomorrow…' The tale of Maggie Rizer, her rise and fall (and rise again), is a cautionary one, certainly – but one with an optimistic conclusion, for it's clearly a career that is far from over.

Its start in 1997 was meteoric: her first editorial job was for Steven Meisel at Italian *Vogue*, a cover and 20 or so pages of couture. She had to be taught *in situ* how to walk in high heels, something the long-legged hockey star had never worn. And it all came pouring in quickly: campaigns for the big names, Gap, Louis Vuitton, Tommy Hilfiger, Calvin Klein, Viktor & Rolf; shoots with *Vogue*'s great names: Irving Penn, Steven Meisel, Patrick Demarchelier. She was famously the face of MaxMara as seen by Richard Avedon. In around five years of hard work, Maggie's fortune was estimated at around $7 million and rising.

Maggie was born in 1978 in Staten Island, and grew up in Watertown on the shores of Lake Ontario. Her parents divorced when she was in her infancy, and her mother Maureen married again. John Breen, Maggie's stepfather, was an insurance broker. Maggie was briefly a waitress at a Sackets Harbor diner, where, she told *Vogue*, she was 'the worst. I dropped everything…' Her entrée to modelling was by a recognised route, but one that never appears to bear fruit. Maggie was the exception. On a whim, her mother sent her high-school photographs to the Ford agency and it worked. 'Like fate,' Maggie said.

The Rizer look was mercurial and malleable. She could be freckle-faced girl-next-door for the home market, and then oleander-scented exotic for Japan and the Far East. She was, said her agent, 'a canvas you could manipulate and mould into whatever mood or look you were doing, which obviously made her a very popular model. That and the fact she was so eager to please.' She was also reliable, charming, lived modestly and was fired with a work ethic that would see her leave Watertown for the bright lights of Manhattan but keep a room at home. And the lights twinkled brightly. At the height of her career she received $20,000 per catwalk show and her advertising day rate was $30,000. There was so much coming in, she hired a manager to oversee her finances.

It all began to unravel back home when her stepfather John Breen persuaded her to drop her financial adviser in favour of him (he was still in insurance). Proud of his stepdaughter's soaraway success and her considerable earning power, he concealed a desperate pair of addictions: alcoholism and gambling. The former was containable for a while, but the latter spiralled out of control. Before long he was financing his lottery habit with the contents of Rizer's overflowing bank account. Nearly all of the $7 million had gone. 'I remember feeling like someone took a bowling ball and knocked me in the head with it,' she said some years later. Breen was jailed, and the distress caused Maggie to withdraw from modelling.

Back in the early days, *Vogue* noted that Maggie, smart and perspicacious, 'needs something more challenging than learning how to walk in high heels'. She has since become well-known – and as hard-working as ever – as an HIV/Aids activist and as a roving ambassador for 'Operation Smile', the not-for-profit medico-dental organisation. She has also started modelling again.

Maggie Rizer (b. 1978, USA)

Right:
'The Frock of the New',
May 2003,
by Thomas Schenk

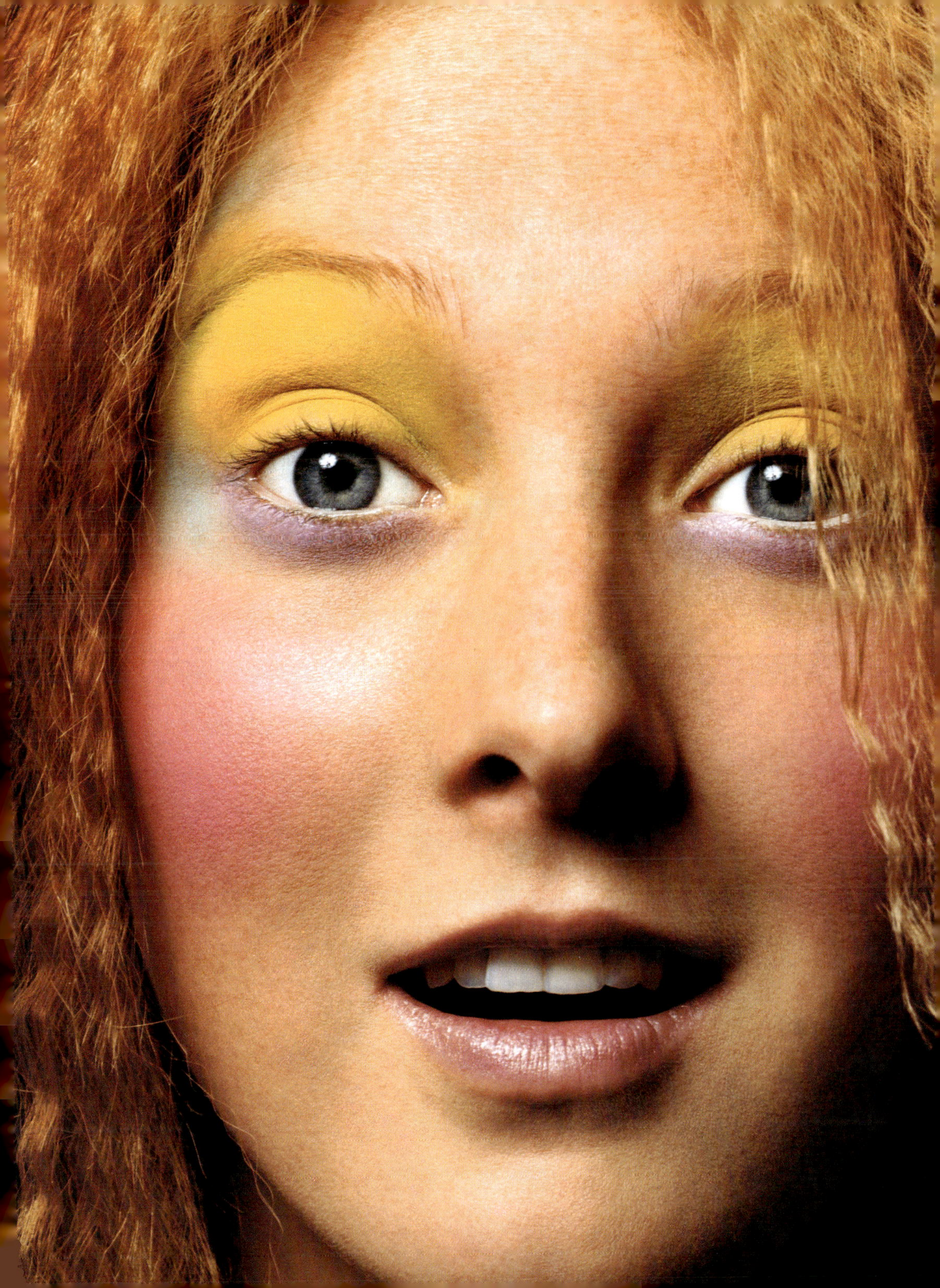

Malgosia Bela

'Another round of shows, another clutch of new models,' announced *Vogue* in 1997. 'They are already developing their own look, which is radically different from the designer labels favoured by the supermodels earlier this decade… and they posses an attitude light years away from prima tantrums.' It was therefore all about enjoying the moment while it lasted. Out of the eight girls *Vogue* showcased, only two made it into the next century with any sort of success, and only one went far: Malgosia Bela.

Born in Krakow in 1977, Malgosia was initially a catwalk star, making the transition effortlessly to the magazine page. Her androgynous look was perfect for the times – an outdoorsy breeziness had given way to a more contemplative look, a 'thrift-shop finish', as one commentator put it. As Malgosia started out, Gianni Versace insightfully remarked: 'Things have got very natural, very undecorated, and these girls suit that. They may not replace Claudia or Carla, but they signify more diversification…'

They were also perfect for the photographers of the time, who saw their medium as a vehicle for expressing opinions which went far beyond the mere depiction of clothes. There were those, for example, who embraced the documentary tradition and hoped to tell it like it is, accentuating the 'real' or the monotony of life, where clothes play only an incidental part. Casting almost from real life gave their photographs a more universal appeal.

'I try to enjoy all the shoots I do,' said Malgosia, 'but if I had to pick a favourite it would be working with David Sims for four days in London doing the Jil Sander campaign.' Jil Sander was pivotal in promoting the new real – 'It's too easy to take a safe-looking girl. That isn't the point of my clothes.'

In 2001 Malgosia embarked upon a film career under her real name, Malgorzata Bela, and mostly in her native Poland. Her films appear to have religious connotations: *We Are All Christs* (2006) and *Karol: A Man Who Became Pope* (2006). Her debut, *Ono* (2004), directed by Malgorzata Szumowska, earned her an acting award at the Verona Film Festival.

Malgosia's spirit of adventure has lasted the course. In 2009, she was a memorable constituent of an unusual sitting for 'More Dash than Cash', *Vogue*'s showcase for style on a budget. It demanded of Malgosia that she wear clothes made out of bin-liners and recyclable shopping bags. This was perhaps recessionary chic taken *ad extremis*, but made an effective point nonetheless. Conversely, she was a vital part of that year's Pirelli calendar, photographed by Peter Beard – neither an arena nor a photographer that habitually demanded the ectomorphic or cadaverous. Malgosia, far removed from the introspection of her early days, did not disappoint.

Among Malgosia's other accomplishments, she is also a classically trained pianist.

Malgosia Bela (b. Malgorzata Bela, 1977, Poland)

Opposite:
'Soft Touch', March 2008,
by Lachlan Bailey.
Fashion by Céline

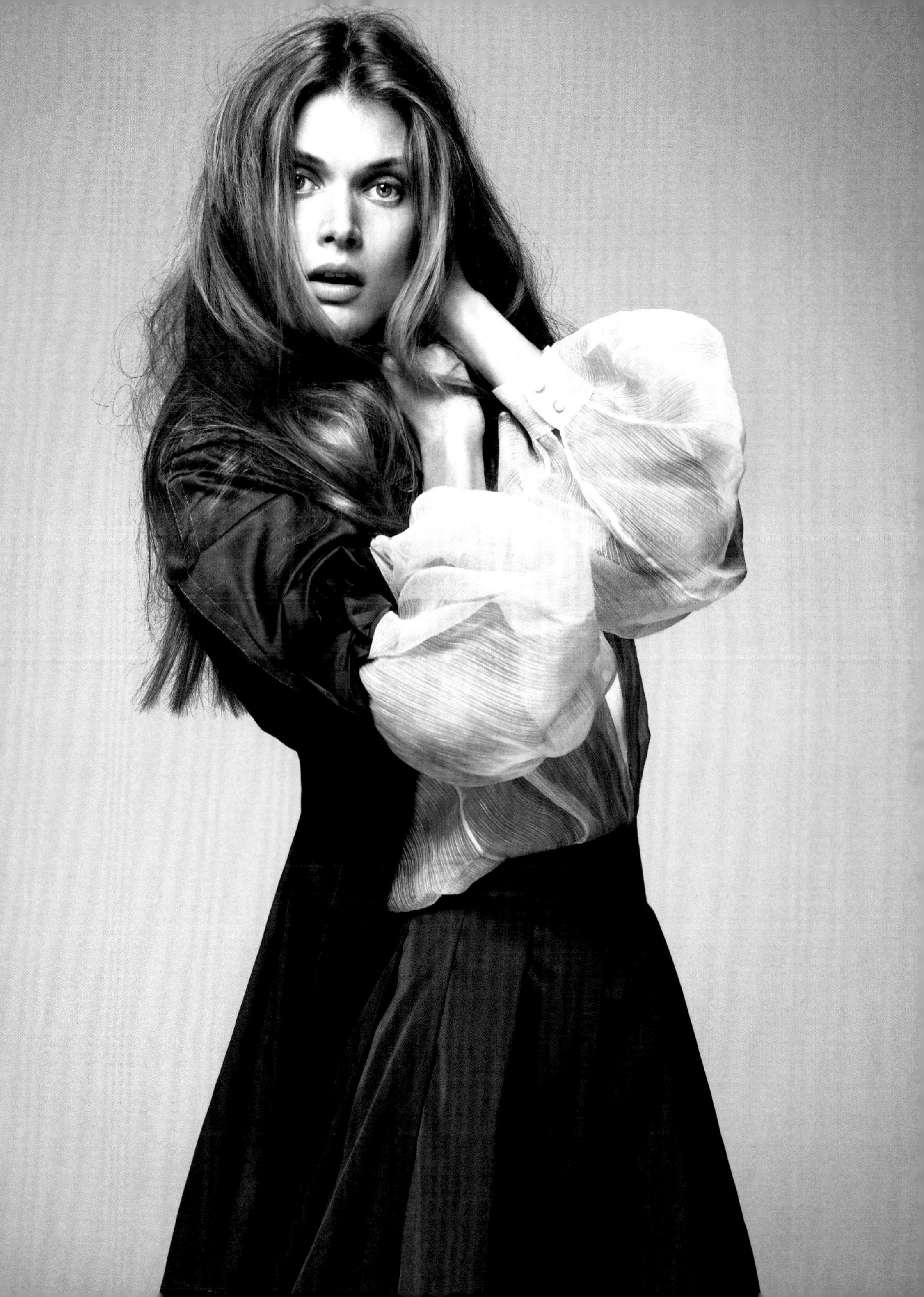

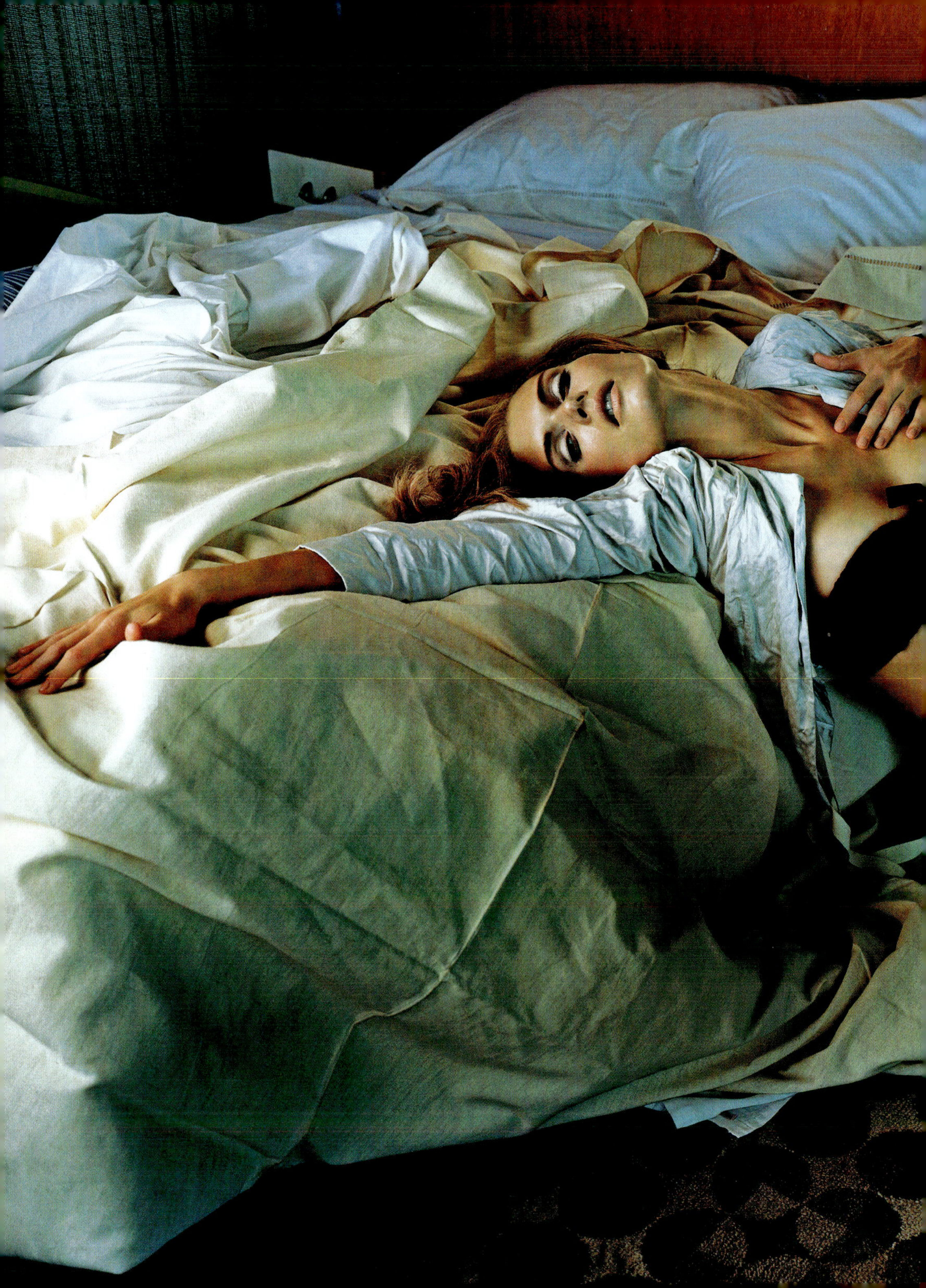

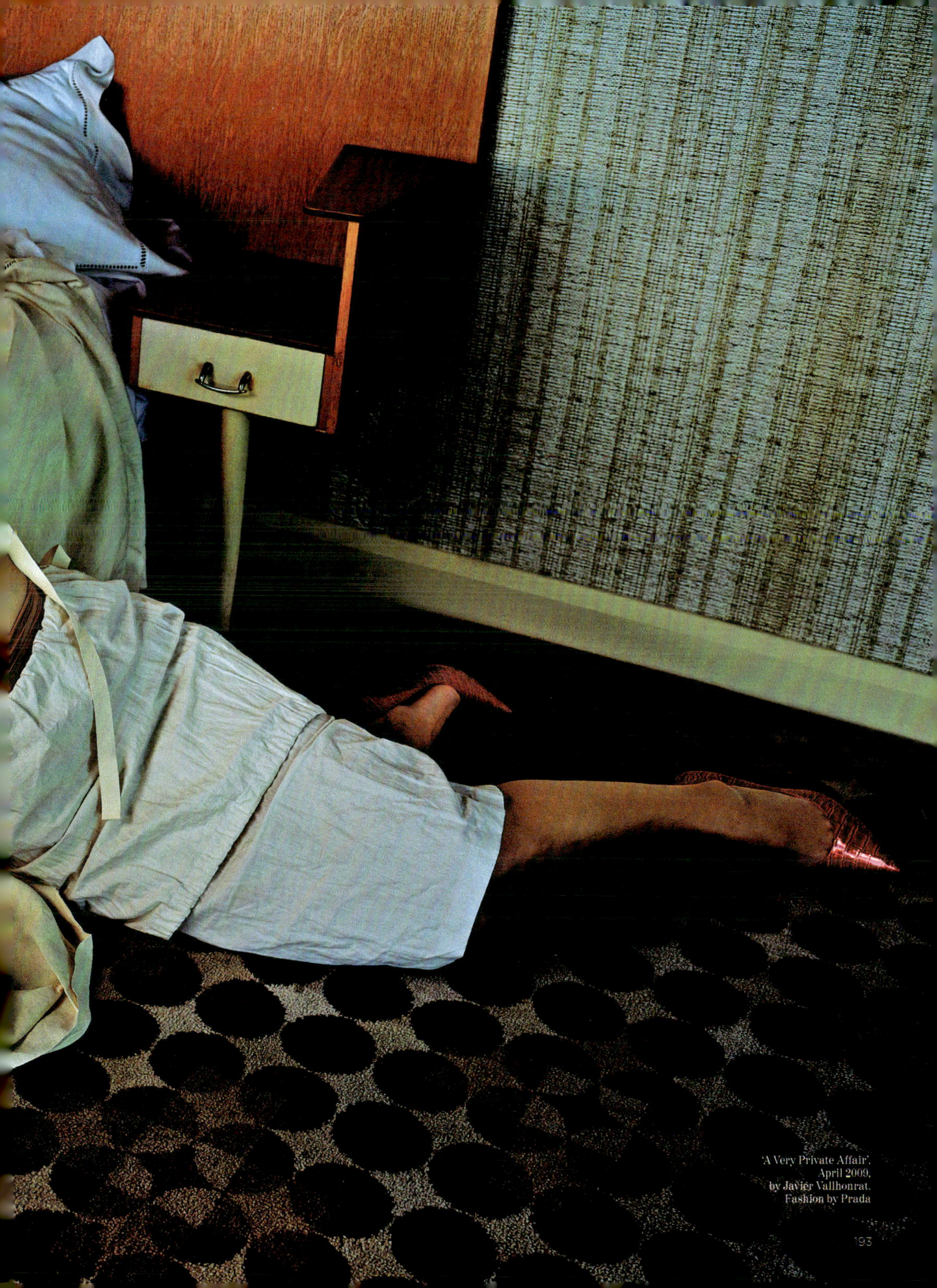

'A Very Private Affair',
April 2009,
by Javier Vallhonrat.
Fashion by Prada

Marie Helvin

The exotic flower Marie Helvin was a staple of the colour-saturated locations much favoured by 1970s *Vogue* and David Bailey. Left in the burning sands of Queensland, perched on the edge of a volcano crater, oblivious to the looming approach of an inflatable turtle – Helvin's selfless collaborations gave *Vogue* glimpses of the world that it might not have experienced had another model been selected. She was also the girlfriend of the photographer, which helped the process greatly.

This same trip to Australia had also taken in Tahiti, where Helvin was required to sport a blonde wig and lime-green tights. 'I felt a fool,' she said. 'It was my first trip abroad for British *Vogue*. I was expecting luxury and first-class hotels all the way. When I arrived in Queensland, I discovered Bailey and I were to be sharing a tiny bedsit with the fashion editor and travel writer. Bailey and I ended up sleeping in the kitchen…' Perhaps the enforced proximity worked, for six months later Bailey and Helvin were married.

Of Japanese and American descent, Helvin was brought up in Honolulu and briefly Tokyo. There she was approached by a representative of the cosmetics giant Kanebo and asked to consider modelling. It turned out to be a three-year contract worth thousands of dollars, which surprised the recipient. 'Of course I had been conscious of my looks and figure, just like any teenage girl,' she wrote later, 'but my self-image had always been that of a gawky, flat-chested stringbean with a frizzy mass of hair. And the length of my leg, which was now being treated as a valuable asset, had always before been a liability…'

The Japanese experience was valuable. Marie learnt the value of courtesy, pleasing other people, a determination to avoid offence, an understanding of the rigid order of things and a fierce work ethic. As important was learning to overcome any inhibitions about nakedness. This would be vital to her years with *Vogue*, as she spent a disproportionate amount of them in bikinis in foreign places for David Bailey. Luggage for their trips was commendably easy: 'Bailey had his cameras,' she explained. 'I had one drip-dry dress for emergencies…'

Her first sets of *Vogue* pictures were taken by Clive Arrowsmith and Barry Lategan and were distinctly oriental in flavour. Helvin had modelled the first London show of the designer Kansai Yamamoto, whose clothes were influenced by Kabuki theatre. This had necessitated Helvin shaving off her eyebrows and playing up the Japanese part of her heritage. She was admonished not to spoil the mystique by revealing she was more than a little American. Thus, throughout these early shoots she barely spoke and if required to, did so in an impenetrable Japanese accent. She was, anyway, already perturbed: Arrowsmith had appeared in an outsize sombrero and twirling two cowboy pistols. Lategan she found, on the contrary, focused and Zen-like.

But it was with Bailey that her reputation escalated. From eyewitness accounts, one might have gleaned that much of the 1970s passed Bailey and Helvin by. Their domestic life was unconventional. They shared their home with the stylist Michael Roberts, 60 parrots, several dogs, a majordomo called César and whoever happened to pop by. Bailey reportedly sat in front of the TV, throwing apple cores and old Coke cans over his shoulder. This was utterly misleading. We can see now that Bailey was almost hyperactive, spending much of the decade escaping the restrictions of studio photography to discover the colours of the world outside in the company of a model herself highly adventurous. He was aided by the competitive nature of all the *Vogue*s in flinging their photographers furthest to see whose pages might first reap the exotic rewards. Within the narrow parameters set by the fashion magazine, Bailey's artistic integrity somehow remained intact.

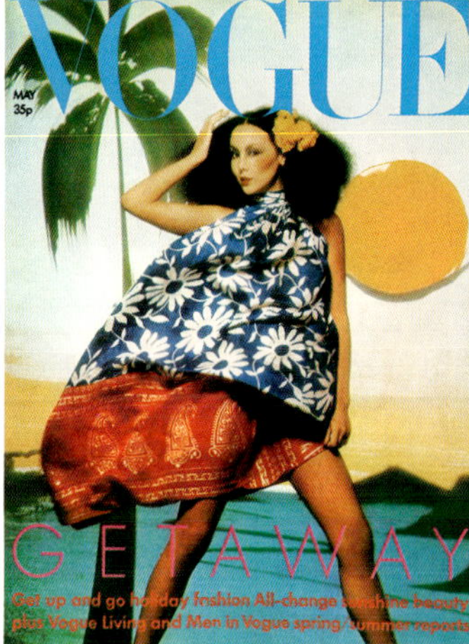

Whatever the magazine presented as a guideline, Bailey with Helvin in tow would find the means to flout it, giving rise to one of the most sustained fashion oeuvres of the 1970s and beyond. He also found time to direct three TV documentaries, co-founded *Ritz*, a glossy newspaper, and published three books of his photographs, including an unconventional book of uxorious portraits of the then Mrs Bailey, *Trouble and Strife* (1980).

Marie Helvin, (b. 1952, Japan)

Above:
'Getaway', May 1974,
by David Bailey.
Fashion by Jean Muir

Opposite:
'Sun', May 1976,
by David Bailey.
Fashion by Pascal

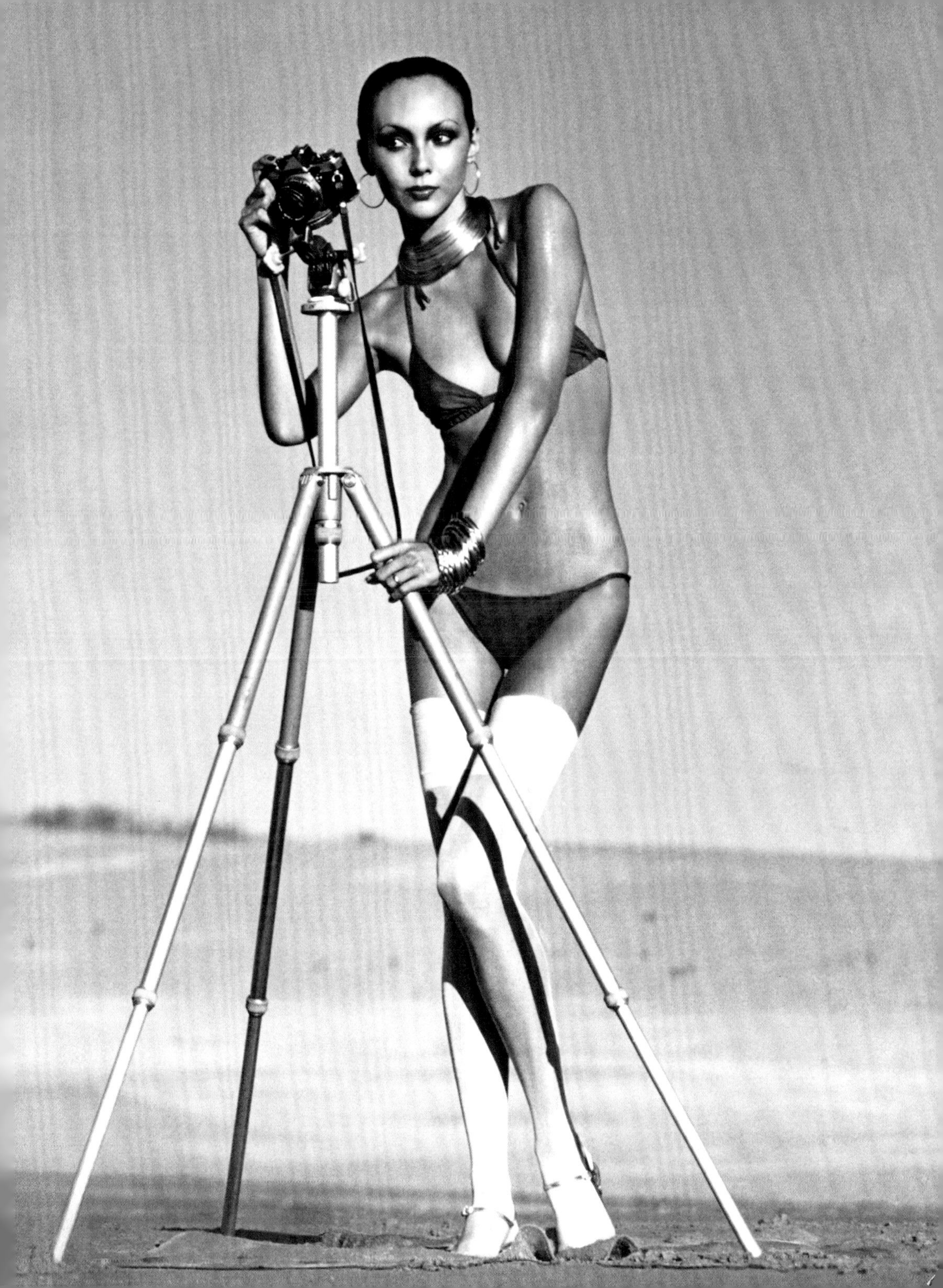

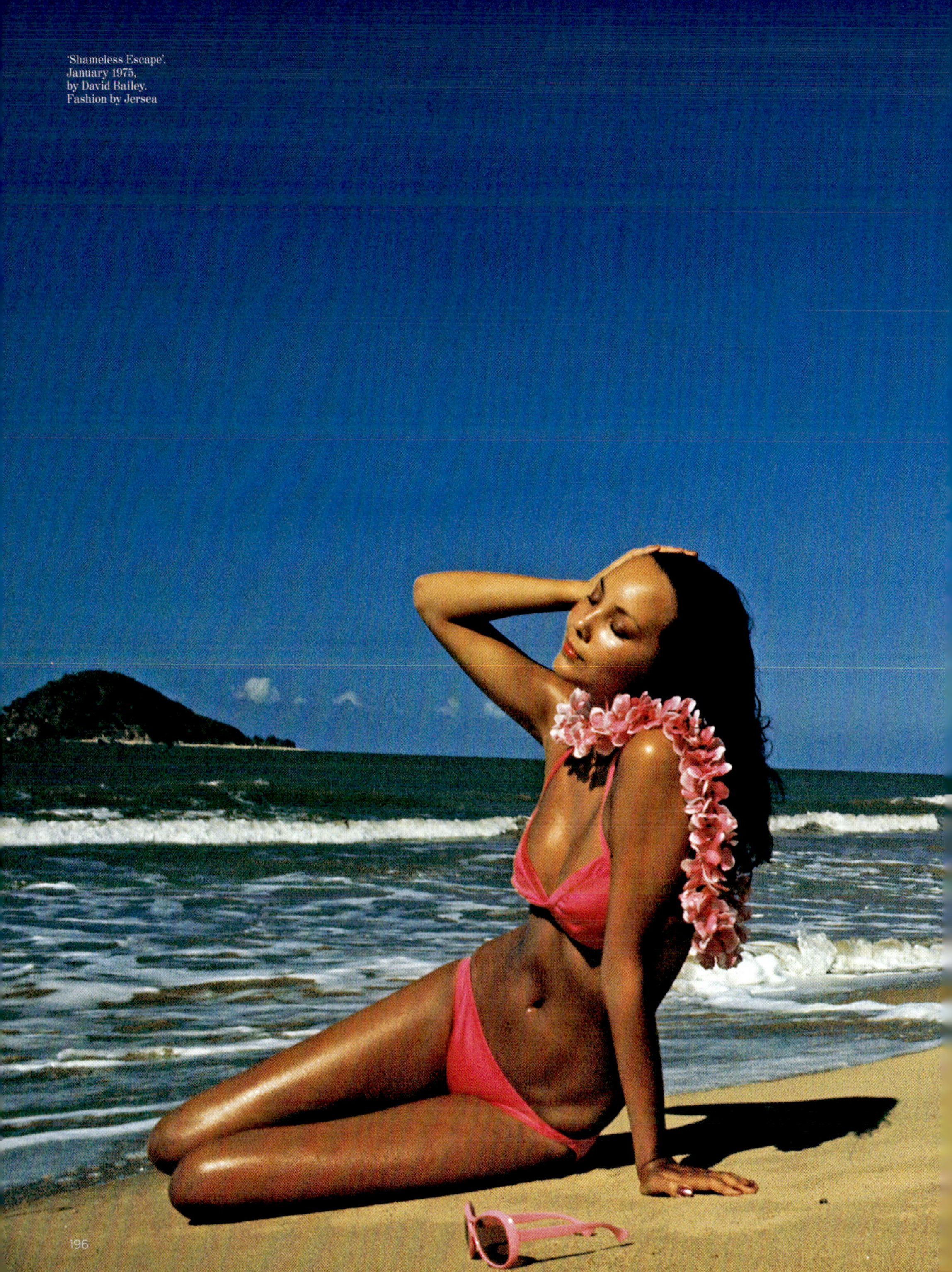

'Shameless Escape', January 1975, by David Bailey. Fashion by Jersea

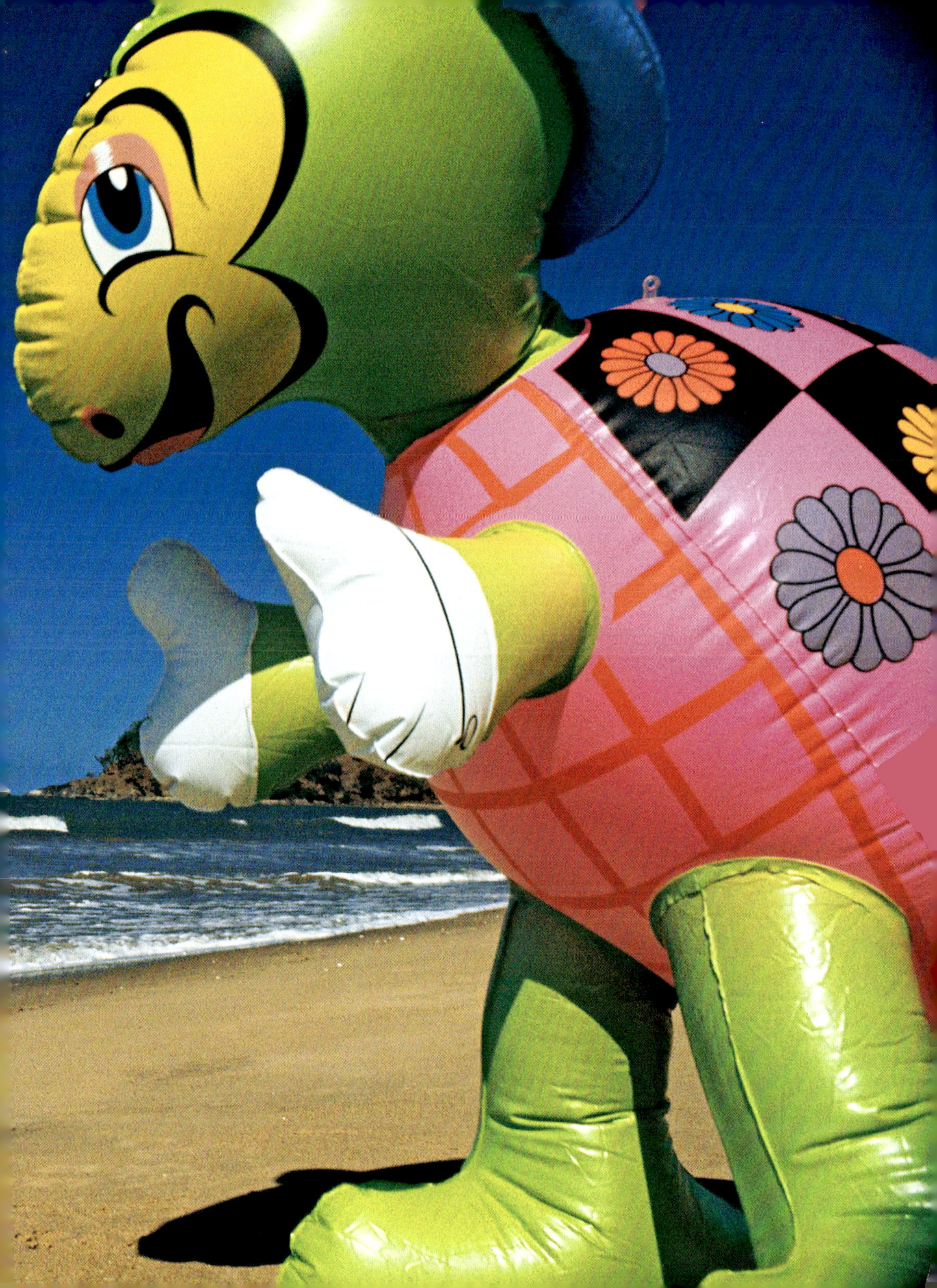

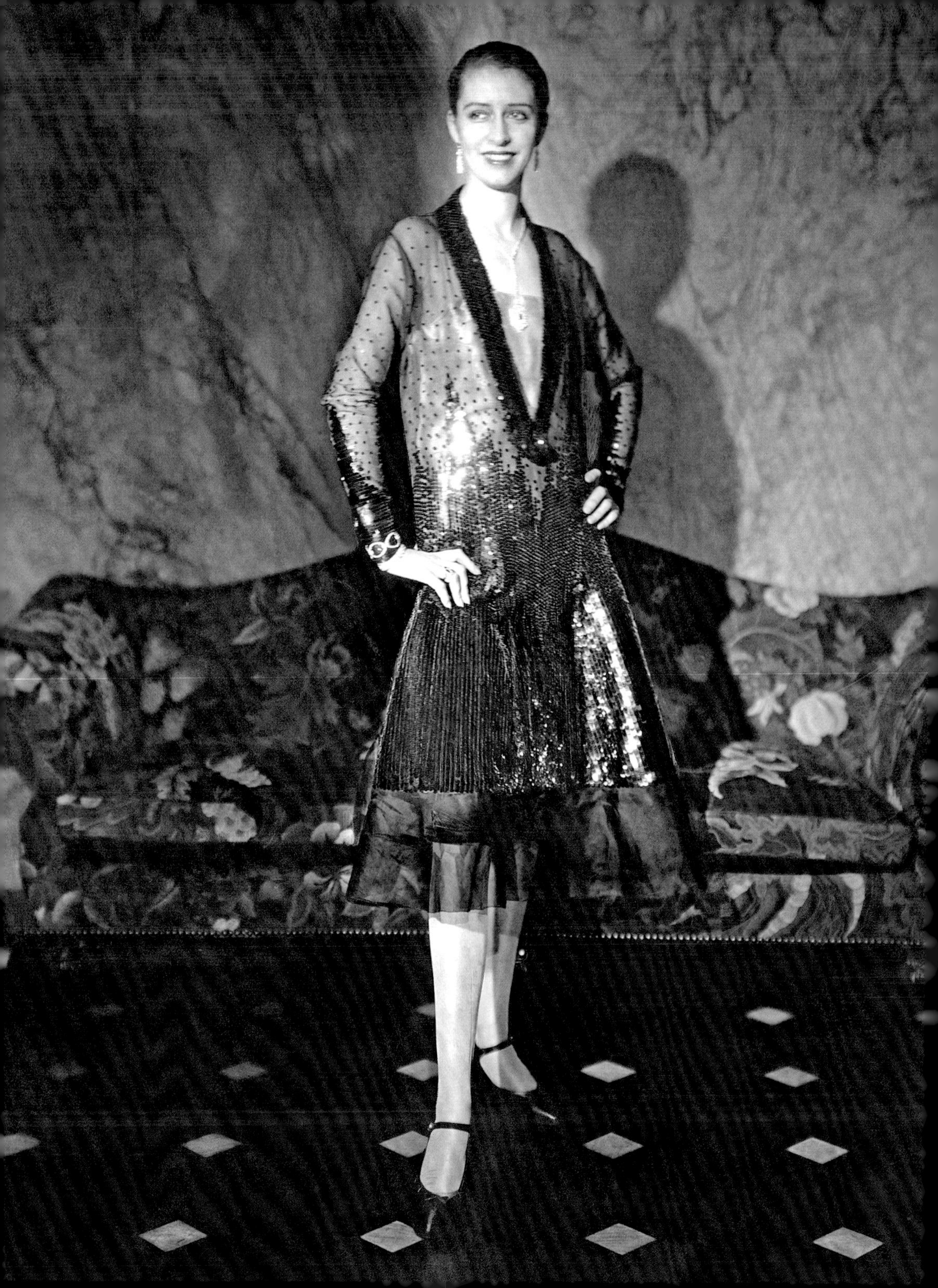

Marion Morehouse

The partnership of Marion Morehouse and Edward Steichen changed the course of fashion photography. 'She gave real distinction to every dress she wore,' observed Cecil Beaton, while Steichen was, *Vogue* trumpeted in 1923, 'the world's greatest living photographer'. This was no idle or polite observation. Steichen remains a giant figure in the history of photography for his crepuscular Pictorialism – he had established the Photo-Secessionist movement with Alfred Stieglitz in 1902 – and then, aged 45, he embarked on a genre-defining career at magazines. As chief photographer for *Vogue* and *Vanity Fair*, he propelled both into the age of Modernism. And they came no more modern and streamlined than Marion Morehouse, with her sleek head, attenuated limbs and ramrod back all revealed by Steichen's dramatic high-key lighting. At a stroke, his predecessor Baron de Meyer's soft-focus aesthetic, a last gasp of High Edwardianism, looked outmoded and trivial. *Vogue*'s proprietor Condé Nast told Steichen: 'Every woman De Meyer photographs looks like a model. You make every model look like a woman.'

It worked because, as Steichen put it, 'Miss Morehouse was no more interested in fashion than I was. But when she put on the clothes that were to be photographed, she transformed herself into a woman who would really wear that gown or that riding habit…' She was the epitome of modernity: chic but wholesome, unassuming yet glamorous. Like a highly responsive thoroughbred, she reacted faultlessly to the vaguest hint of direction and, trained to perfection, second-guessed what might come next. Beaton considered her 'a joy': she was 'the first famous model with whom I had worked, and suddenly I was breathing pure oxygen…'

It is often laid at Marion Morehouse's feet that photographic models became so recognisable that they began to exert a fascination over the public. And with justification. She was not an actress, a music-hall star or a society figure, but something new entirely – a model girl. *Vogue* began to use her name in credit lines as it might Ina Claire from the stage or Princess Youssoupoff, lately of Russia: 'Two mink-trimmed bias panels fall from this gown of green-and-gold lamé – a gown of great elegance and richness obtained by its gleaming fabric and intricate cut; posed by Marion Morehouse.'

She was equipped with a *joie de vivre* and, as Steichen revealed later, a keen sense of adventure too. He had suggested that they do a series of experimental nude photographs and his model readily agreed. On learning that she was a married woman, Steichen destroyed the negatives, to spare her any future shame. However, she was married to the avant-garde poet EE Cummings – he, of all husbands, Steichen later surmised, might have applauded the results of their innocent experimentation.

Marion Morehouse (b. 1906, USA; d. 1969)

Opposite:
'The Paris Mode, as New York Likes It', May 1927, by Edward Steichen. Fashion by Chéruit

Marisa Berenson

'The 1960s wasn't an era of classic blonde blue-eyed beauties,' Marisa Berenson told *Vogue*. 'We were all very different-looking with strong personalities.' None came stronger in this respect than the majestic Veruschka, but Bailey confided (some years later) that 'she didn't have the mystery I like. I much preferred Marisa Berenson...'

Berenson's influence on her peers was considerable: 'I remember sitting in the hairdresser's with my mum,' recalled Marie Helvin, 'and reading *Vogue* and seeing a picture of a woman with huge eyelashes and her hair scraped back. It was all so glamorous and so alien to me. I found later she was Marisa Berenson... We all idolised Marisa – to us she was so beautiful.' *Vogue* could barely get enough of the raven-haired, dark-eyed beauty, and made her, along with Jean Shrimpton, Twiggy and Penelope Tree, one of the few models to be identified by name.

Born in 1947, Berenson's fashion heritage was beyond reproach, so too her aristocratic antecedents: her maternal grandmother was the couturier Elsa Schiaparelli; she was the great-niece (paternally) of the art historian Bernard Berenson – *Vogue* had much admired his fascinating gardens at the Villa I Tatti – and (maternally) of Giovanni Schiaparelli, the gentleman astronomer who first posited that Mars might have canals. Further, her great-aunt Senda, a renowned athlete, achieved immortality of a kind, being one of the first women elected to the Basketball Hall of Fame. Her stepmother was the aristocratic Marchesa 'Gogo' Cacciapuoti di Guigliano, a fashion leader in her own right, and Marisa's best friends included Diane von Furstenberg, Andy Warhol, Jack Nicholson and Yves Saint Laurent, who labelled her the Girl of the 1970s. The whiff of privilege and privileged access made her a firm fixture in the society pages. Her Beverly Hills wedding to James H Randall in 1977 was the party of the year, so stunning that one guest confided 'No-one can get married for at least a year after this!' Another remarked 'If there was ever such a thing as a groovy wedding, this was it...'

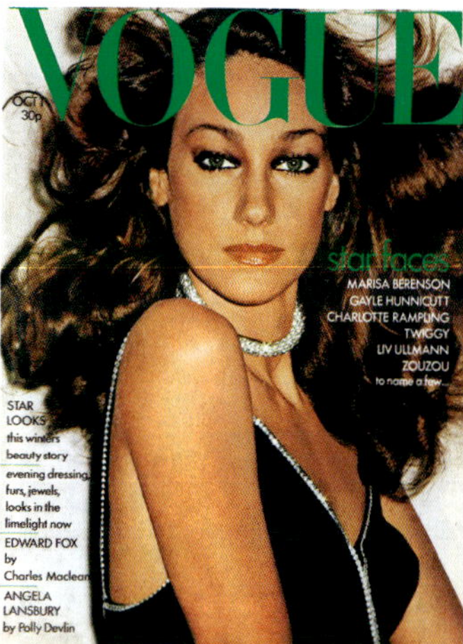

Marisa was first photographed for *Vogue* by David Bailey ('I was terrified. The room was dark, the music was blaring') but something clicked and she worked with all the great names: Horst, Henry Clarke, Avedon and Penn. ('He could always get the most amazing things out of me.') Her modelling career stopped because an acting one had started and presumably her peripatetic, jet-set lifestyle and lively social life could not contain it all.

A few bit parts in the late 1960s led to Luchino Visconti casting her in *Death in Venice*. She played opposite Ryan O'Neal in Stanley Kubrick's lavish period drama *Barry Lyndon*, in which the director's legendary attention to detail led to the acquisition of wardrobes of antique clothing, which were replicated by a team of 35 seamstresses in the six months of pre-production. She was heartbreaking – and award-winning – in Bob Fosse's *Cabaret* as the Jewish fiancée who comes to Liza Minnelli's Sally Bowles for advice in matters of the heart.

Marisa Berenson (b. 1947, USA)

Above:
'Star Faces', October 1973,
by Helmut Newton.
Fashion by Chloé

Opposite:
'The Life that's in British Fashion', September 1968,
by David Bailey.
Fashion by Austin Garritt

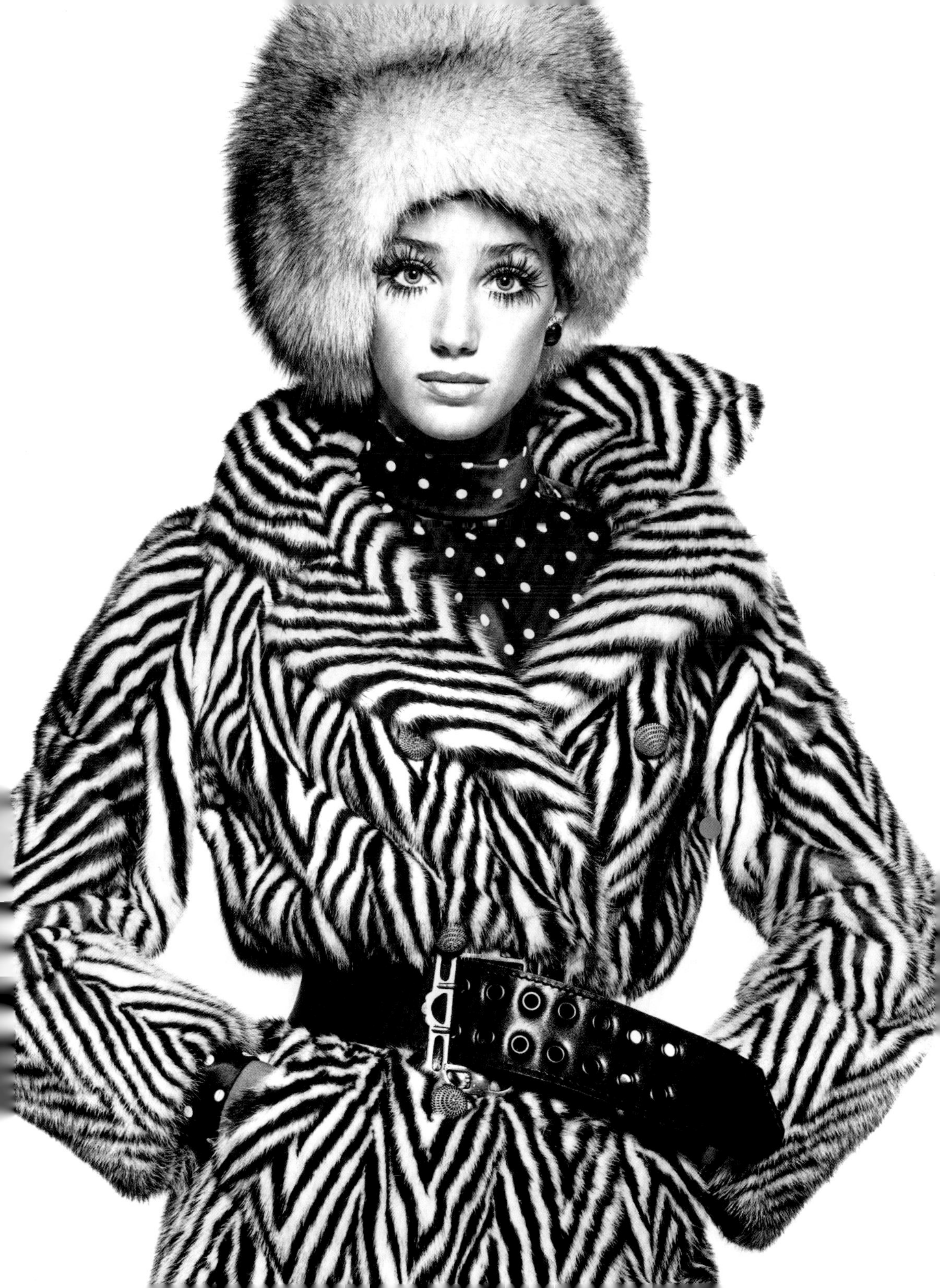

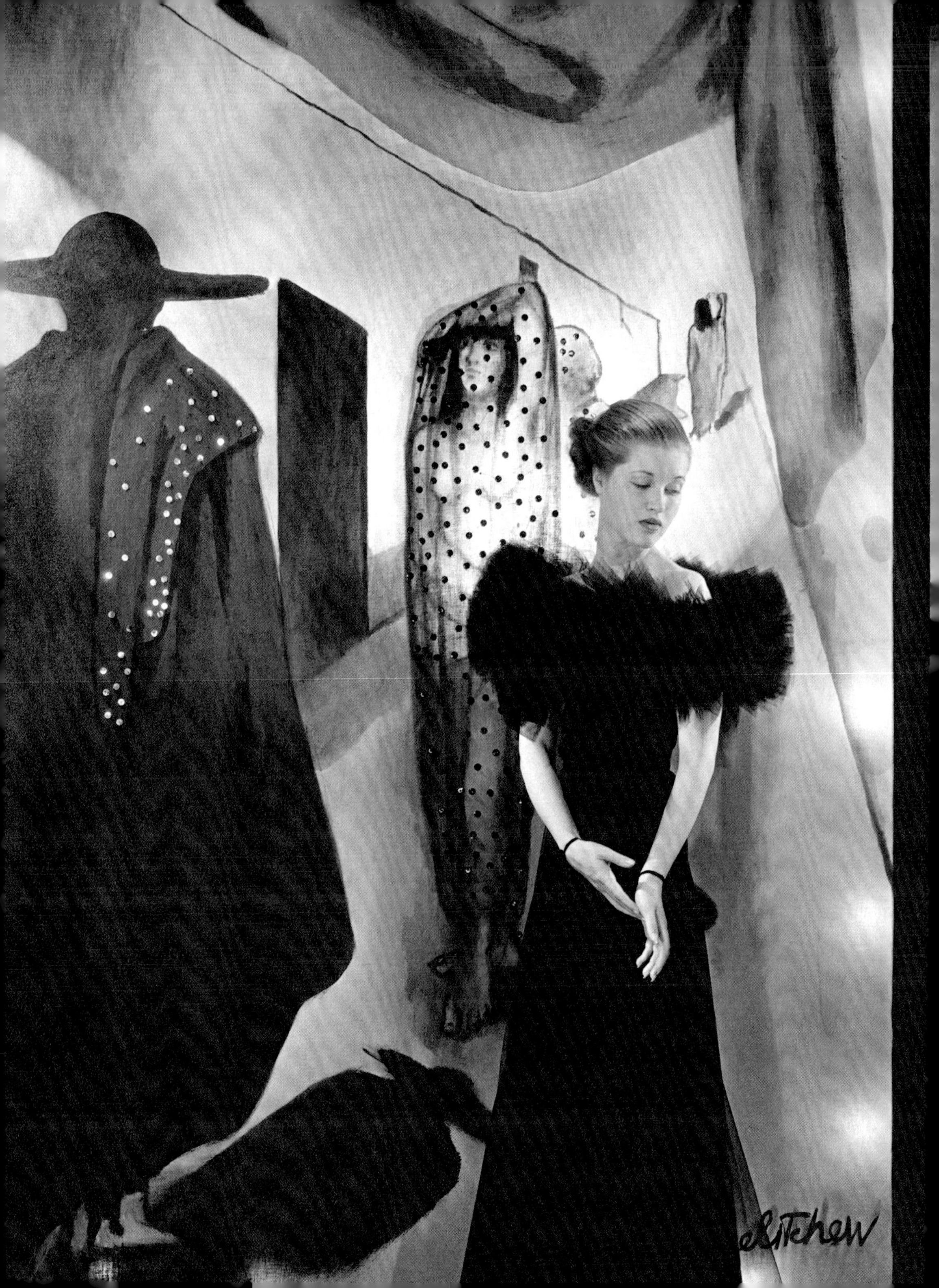

Mary Taylor

Into *Vogue*'s pages strode Miss Mary Taylor, in 'Schiaparelli's hunting-pink jacket, black shirt and fringed fascist cap'. Well, it *was* the mid-1930s, and *Vogue*'s window was open to the world. The connotations would have appalled Taylor in later life, as she became a leading crusader against the anti communist Hollywood blacklist. But back then in Manhattan, 'Mimsy' Taylor was the society girl *du jour* and subject to *Vogue*'s enthusiastic, close inspection. Her sleekness and her aristocratic hauteur – which could also pass as disdain and discrimination – made her in great demand. She was delighted to comply.

Her chic was carefully studied. Off abroad on a shoot, the magazine marvelled at Mimsy's passport photograph – most likely a cut-down, pasted-in test shot by Horst – and in so doing remarked upon her courtesy to the tired eyes of the Department of Immigration. *Vogue*'s eagerness for intimacy reached an apogee in 1935 when the magazine reported on what her dog, a standard poodle, liked to do when Mimsy lunched at the Colony with Niki de Gunzberg. (Unsurprisingly, the poodle slept.)

As a model (chiefly for Edward Steichen and Cecil Beaton), she was tireless. She had suffered from bone-marrow cancer as a teenager, and when her doctors gave up hope, her last wish was to go into fashion. The successful treatment likely gave her great depths of patience. Her oval face, full lips and slanting eyes, remarked *Vogue*, were 'exotic, totally unclassic, more like a Balinese mask than anything else'. Beaton was enchanted and photographed her as a butterfly caught in cobwebs of net and tulle and as a sylph, pale and demure, against backdrops by the Neo-Romanticist painter Pavel Tchelitchew.

Perhaps that aristocratic disdain did not endear her behind the scenes. In her memoirs, fashion editor Bettina Ballard damned Taylor's sophisticated and snobbish elegance with faint praise: 'She never smiled and expressed bored indifference to the affected poses directed by Beaton. Sometimes her hand would be held out to a stuffed white dove, sometimes caressing a flower or gesturing to thin air – all equally meaningless, but with some innate instinct for fashion... It was a ridiculous period of posing – the dying-swan era – to which she added a Pavlova touch.'

Mimsy did not go unnoticed by *Time* magazine too, which noted that she was careful to avoid posing for 'any of the more intimate feminine accessories' and approved of her sensible business brain – her fee was $50 an hour in 1934. Most of this, *Time* told readers, she spent on drama lessons, and in due course Mimsy made the transition to the movies with a degree of success. *Vogue* noted her Hollywood debut in 1936's *Soak the Rich*. She married the producer of her second film, *Lady of the Tropics*; Sam Zimbalist was her devoted husband for 20 years. His death of a heart attack in Rome on location for the epic *Ben-Hur*, of which he was producer, is often attributed to stress as the budget spiralled. She picked up his posthumous Oscar in 1960.

Much later, looking at Beaton's photographs of Mimsy, the toast of the town, Diana Vreeland wrote: 'There isn't a boy in the world who wouldn't fall in love with her. And there isn't a girl who wouldn't want to look like that *today*.'

Mary Taylor (b. 1915, USA; d. 2008)

Opposite:
'Night Mists', July 1935, by Cecil Beaton. Fashion by Bergdorf Goodman

Maxime de la Falaise

As early as 1949, the Comtesse Alain de la Falaise was, according to *Vogue*, 'a prompting spirit in Paris couture'. She was one of the earliest higher-born women to sport the cropped gamine hairstyle, previously sported by women working in factories or on the land. This she contrasted greatly with the boldest designs of couturier Colette Massignac at the Maison Paquin, which tended to taper and spiral into ankle-constricting narrowness. Her mermaid dress was almost too much to stand up in, let alone move about, so Cecil Beaton photographed her sitting down – the better, as it turned out, to view its fishtail train.

Despite her Francophilia and her Gallic-sounding name, she was born Maxine Birley (in time she changed it to the more masculine Maxime) to the English society portraitist Sir Oswald Birley and Rhoda Pike, a celebrated Irish beauty. The domestic circumstances of the Birleys were comfortable and – to their social equals – relaxed to the point of recklessness. Sir Oswald and Lady Birley gravitated *de haut en bas*, encouraging writers and artists to share their homes and good fortune. It was, recalled one observer, 'haute bohemia at its hautest' – the Ballets Russes and Rudyard Kipling might dine upon Lady Birley's legendary lobster curries, with which she also composted her rose garden.

After an undistinguished childhood (much of it spent at school in cast-off Poiret or Schiaparelli – 'I could have charged other pupils to look at my clothes. They were absolutely in awe of them'), as a WAAF Maxime was recruited to the codebreaking centre at Bletchley Park. She distinguished herself by rampant kleptomania and was invalided out, on the grounds of nervous exhaustion. In time, she found herself in Paris as the couture reawoke from Occupation-era hibernation. She modelled for Elsa Schiaparelli, whose designs had a brief renaissance in the early postwar years, and became a stylish *vendeuse* and ambassador for the label, as well as for Christian Dior in his ascendancy and, especially, for Paquin before it closed its doors in 1956.

Apart from her modelling for Horst, Beaton, Clifford Coffin and others, the Comtesse (she married Comte Alain de la Falaise in 1946, but was divorced from him by 1950), she was a decorative ornament in *Vogue*'s society pages, customarily in Paquin's more adventurous creations. In the magazine's food pages she was given free rein with an aphoristic style: 'Lemon is the speed of cooking.' For a time she was the unofficial house caterer to Andy Warhol's Factory.

When her modelling days were well behind her, she kept herself financially afloat (the Comte had been penniless) by writing, selling furniture and being a slightly older muse to Yves Saint Laurent, whom she had known from his early days at Dior and for whom her daughter Loulou was muse *de plus importante*. For Beaton, Maxime was 'the only truly chic Englishwoman of her generation' – and on the evidence of *Vogue*'s fashion pages, which she enlivened for several decades, she was certainly among the most adventurous.

Maxime de la Falaise (b. Maxine Birley, 1922, UK; d. 2009)

Opposite:
'Elegance', January 1950,
by Cecil Beaton.
Fashion by Paquin

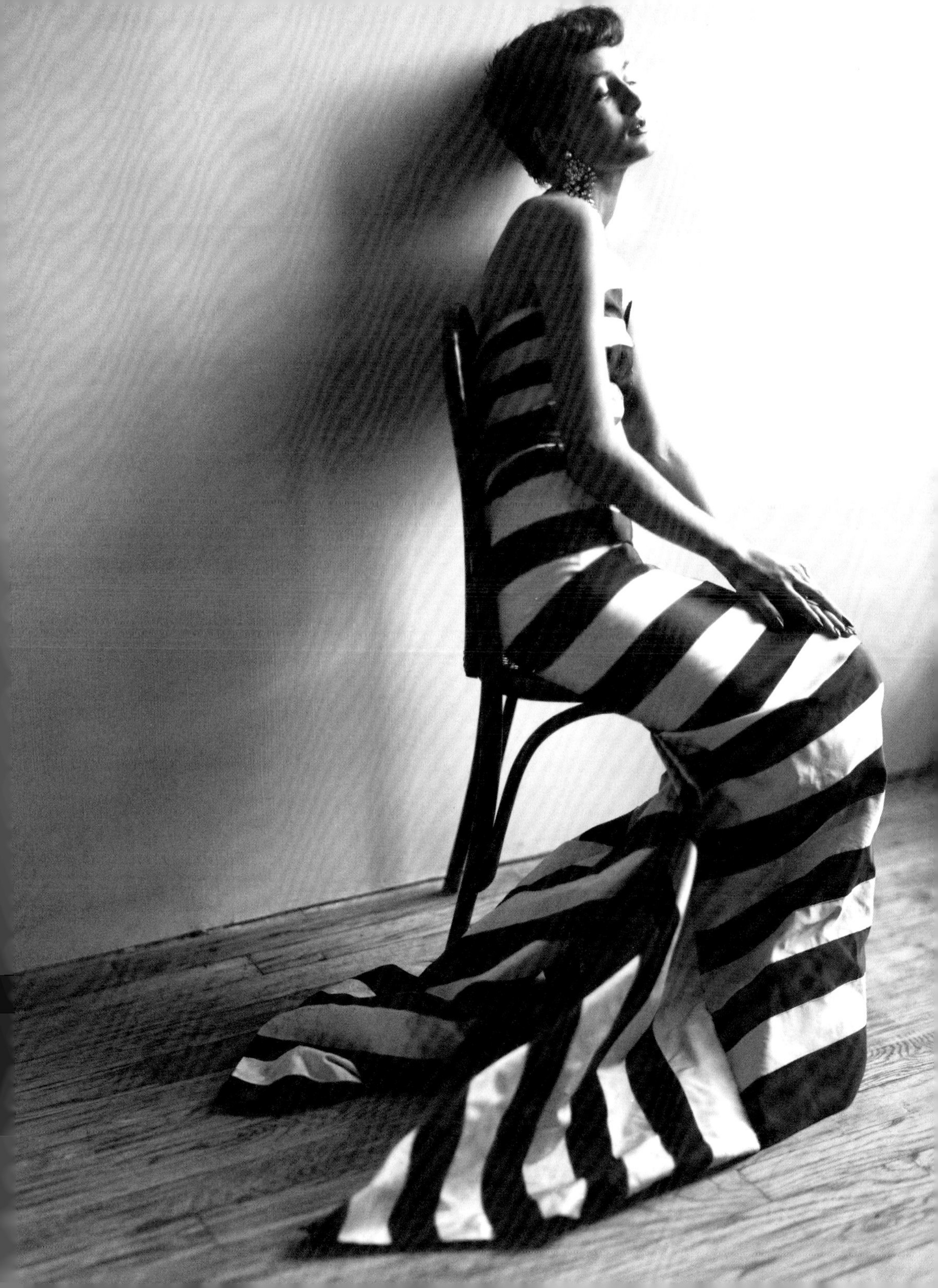

Nadja Auermann

The new season always dazzled best on Nadja Auermann, *Vogue*'s 'platinum-blonde powerhouse', 5ft 11½in with legs measuring 45in. Nadja was a rarity to be prized, polished and put on show, the last vestige of a diminishing tribe, the last of the first wave of supermodels. 'I started modelling at the height of the supermodel era,' she remembered for *Vogue*. 'The shows were crazy backstage. People screamed your name, wanted your autograph. You felt like a rock star.' And you could see why: as American *Vogue*'s Katherine Betts put it, 'with her halo of freshly peroxided albino-white hair, crystal blue eyes, well-built frame, absurdly long legs and Brancusiesque oval head, it was all over for the undernourished look...'

Although she was discovered in Berlin in 1990, it was in Paris that she secured her first assignments. The icy Teutonic demeanour coalesced only when she bleached her hair blonde the following year. In September 1994, she appeared on the cover of British *Vogue*, US *Vogue* and *Harper's Bazaar* too – all of them fat, new-collections issues, the highpoint of the magazine year. That the same model should appear on each simultaneously was a fashion moment eagerly anticipated but rarely seen.

Less anticipated, and usually a shock when they appeared, were Auermann's photographic narratives with fellow Berliner Helmut Newton, now keenly collected. Model and mentor satirised in photographs her statuesque, impossibly Aryan physique: a story on high heels found Auermann in a wheelchair and callipers; for a play upon the Greek myth of Leda, readers were shocked to find her all but ravished by a swan. 'Helmut had a great sense of humour – very dark, very... Berlin.'

German photographers were quickest to appreciate her idiosyncratic charm. For the photographer Peter Lindbergh, when they worked together it was 'an adventure to see [her] stepping out of her bus in the morning'. Similarly for Ellen von Unwerth, whose models were far removed from the then fashionable droopy waifs. Von Unwerth shot her first published pictures for British *Vogue*, an acknowledged homage to Newton, recognising an aggressive sexuality. In fact, she was the first photographer to hire Auermann at all: 'Nadja has lots of different sides to her. Most girls you think of for specific roles, older, younger, retro or very modern, but Nadja can be any woman.'

Auermann's discipline fitted the roles perfectly: 'I am very German, yes,' she told American *Vogue* matter-of-factly. 'When I first moved to Paris I wanted to put my head through the wall.' This was not a preparatory psych-up for a Newtonesque scenario, but because 'they take two-hour lunch breaks, never stop talking. I was like, "I want to work!"'

Back home in Berlin, Auermann had wanted initially to be a tightrope-walker or, failing that, Chancellor of Germany. Then a level head prevailed and she considered architecture; but fate helped make up her mind. A talent scout saw her in a café (it was all about the crossed legs) and within a week she was in Paris. She was not an overnight success – she was, by her own admission, too freakish and too fat. The steeliness kicked in. She lost weight (dramatically, according to one eyewitness, who guessed it might have been half her body weight), changed her hair to platinum/plutonium, and the world took notice.

'She is the product of her iron will,' fellow German Karl Lagerfeld told *Vogue*. 'The body and the look were built by herself. When she made her hair white-blonde the career boomed; she became like a woman from another planet.' The alien landed, strode by on her unfeasibly long legs and began to lay waste to whatever pre-existing conceptions of beauty she encountered. No reedy, panda-eyed grunge girl was safe again.

Nadja Auermann (b. 1971, West Germany)

Opposite:
'She is an Enigma', October 1991, by Ellen von Unwerth. Fashion by Philip Treacy

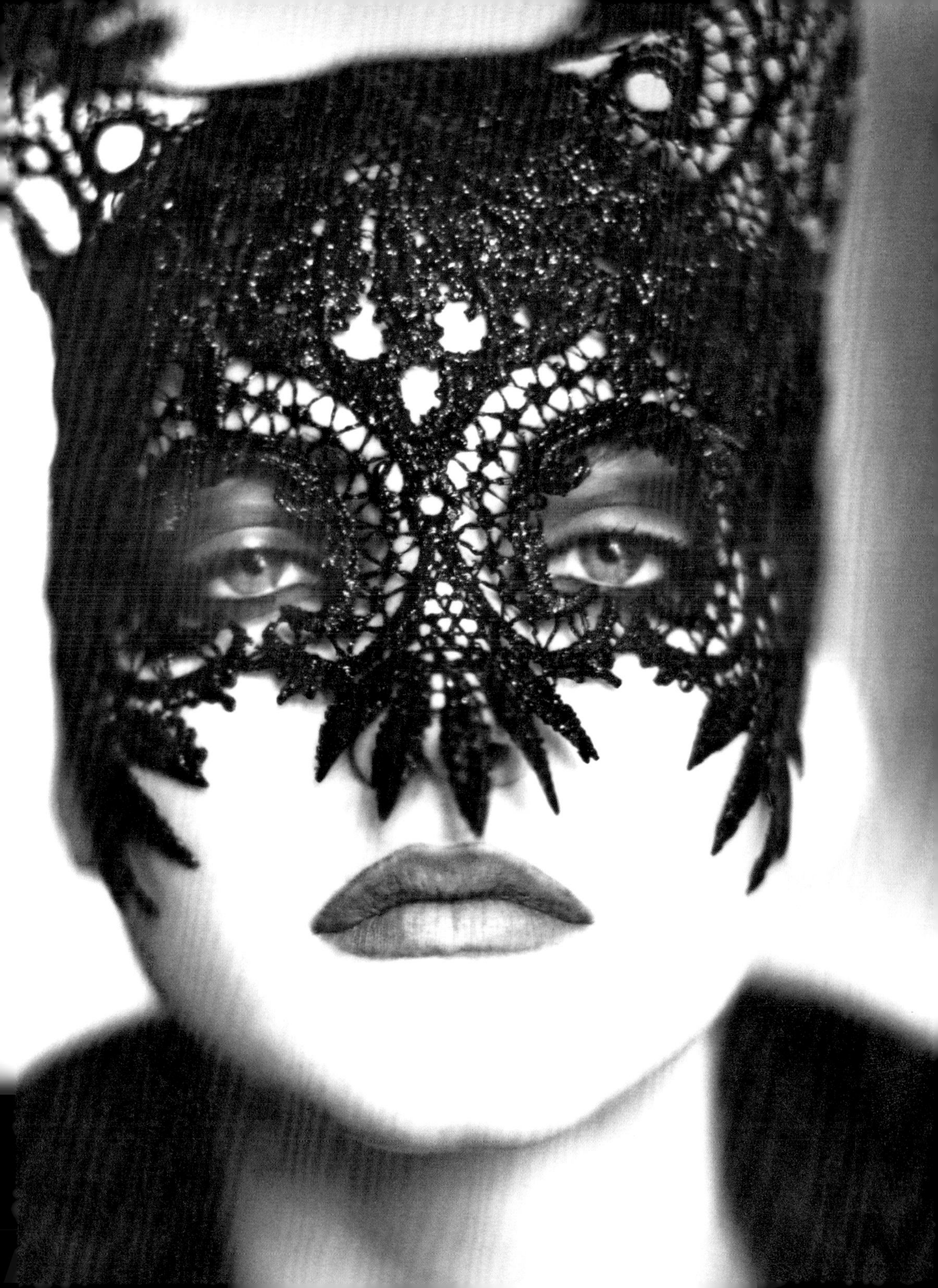

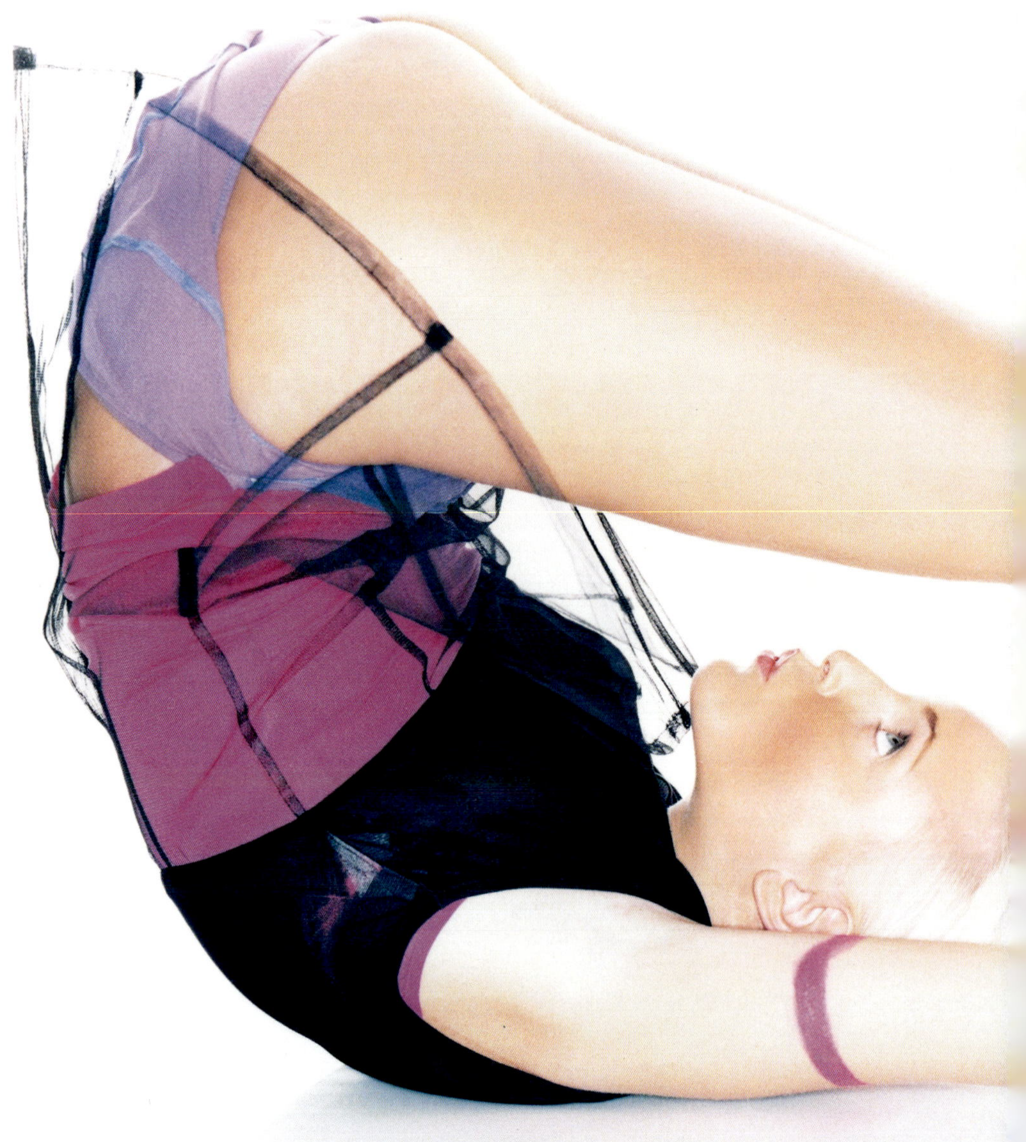

'Punk's New Clothes',
March 1994,
by Nick Knight.
Fashion by Yohji Yamamoto

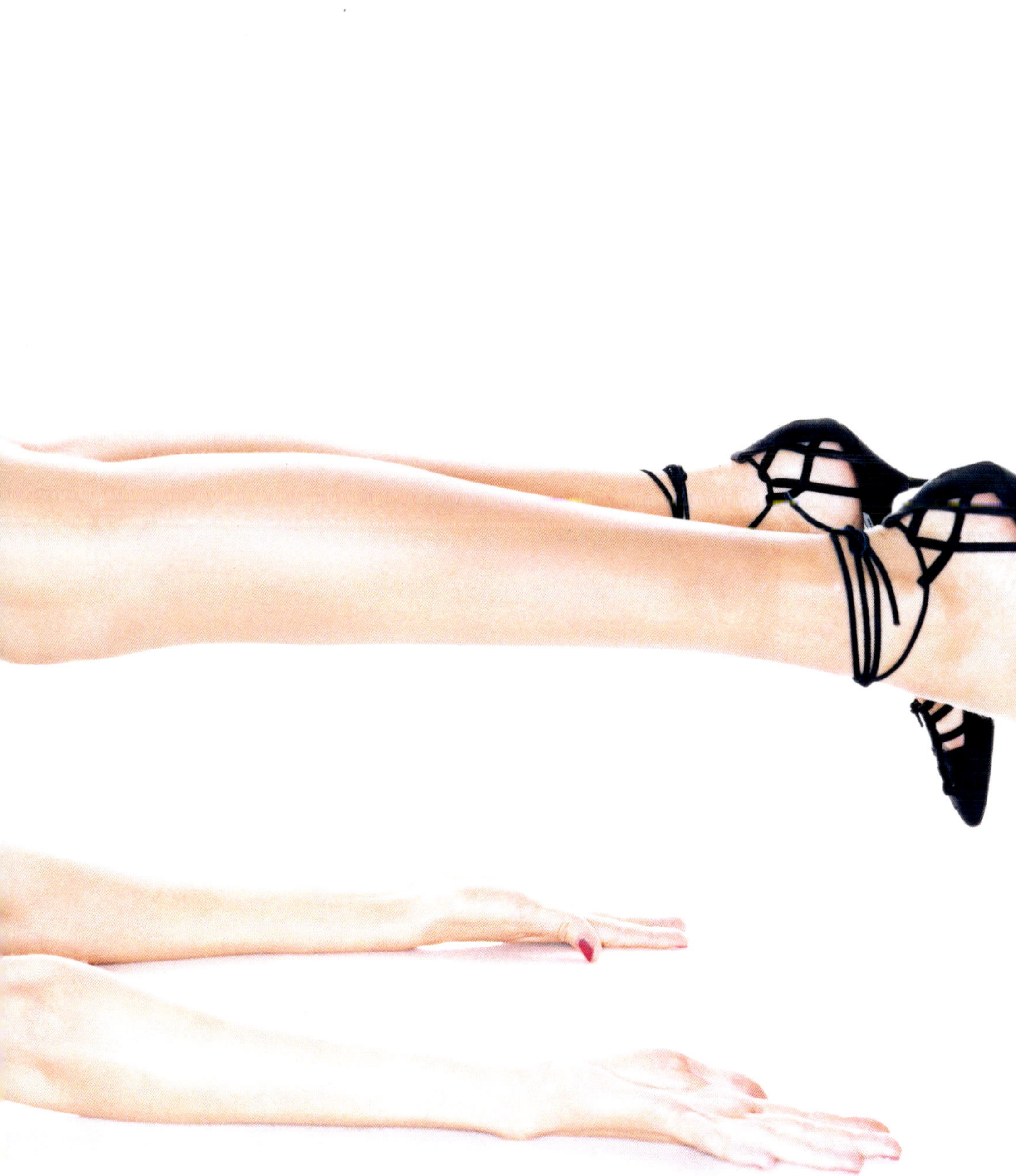

Naomi Campbell

Born in 1970 in Streatham, Naomi made the journey from bright-as-a-button south London teenager to supermodel of extraordinary grace to diva of unpredictable overconfidence in a relatively short time and with great ease. She has now been a star for well over 20 years, and her fame appears not to have waned in the slightest. Nor has her ability to generate breathless tabloid headlines – especially if they happen to involve her personal staff and electronic personal organisers.

It is likely that life ceased to be pedestrian for Naomi at 15, when a talent scout spotted her, though before that, as a pupil at a London stage school, she had already tasted fame of a kind as a dancer in music videos. Since then, she has lived her life as much on the front pages of newspapers as of magazines. She appeared on the cover of French *Vogue* at the suggestion of an early champion, Yves Saint Laurent. Her British *Vogue* debut preceded that, an iridescent Christmas cover by Patrick Demarchelier.

'You have to remember,' observed *Vogue*'s Lucinda Chambers, who first hired Naomi for a fashion shoot, 'she has lived in a bubble and within that bubble she can get away with anything. And sometimes she has. But I think now she wants to find a way back out of that bubble.' Chambers also recalled that first shoot: 'The day before the shoot, Veronica Webb cancelled. I specifically wanted a black model and her agent said "We've just found this girl." When Naomi walked into the offices I thought she was the most beautiful girl I'd ever seen – and she carried all the suitcases.'

Her longevity has seen several personal projects come to fruition, not all successful, but all guaranteed of a certain level of attention. *Swan*, her debut novel, appeared in 1994, but it merely bore her name above the title, being the product of a ghost-writer. The following year, her pop album *Baby Woman* was released; although unsuccessful in her native country, it sold well abroad. Far more profitable have been her fragrance lines, with memorable names such as Naomagic and Cat Deluxe at Night. Her charity work, which rarely attracts the attention it merits, brought her into close proximity with Nelson Mandela, revered by Naomi as a great leader and as something of a father figure.

Mario Testino has reinvigorated a career that had started to decline just a little. 'She exemplifies,' he says, 'a lot of what I like about women. She believes that she is beautiful. She dresses up when she goes out. She loves the glamorous life.' Testino stops short of calling Naomi a diva, in the very positive sense of the word – larger than life, dignified, head-swivellingly sensational.

Naomi does have a slight reputation for erratic timekeeping, and few are exempt; however, she is always forgiven, because when it works with Naomi, it really works. This is *Vogue* editor Alexandra Shulman's affectionate take on waiting for her in Paris: 'The fact that Naomi is late is not, of course, news. Big news would be if Naomi were on time. But the minutes are now turning into hours…'

'What is there left to say about Naomi Campbell?' asked *Vogue* some time ago, before answering: 'She, along with Linda, Christy, Cindy *et al*, personified the age of the supermodel. She dated actors, boxers and rock stars. She got engaged. She got unengaged… She endured the slings and arrows of the critics. So all that's left to be said,' the magazine concluded, 'is that she is still one of the best models around. Model-actress-whatever? More like model-icon-whatever.' And that was 1997. It still holds true another decade down the line.

Watching her as a shoot with Corinne Day unfolded (four and a bit hours after its intended start), Shulman observed: 'She's happy to just sit there and be made into whatever we make her into. Naomi might be a 1970s Black Panther goddess today, but she's been a rock chick, a T-shirted girl from south London, a walking, talking glamour doll and any number of guises we've wanted to squeeze out of one of our few famous black-skinned beauties…'

Naomi Campbell (b. 1970, UK)

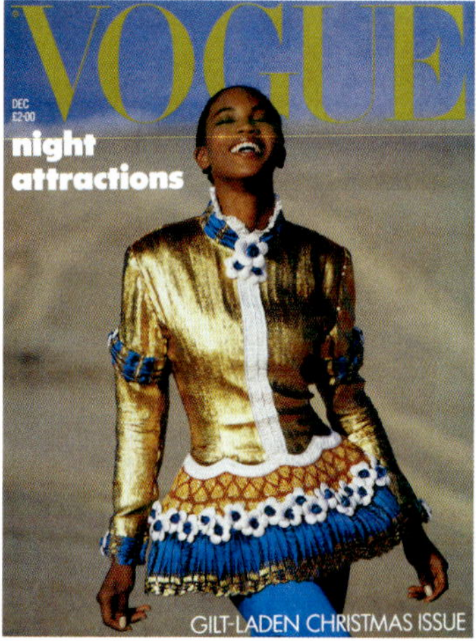

Above:
'Night Attractions', December 1987, by Patrick Demarchelier. Fashion by Chanel

Opposite:
'Heavenly Bodies', December 1990, by Herb Ritts. Fashion by Norma Kamali

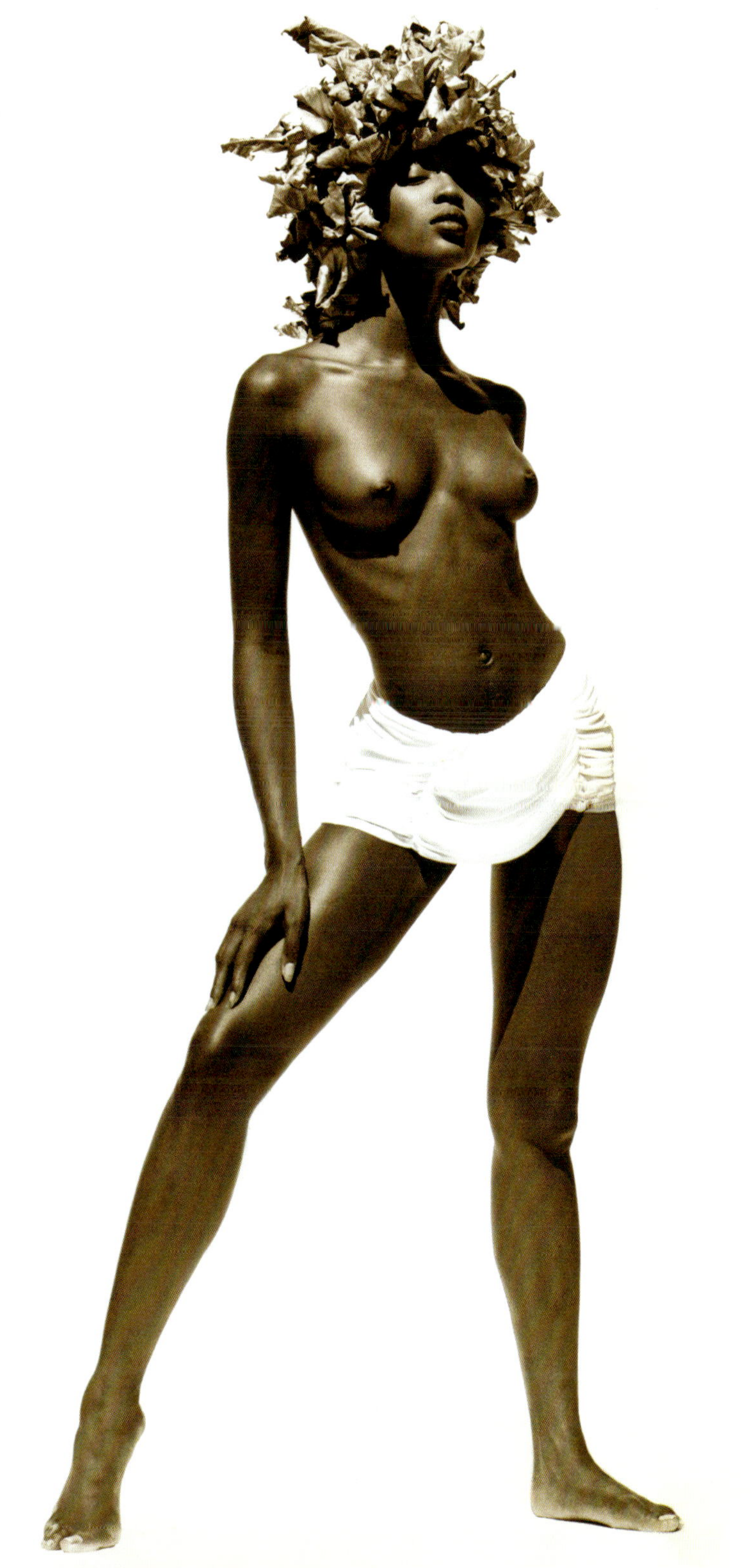

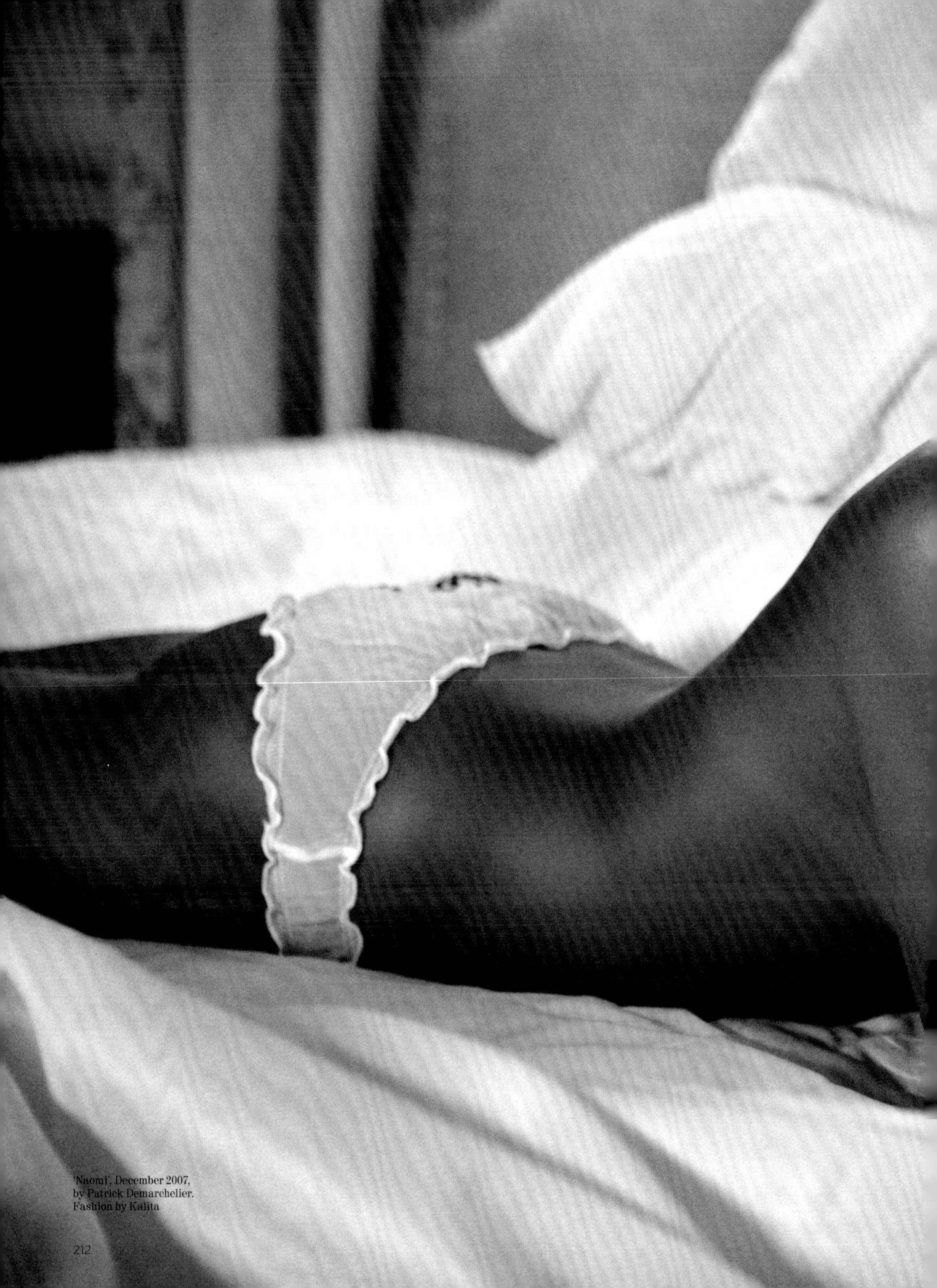

'Naomi', December 2007,
by Patrick Demarchelier.
Fashion by Kalita

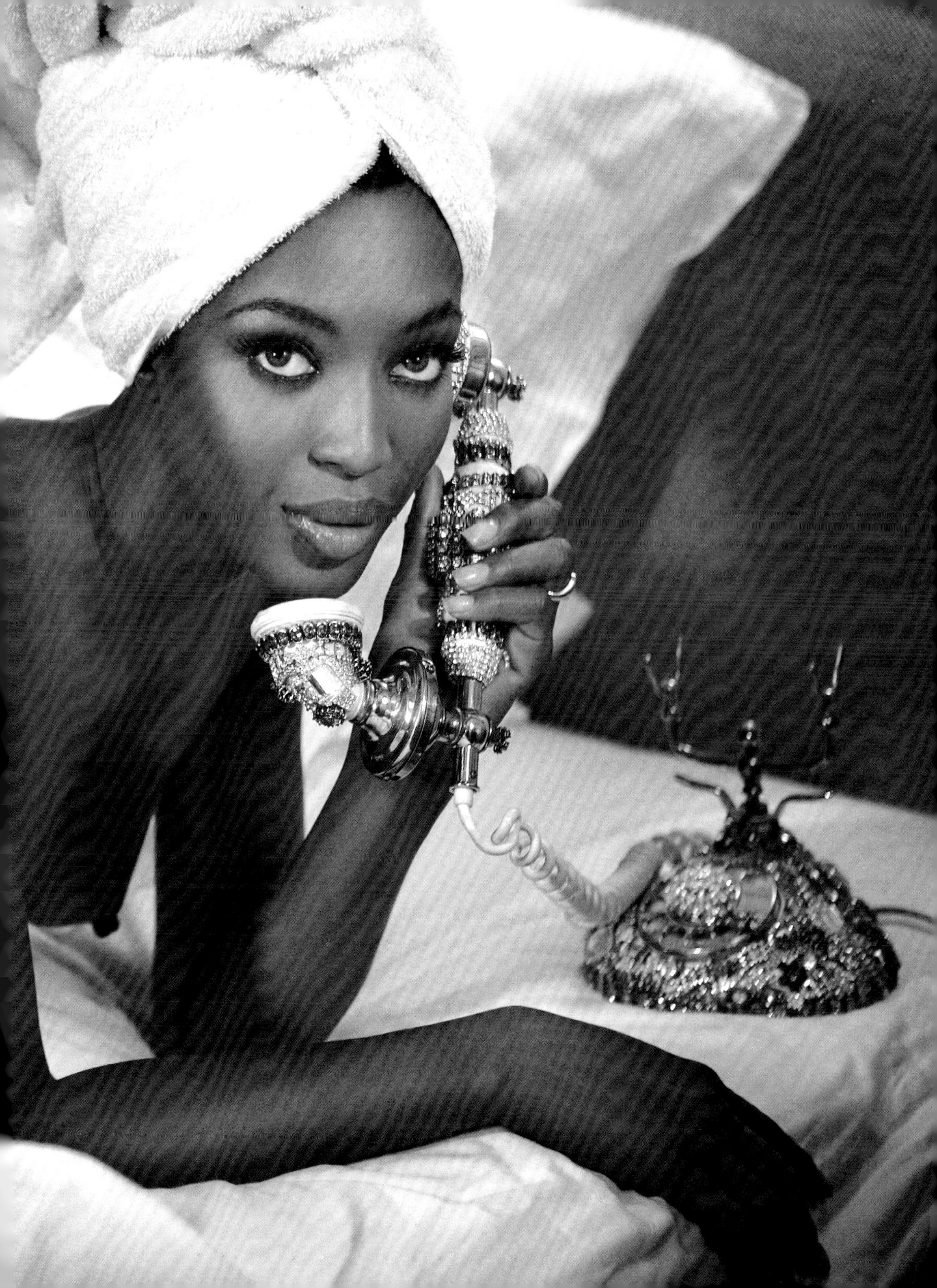

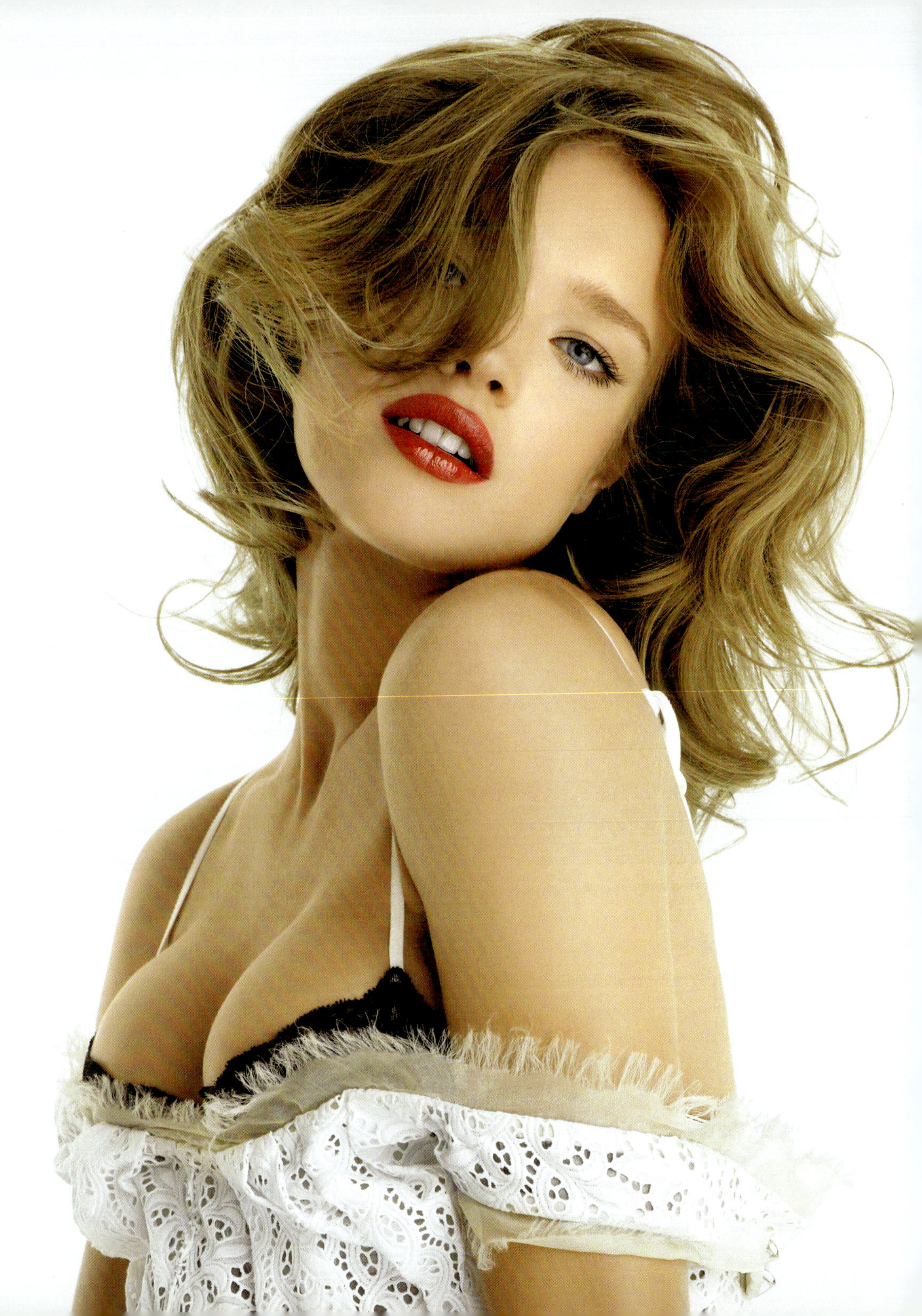

Natalia Vodianova

Of all the rags-to riches stories in fashion – and they proliferate – Natalia Vodianova's stands alone. And, as for all great folk tales, embellishment is pointless. The truth is strange enough. Married into British aristocracy, she is now the Hon Mrs Justin Portman, with three children and houses in London, Uruguay, New York and West Sussex. This is, to put it mildly, a far cry from her upbringing in the Russian city of Gorky. (Its name flutters back and forth over the centuries, depending on who is in power; currently it is Nizhny Novgorod.) The novelist Maxim Gorky was born there, and famously depicted life on its down side (there never appeared to be an up).

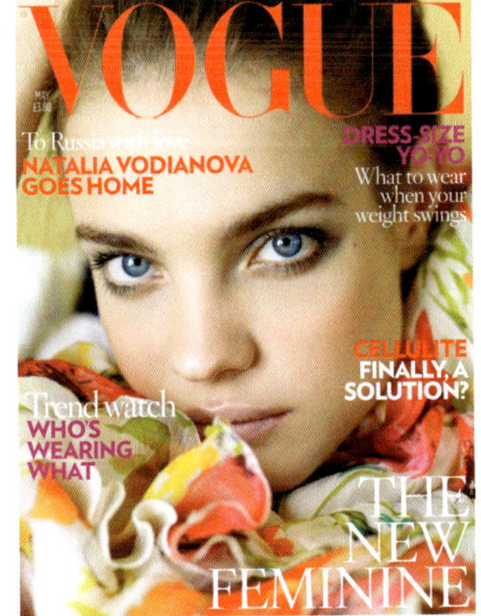

And bleak though it presently is, it was considerably bleaker in the Soviet era; there and then, in its bleakest part, you would have found Natalia, her single mother, and Natalia's brain-damaged sister, Oksana. Natalia sold fruit from a stall to support the family. By the age of 12, she was driving long distances to wholesalers and returning to sell whatever she managed to get. By 14 she was well known for her shrewdness and hard bargaining. She was also the one who dealt with the local crime syndicates. 'I would have to wake up and survive that particular day,' is what she says to enquiries. 'I would never look into the future.' Despite it all, it was not, she says, an unhappy childhood – just a hard one.

Three years later, in 1999, Natalia was talent-spotted by a visiting model agency (though Nizhny Novgorod must be near the bottom of any scout's list), who suggested she learn English. She stopped selling fruit in sub-zero temperatures, but applied her fruit-seller's work ethic and spoke it well in under three months. She moved to Paris, signed up to an agency and after that it all happened fast. She became the Supernova, a name given to her by Mario Testino that has stuck. So did Baby, given to her by Steven Meisel, chiefly because at just 19 she was the youngest of the current crop.

By 2001 she was married to Justin Portman, a then Paris-based artist and scion of a landowning family (large chunks of central London comprise the Portman Estate). Within a further two years, the Supernova had gone stratospheric, one of the world's highest-paid models, the face of Calvin Klein (in a deal said at the time to be its most lucrative ever) and something similar for L'Oréal. The work came pouring in. It was inexhaustible, and so was she. A youth spent scrabbling for lemons on cold streets in order to survive put paid to any hesitancy here. 'My agency has a Polaroid of me from the day I arrived in Paris,' she told the writer Yasmin Mills. 'And it's frightening. It says, "If you come anywhere near me, you're dead."'

Natalia's endless capacity for hard work and a productivity rate outstripping any Five-Year Plan has been applied with grace, guile, charm, style and tirelessness to her fundraising for the Naked Heart Foundation. The charity, her brainchild, aims to provide playgrounds and other recreational facilities – and hope and inspiration too – for children trapped in Russian cities with little to look forward to. So far she has opened 39 play parks, with the prospect of many more to come. The first was in Nizhny Novgorod, formerly known as Gorky.

Natalia Vodianova (b. 1982, USSR)

Opposite:
'Kiss Me Quick', May 2006,
by Patrick Demarchelier.
Fashion by Dolce & Gabanna

Above:
'The New Feminine',
October 2008,
by Mario Testino.
Fashion by Ralph Lauren

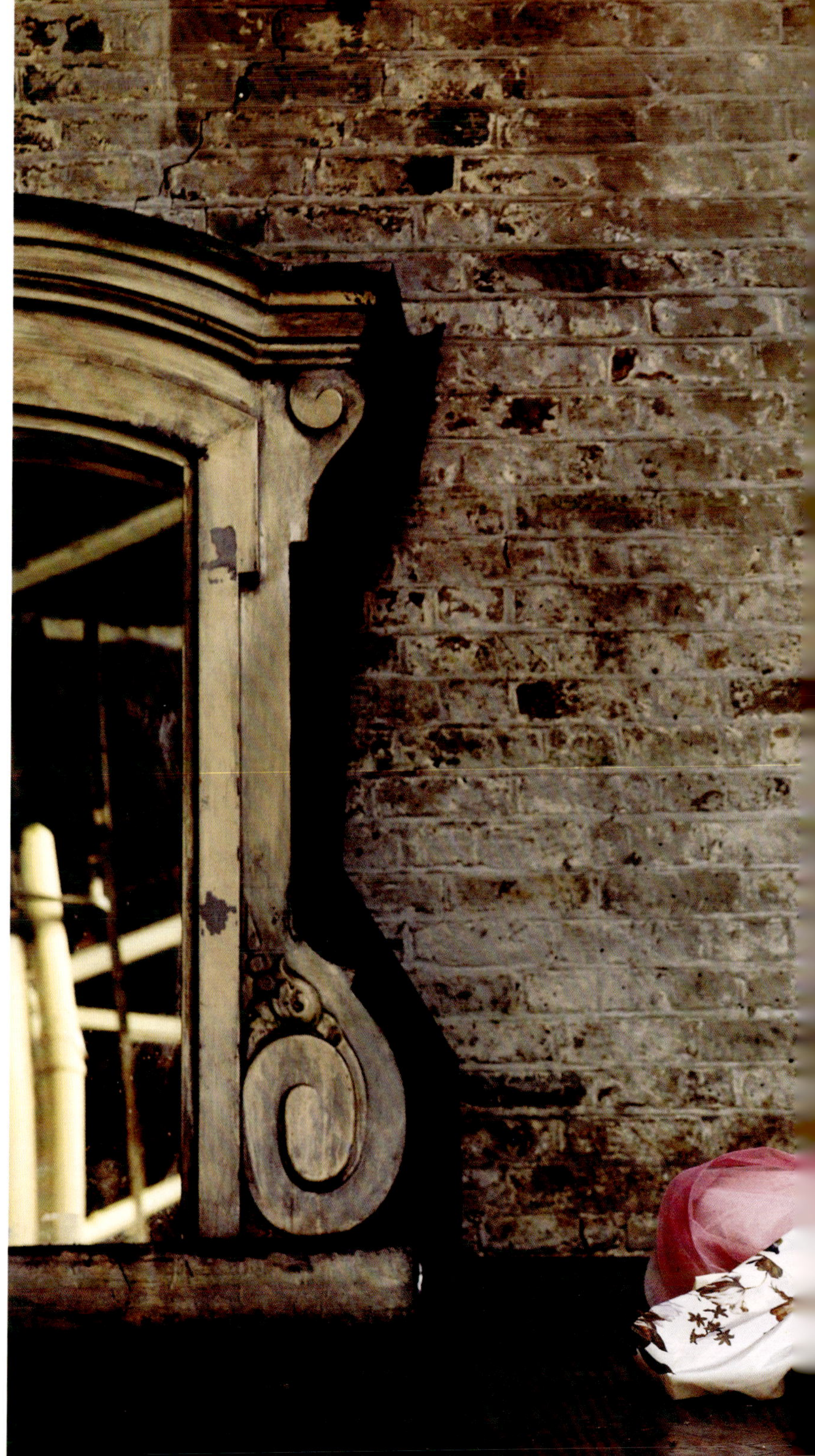

'State of Grace', May 2009,
by Mario Testino.
Fashion by Dior

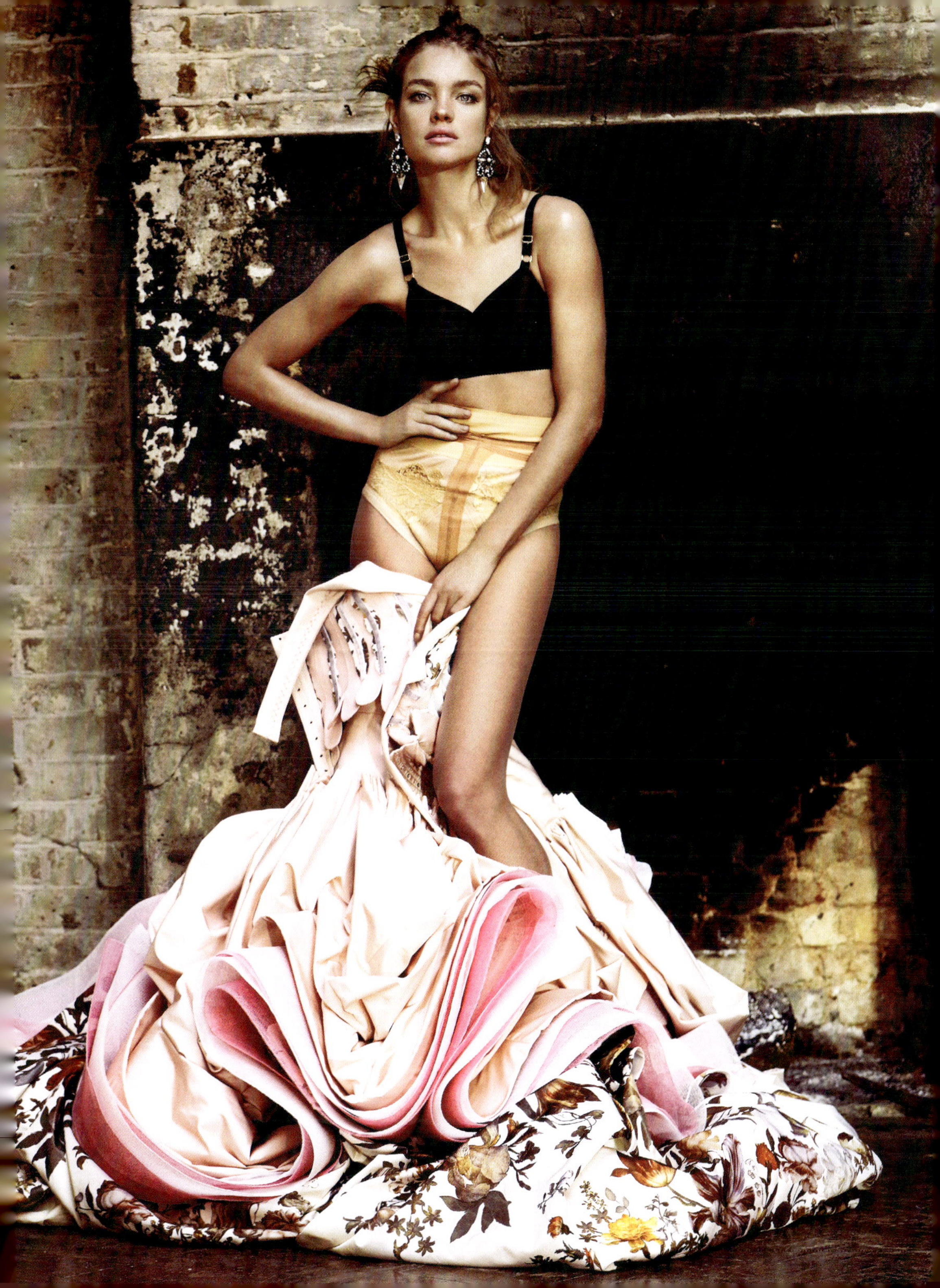

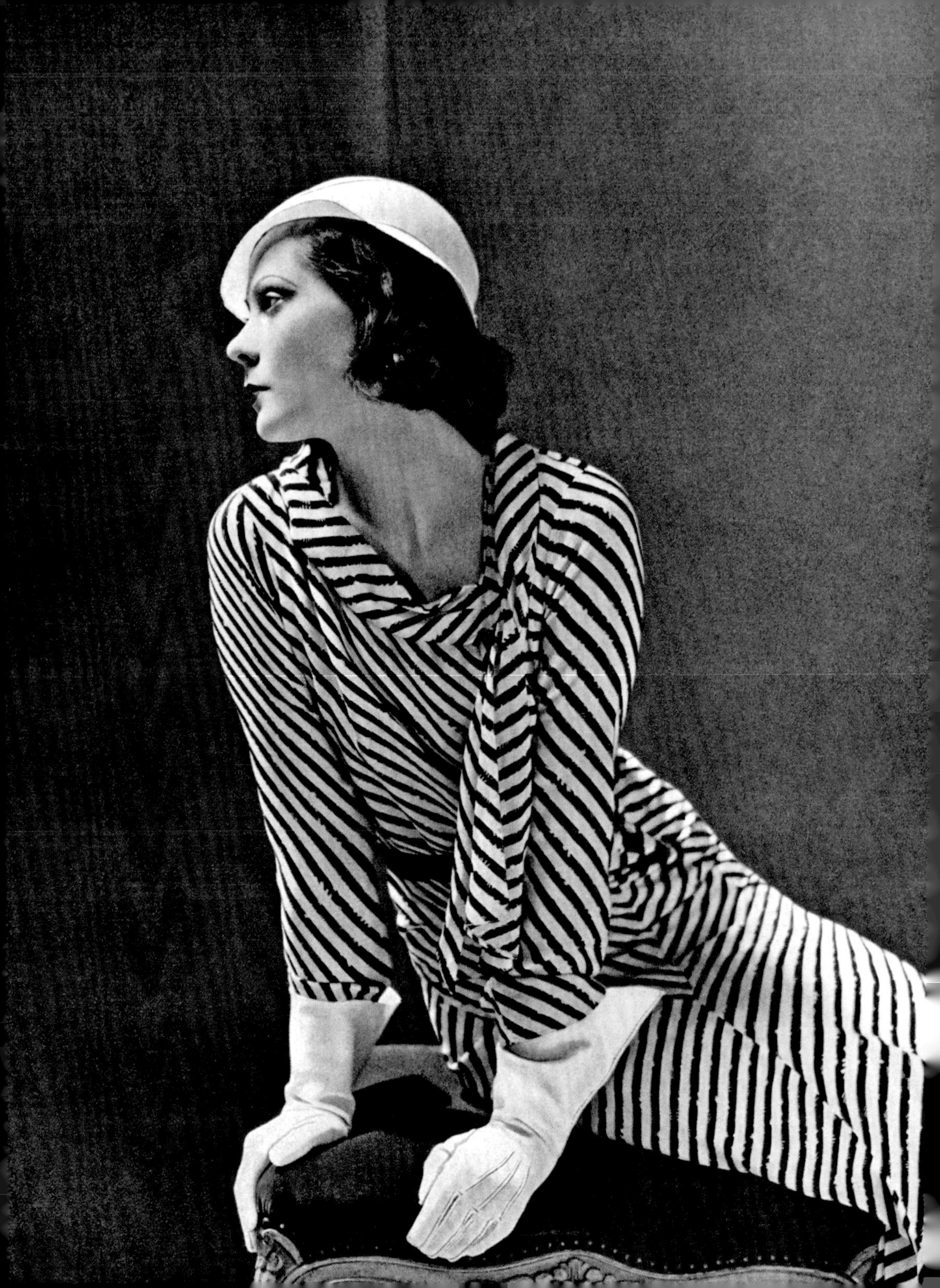

Natalie Paley

One of the most elegant women of her generation, married to couturier Lucien Lelong, and counting Jean Cocteau, Horst, Noël Coward and Cecil Beaton as close friends, Princess Natalie Paley was, unsurprisingly, a fixture in *Vogue*: 'One of the chic women who have *tremendous* influence on contemporary fashion,' it declared. Cocteau's devotion was unflagging – he claimed to have been her lover during the Occupation of Paris, which those who knew both of them considered wildly improbable. Horst was awestruck: 'We walked into Maxim's and everyone turned to look at her. The elegance and *noblesse*! She was astonishing…' Beaton was moved to rhapsody: 'Her eyes are star-bright and her laughter tinkles like a mountain stream over pebbles.' A granddaughter of Tsar Alexander II, she possessed stunning looks and the capriciousness of a thoroughbred. In her husband's sculpted creations, Princess Paley became the focus of many of early fashion photography's greatest moments.

Her blue-blood heritage was clear from her bearing and hauteur, but in pure genealogical terms it was complicated to work out. Unwilling to dissemble, *Vogue* did the calculations for us. She was a daughter – one of several – of Alexander II's eighth son, the Grand Duke Paul Alexandrovich, by his second marriage. Natalie's mother, Olga, was a commoner and her parents' marriage scandalised the Romanov court. The Grand Duke was dismissed from the army, his assets seized and the couple went into exile. Quite where the Paley comes into it, *Vogue* was at a loss to explain, though it is commonly supposed that Nicholas II pardoned his brother Paul and recognised the marriage with the Paley title.

This did not greatly improve the family's fortunes. The Revolution broke out and the Grand Duke and his family were placed under house arrest. In July 1918, the Tsar and his immediate family were killed. The Princess's brother Vladimir, a talented poet, was thrown down a mineshaft with the Tsarina's sister and finished off with a hand grenade. Another younger brother was shot. Six months after that, Natalie's father was shot. The remaining Paleys escaped, penniless, to Finland. (They walked.)

Perhaps as a result of these early vicissitudes and uncertainties, the Princess felt she never truly belonged anywhere, though she called Paris home. *Vogue*'s Paris-based photographer George Hoyningen-Huene made a Surrealist movie with her in 1933; as his collaborator Horst recalled it, it was not merely underground – it had no title, no plot and was never shown.

Her marriage to Lelong was one of convenience to both and each retained their own circle of intimates, though Lelong kept his wife in glamorous accoutrements. Hoyningen-Huene and Horst managed to be close friends with both, but photographed Natalie the most. Hoyningen-Huene had met her as a child at ballet class, as his father was equerry to the Tsar. Horst was sensitive to her warmth and lack of pretension. *Vogue* sensed a refreshing lack of formality too: 'Princess Paley is constantly being photographed in settings of incredible magnificence, but she really likes shorts or the briefest of bathing suits…'

Cecil Beaton considered that the Princess's sole rival in looks was Greta Garbo, and it was only a matter of time before a film career was given due consideration. That a couturier's wife and muse might also be a film star *manqué* was thrilling for *Vogue*: 'With Hollywood and a stellar role in *Les Folies Bergères* awaiting her, Princess Paley stopped in New York just long enough to pose for *Vogue* in two costumes designed in Paris by Lucien Lelong.' Their marriage dissolved as her film career took off, though it would ultimately be short-lived. She was cast in Alexander Korda's *The Private Life of Don Juan* as 'jealous husband's poor wife' and played an uncredited role in George Cukor's *Sylvia Scarlett*. She did, though, become a close friend of the film's leading lady, Katharine Hepburn.

The roles stopped and by 1937 she had married the impresario John Chapman Wilson, who had directed several Noël Coward successes. Though not a loveless marriage, the couple led separate lives, keeping their own *petit clan*. Princess Paley's appearances in *Vogue* diminished, but she never entirely disappeared from fashion circles. For many years she was a PR consultant to the couturier Mainbocher. She died in 1981. Natalie's friend Diana Vreeland recalled the tiny picture of her brother she always kept with her: 'one of those pathetic pictures you have of someone who's dead because you never thought of collecting pictures of your brother who was nine when you were 15.'

Princess Natalie Paley (b. Countess Natalia von Hohenfelsen, 1905, France; d. 1981)

Opposite:
'Madame Lucien Lelong', September 1931, by George Hoyningen-Huene. Fashion by Lucien Lelong

Nena von Schlebrügge

In 1958 – more innocent times – Norman Parkinson was on location in Sweden and scouting for new faces. 'I have managed to find out,' he told the *Vogue* team, 'the name and location of one of the smartest girls' schools in Stockholm, and I'm going to wait outside when the senior girls leave in the evening…' His prayers were answered: 'a shapeless beanstalk blonde who stood head and shoulders above her raincoated friends stepped out; "I'm a photographer; *Vogue* is doing a feature here in Sweden. Have you ever thought of doing any photographic work?"'

This was Nena von Schlebrügge's entrée to modelling. Cool and calm, she did not bat an eyelid at the approach and by 1959 was a favourite of British *Vogue*, becoming the face of its annual model contest. Grace Coddington recalled flicking through *Vogue* and thinking 'This is the most beautiful woman I have ever seen.' *Vogue*, however, damned the young Swede with faint praise: 'Could this be you? Out of the question you may think, but when Norman Parkinson first discovered her she was the unsophisticated girl you see pictured here…'

Parkinson took an especial interest in his discovery. Nena had a mother who cooked well and a German baron for a father. 'I never discovered who smoked more,' recalled Parkinson, 'Nena or her mother. The intake of both was phenomenal. Nena hardly had the frame to absorb all the nicotine…' He despaired, too, of her stylistic prevarications. She was neither hippy flower person nor Chelsea girl, but 'hovered between the two like some half-filled helium balloon'.

She made her mind up in 1964, marrying the icon of 1960s counterculture Dr Timothy Leary, in what was billed as the 'wedding of the Season'. DA Pennebaker intended to document the whole day in his film *You're Nobody Till Somebody Loves You* but the ceremony itself was never recorded, only the build-up and the reactions of the eclectic guest list: Diane Arbus, Charles Mingus and the singer/hairdresser Monti Rock III. The marriage, Pennebaker observed, 'was over before I'd finished editing the film'.

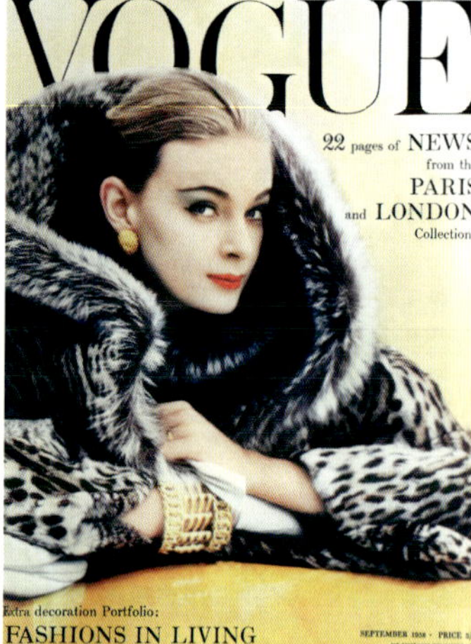

Nena and Leary divorced in 1965 and two years later she married another doctor (this time of Tibetan Buddhist studies), Robert Thurman. Their daughter Uma followed in her mother's footsteps and became a *Vogue* model before trying her hand at acting, with much success.

The last word ought to belong to Parkinson: 'She was an exceptionally beautiful girl and however you lit her always looked wonderful. I do not think many with her innate elegance will appear again – with or without cigarettes.'

Nena von Schlebrügge (b. Birgitte von Schlebrügge, 1941, Mexico)

Above:
'News from the Paris and London Collections', September 1958, by Norman Parkinson. Fashion by Bradleys

Opposite:
'Could This Be You?', April 1959, by Claude Virgin

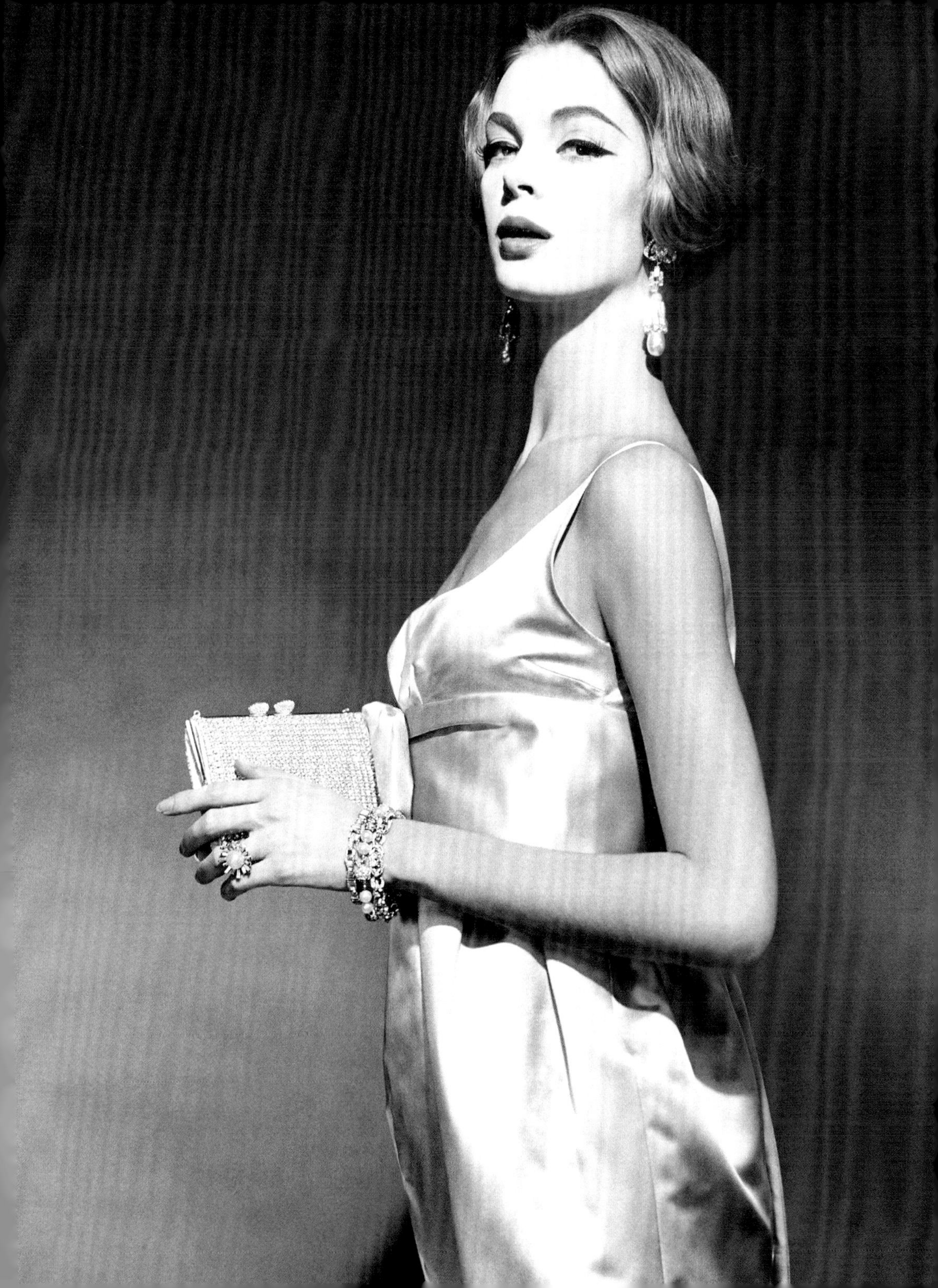

Patti Hansen

'I was always the energetic one – the model they'd hire to leap over fences…' Along with Lisa Taylor and Christie Brinkley, Patti Hansen personified *Vogue*'s fervour for the outdoor life. 'Their looks are the ones changing beauty today,' trumpeted the magazine in 1978. 'It's health! It's vitality! It's fitness!' It was also a lot of cosmetic enhancement by Way Bandy ('He slathered me in make-up,' Hansen recalled. 'But over time my freckles, which I'd always hated when I was growing up, were allowed to appear'), and a lot of primp-and-curl by Harry King, king of hairdressers, whose unkempt look brought 'wind-blown' to even the stillest location day ('My hair grew like a weed,' continued Hansen, 'so I never minded having it cut'). It also took a lot of Californian sunshine at the ocean's edge. Hansen's trademark was running through water with a happy, open-mouthed smile. Later it was shoots with the wind-machine indoors for the late Bill King, whose much-heard request was: 'Get Patti. She'll jump higher than anyone.' Hansen also had the highest, sharpest cheekbones in the business. You couldn't take a bad picture of her.

Hansen was born in Staten Island, the seventh and youngest child of a bus driver who also had a beachside hot-dog stand. For young Patti, the happiness and the proximity-to-water thing started early. There was little else to preoccupy her: 'I was pretty oblivious to the world,' she told *Vogue*. 'I mean, the whole Watergate-Nixon thing was going on but I wasn't really aware of it because I was down at the beach having fun,' she recalled. 'I don't think I even knew there was anything outside Staten Island, except for Brooklyn…'

Hansen started modelling at 16, photographed by a family friend down at the beach (where else?). With her blonde hair ironed long and straight, she channelled Jean Shrimpton – 'those Yardley commercials were absolutely *it*' – thus betraying that she knew there *was* a world beyond Brooklyn. The pictures ended up with Wilhelmina Cooper at her eponymous modelling agency, and she started working straight away, initially for *Seventeen* and *Glamour*, American *Vogue*'s baby sisters. *Vogue* followed on naturally and Hansen became a favourite of fashion editor Polly Mellen.

Her first big story was with Mellen and photographed by Arthur Elgort: 'Eighteen pages! Plus, the clothes were so grown-up – Halston, Geoffrey Beene, Bill Blass.' She was a favourite of Helmut Newton ('I would always be five or 10 pounds overweight, and Helmut would love it') and Chris von Wangenheim, who 'made girls look… *hot*.' Almost literally, as he placed her in front of a car which he then combusted.

Between 1975 and 1978, Hansen was on *Vogue*'s cover on a dozen occasions, but it did not lead to the type of multi-million-pound beauty deals that seemed to go Lauren Hutton or Christie Brinkley's way. Hansen put it down to the freckles or the relentless partying, or both: 'It was Studio 54 every night. Studio was great. It was my home, and I loved it.' This unnerved her parents back home in sleepy Staten Island, but what made them especially jittery was hearing about their daughter and Keith Richards.

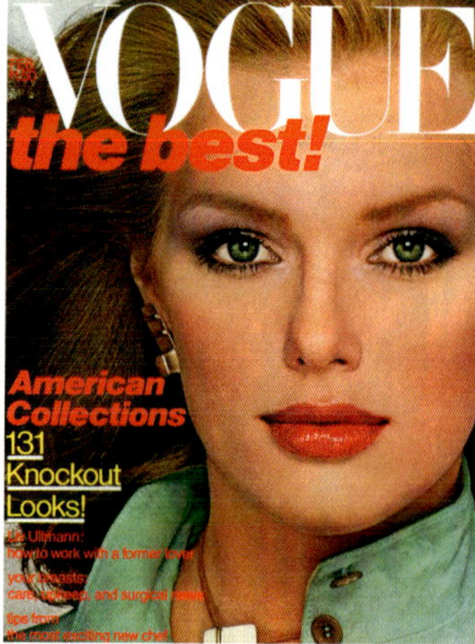

No other rock band behaved quite like the Rolling Stones, or looked anything like them – at once preening and almost effeminate, wayward and half-tamed. Guitarist Keith was said to pack a .38 to shoot out the lights, if need be, on riskier nights out. 'So on 18 December 1979, I drank a bottle of vodka, grabbed my gay friend Billy and went to Keith's birthday party,' Hansen told *Vogue*, 'and that was it. Keith and I spent the next five days together. And I haven't been with anyone since.' At that point, or not long after, she walked away from modelling full-time, right at the top, with her freckles now worn like a badge of honour.

Patti Hansen (b. 1956, USA)

Above:
'The Best!', February 1977,
by Albert Watson.
Fashion by Bill Kaiserman

Opposite:
'American Beauty Now',
February 1976,
by Arthur Elgort

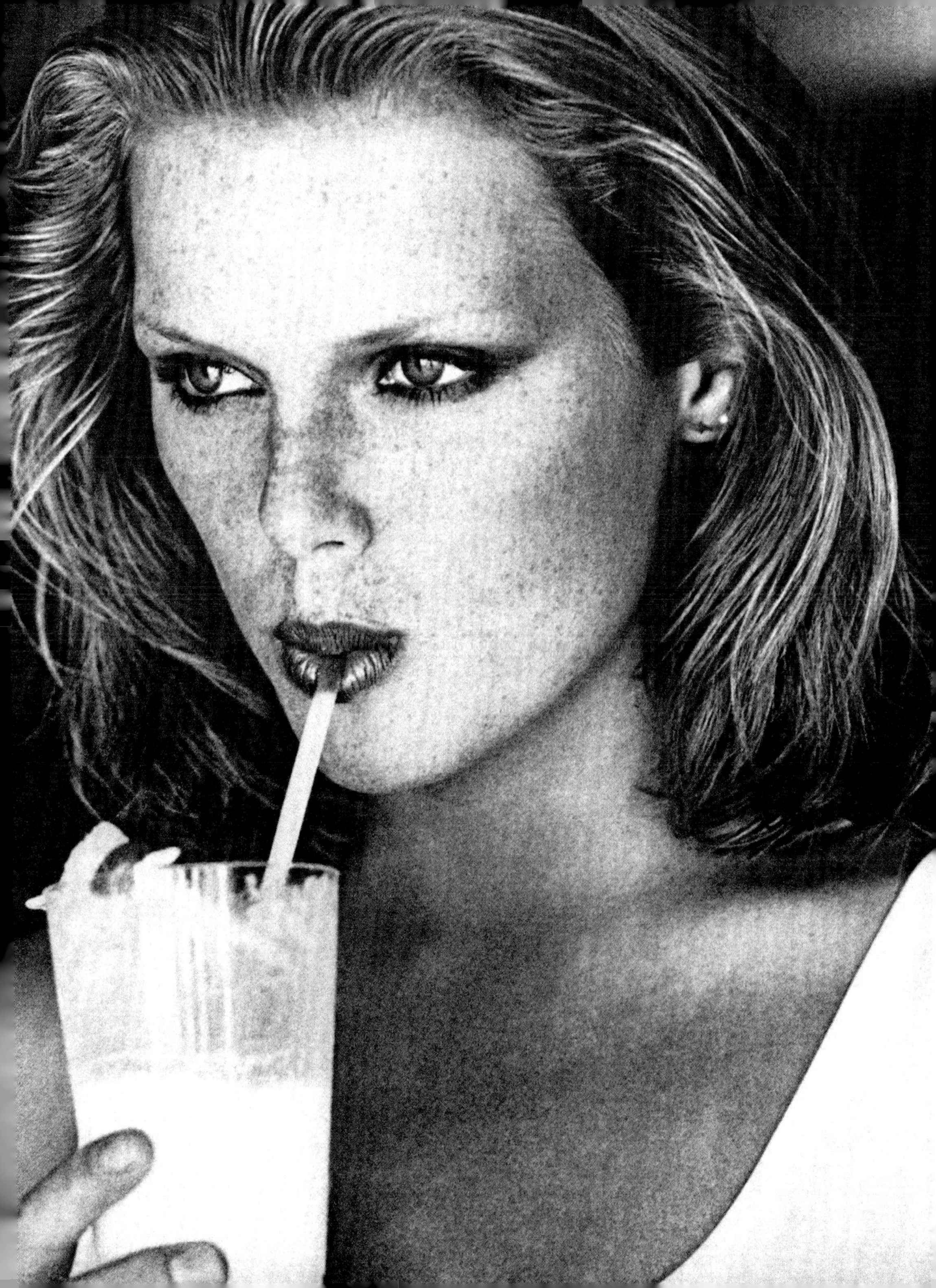

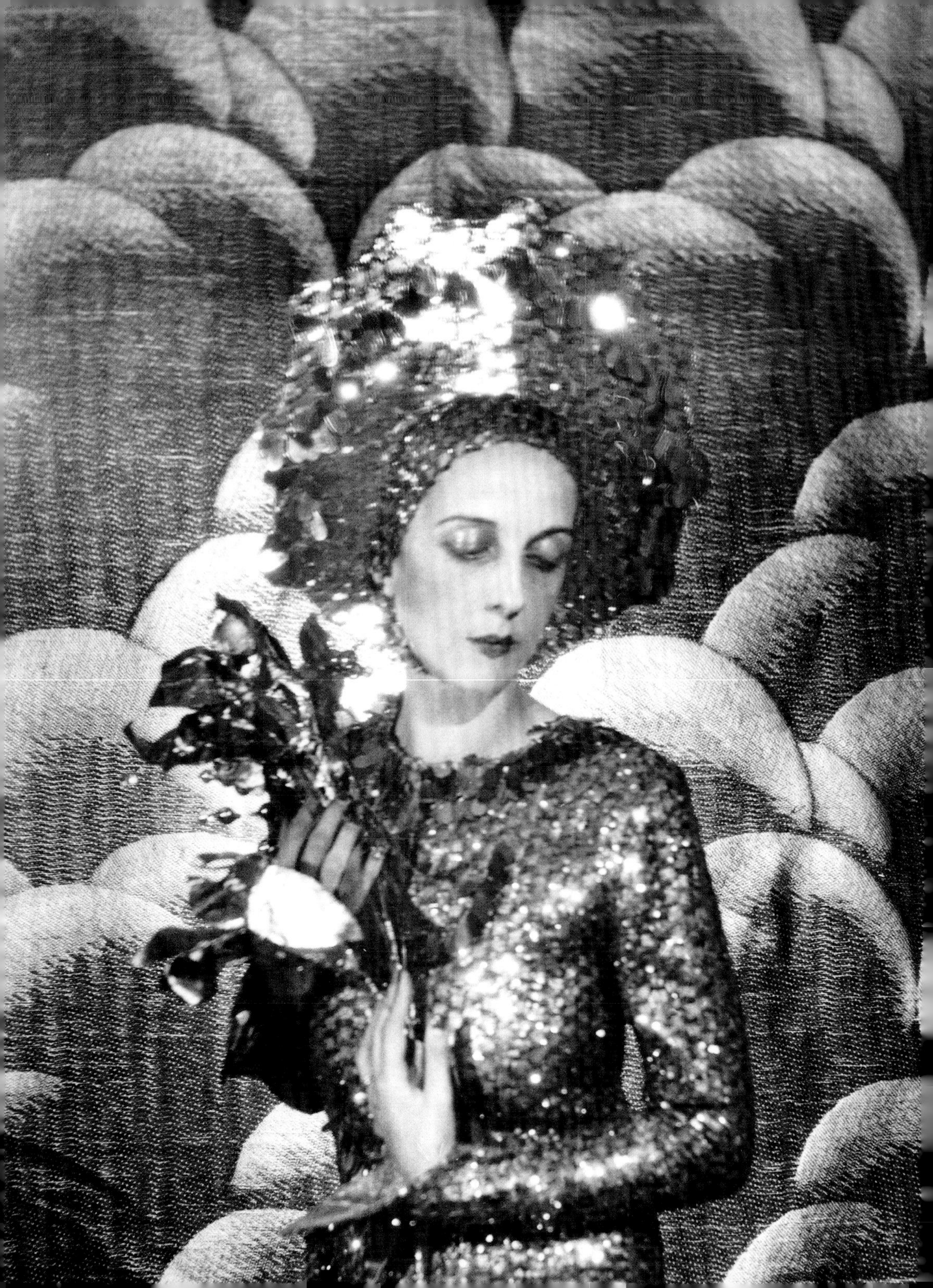

Paula Gellibrand

'The first living Modigliani I ever saw,' remarked Cecil Beaton of the orchidaceous Paula Gellibrand. 'Her enormous blue eyes were surrounded by a halo of dark mushroom-coloured fatigue, giving her the appearance of always being heavily made up... her hands were of an extraordinary flexibility and length.' Though Gellibrand was, according to many accounts, a perfectly ordinary upper-middle-class Home Counties girl (boarding school, hockey, riding to hounds), from early on she was something of a *femme du monde*, possessing a preternatural look of languid sophistication that spoke more of the Bois du Boulogne than Basingstoke.

A childhood friend was the equally astonishing Baba d'Erlanger, born and brought up by her flame-haired mother in Byron's former home in Piccadilly. When both girls promenaded in St James's Park, they were accompanied not by a nanny but by a turbaned Mameluke. Under the tutelage of the d'Erlangers, Paula Gellibrand made the most of her extraordinary appearance, dressing with a severity which showed it to fullest advantage: austere wimples, close-fitting skullcaps, unadorned linen shifts. Later, she introduced a trend by applying Vaseline to her eyelids to accentuate their natural sleepy droop. Her hair (when it could be glimpsed) was golden, and her face deathly pale.

Hostesses had to tread carefully if they were thinking of inviting Paula (who married the Spanish-Cuban Don Pedro Mones de Casa Maury and became a marquise) and Baba (who married Jean-Louis de Faucigny-Lucinge and became a princess). They had to fight shy of the pair's vast and ever-changing 'displeasure list' of socialites and style leaders. Bettina Ballard, American *Vogue*'s fashion editor-at-large in Paris, found them insufferable and their influence on the contemporary mode 'inexplicable'. *Vogue* was equitable, calling the Marquise's taste 'individual and original'.

'Bobby' Casa Maury introduced a streak of the daredevil to his wife's in-built languor. A brilliant aviator, he was also an indefatigable Grand Prix racing driver, usually in a fired-up Bugatti Type 22. Off the track he favoured a customised Bentley, and his wife would occasionally dress to match its pigskin upholstery, clad in what one observer described 'as a coat of honey-beige summer ermine'. Bobby was a friend and confidant of Lord Mountbatten, one of the 'Dickie Birds' who fluttered around the naval commander. In World War II, as chief of combined operations, Mountbatten was in overall charge of the ill-conceived Dieppe raid of 1942 and put Casa Maury in charge of intelligence. This proved an unqualified disaster. A more lasting legacy was Casa Maury's founding of the Curzon cinema in Mayfair.

The marriage did not last. On divorcing Paula, Casa Maury married the socialite Freda Dudley Ward (sometime mistress of the then Prince of Wales), and thereafter *Vogue*'s pages thrilled to two bewitching Marquises de Casa Maury (Paula briefly kept the Castilian title, despite marrying the war hero and diplomat William Allen in 1932). The first Marquise kept up her appearances in *Vogue* briefly but with vigour, shimmering in gold lamé. She caused another brief sensation by accompanying the Prince of Wales rather too frequently – to the theatre, to the races and to an appointment with a phrenologist.

Paula was immortalised early on as the eponymous heroine of Enid Bagnold's novel *Serena Blandish, or the Difficulty of Getting Married* (1924): 'When I talk to you,' says an ardent suitor of Miss Blandish, 'I feel myself endowed with your sparkle, your health, your hope, your vitality...'

Paula Gellibrand (b. 1898, UK; d. 1986)

Opposite:
'The Marquise de Casa Maury', February 1928, by Cecil Beaton. Fashion by Worth

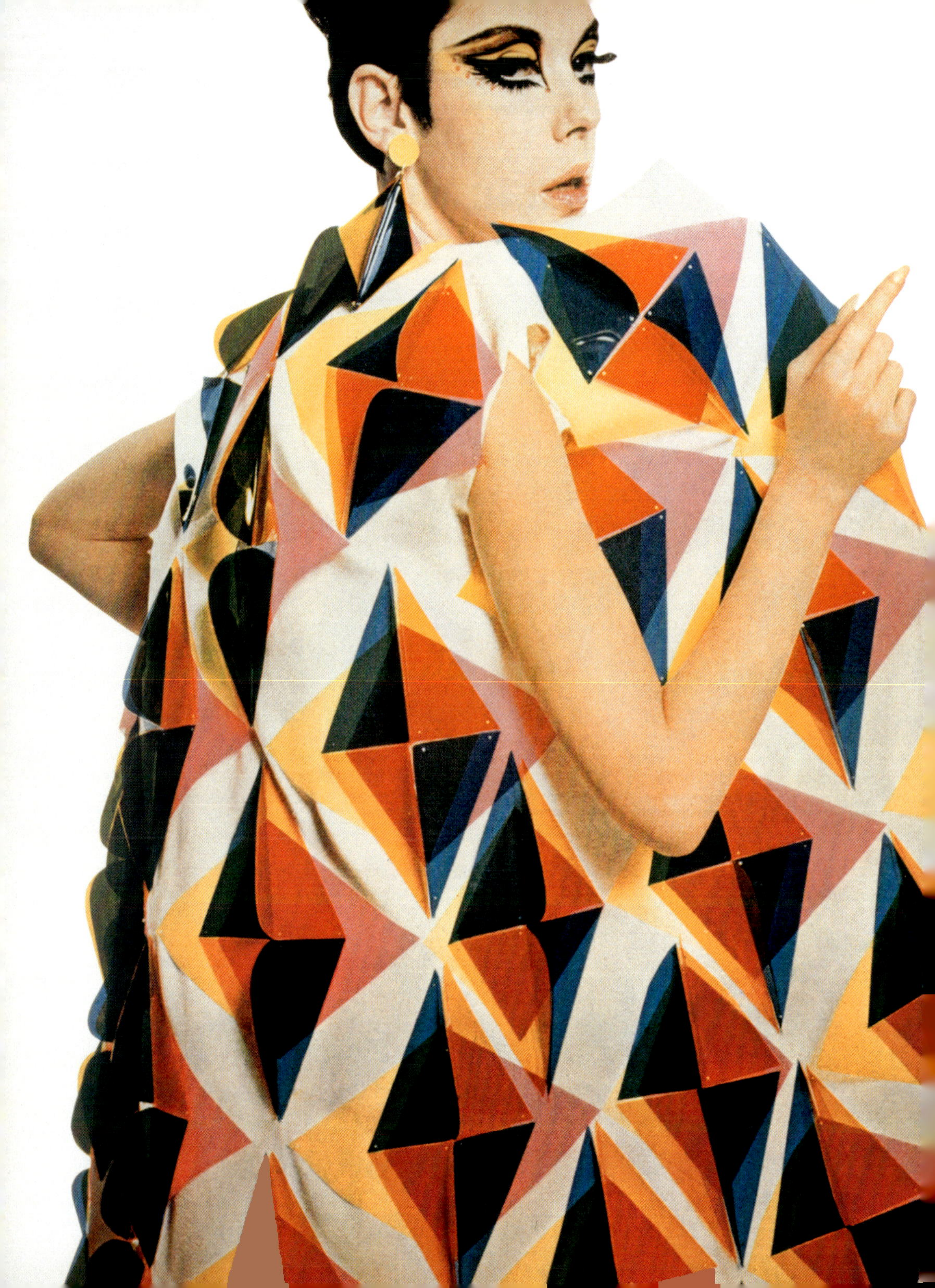

Peggy Moffitt

Once Swinging London had passed its peak, out they came kooky and krazy instead. Peggy Moffitt was the oddest, most off-kilter of all. A true fashion original, her angular bobbed hairstyle (the 'Five Point'), death-white pallor and unnaturally spidery false eyelashes spawned few imitators. She was the avant-garde personified, a difficult look to ape convincingly. For *Vogue,* the future of fashion was embodied by Venet's Neon-Lit Kite coat, enhanced by Paco Rabanne's plastic diamonds – a space-age design that was mostly unwearable. Together with Rabanne, Pierre Cardin and André Courrèges were able – briefly – to find a market for such futuristic designs. And Moffitt, with her geometric hairstyle, was a suitably otherworldly model.

She was the muse to avant-garde fashion designer Rudi Gernreich and, in conjunction with photographer William Claxton (later her husband), consistently brought his architectural patterns to a wider audience. 'Think of something in your life that took one-sixtieth of a second to do. Now imagine having to spend the rest of your life taking about it…' lamented Gernreich. This was his topless swimsuit, the Monokini, banned by the Pope and modelled by Moffitt.

'There are few models so identified with one designer and one milestone design in fashion history,' wrote Harold Koda in *The Model as Muse,* 'that they transcend the normal process of editorial validation.' Moffitt conceded that her job would have been more boring if it hadn't been for Gernreich's all-but-unwearable items: the Pubikini; the transparent-strap bra; the 'no-bra' bra; the Nightrider coat and dress. Moffitt looked curiously feminine, despite the clothes (or lack of them). Otherwise she was cast, often in the company of the equally angular Donyale Luna, as an otherworldly exotic, a handmaiden straight off a pharaonic tablet.

Moffitt started out as an actress, appearing in the Dean Martin and Jerry Lewis vehicle *You're Never Too Young* (1955) and with Cyd Charisse in *Meet Me in Las Vegas* (1956). She was an ornamental addition – along with Luna – to William Klein's satire *Qui Etes-Vous, Polly Maggoo?* (1966) and had an uncredited role in the *ne plus ultra* of the 1960s scene: Michelangelo Antonioni's *Blow-Up*. Gernreich died in 1985, bequeathing the rights to his designs to his muse, and in 2003 she created, in collaboration with Comme des Garçons, a collection inspired by his work.

Peggy Moffitt (b. 1939, USA)

Opposite:
'Looks with a Future in Paris', March 1966, by David Bailey. Fashion by Venet

Penelope Tree

One of the last century's legendary parties took place at the ballroom of New York's Plaza Hotel in November 1966. This was Truman Capote's black-and-white masked ball for the 'people I like' – all 500 of them. One of the guests dashing in from the torrential rain outside was 16-year-old Penelope Tree, who was surprised to be asked alongside Tallulah Bankhead, Norman Mailer, Frank Sinatra and Mia Farrow. Daughter of the socialite Marietta Peabody and Ronald Tree, the Conservative MP for Harborough, Penelope had first been photographed three years previously by Diane Arbus. The results only saw the light of day much later, as her father had threatened to sue if they were published.

At the ball Penelope met Richard Avedon and Diana Vreeland, his editor at *Vogue*. (Capote she already knew.) 'They both called up next morning,' Tree recalled. 'I didn't know Vreeland, but I loved her as soon as I met her – I think that's the reason I was attracted to working as a model. I was fascinated by Vreeland and Avedon.' The feeling was mutual. By the autumn of 1967, Penelope Tree was a star, winking with one impossibly long-lashed eye – the 90.38-carat Briolette of India diamond masked the other. 'She projects the spirit of the hour,' trumpeted American *Vogue*, 'a walking fantasy, an elongated exaggeratedly huge-eyed beautiful doodle drawn by a wistful couturier searching for the ideal girl...'

Avedon was entranced by 'the Tree', a counterpoint to Twiggy ('the Twig'), whom he had already launched into superstardom. 'Penelope,' he breathlessly announced, 'is never only of today; to each gesture she brings a sense of all the things that have ever interested her.' And this was typical of the epithets and descriptions that trailed after the quirky, ethereal Penelope Tree. Asked to sum her up in three words, John Lennon replied: 'Hot, hot, hot. Smart, smart, smart.' British *Vogue* was not immune to the hyperbole, declaring her its own 'home-grown flower-child' with 'weeping-willow hair, legs as long as sunflower stalks and eyes that see and know everything.' David Bailey called her 'an Egyptian Jiminy Cricket', which seemed at that time a fair summation of her exotic, huge-eyed look.

Bailey photographed her first for *Vogue* in 1967 and was on a strict warning: no swearing and no pouncing. Of course, he immediately did both, and Tree and Bailey made for a time a striking couple. They embraced the spirit of the era. (Tree installed a UFO detector in their London home.) 'In terms of fashion,' Bailey recalled of their seven- to eight-year liaison, 'she did lead me up the garden path a bit. She made me grow my hair long and dye it blue. And to wear things like a purple leather jacket that she had Ossie Clark make.'

Tree's looks were not what might be termed commercial, as she acknowledged herself – 'I was rather *gothic*' – and her career paled as the prevailing penchant for the unusual diminished. And she was not entirely upset about it. 'In some ways I felt like an imposter,' she recalled, 'like I'd made myself up to look interesting whereas the others were natural beauties. I was a kind of sham.' Like the Briolette diamond, she was for a time an exotic, enigmatic ornament.

Penelope Tree (b. 1950, USA)

Right:
'The Blossoming of Penelope Tree', November 1967, by David Bailey. Fashion by Kenneth Kemsley

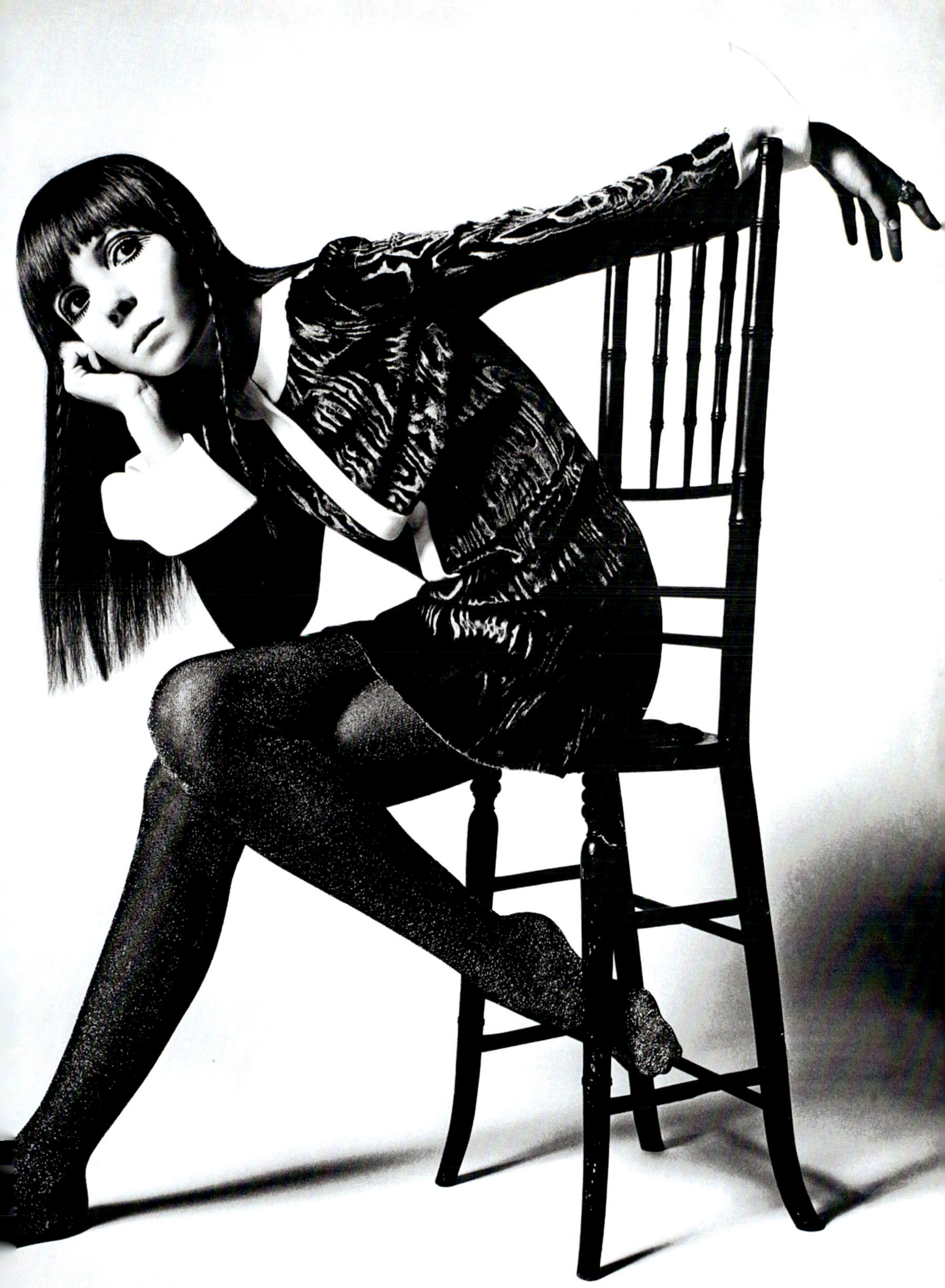

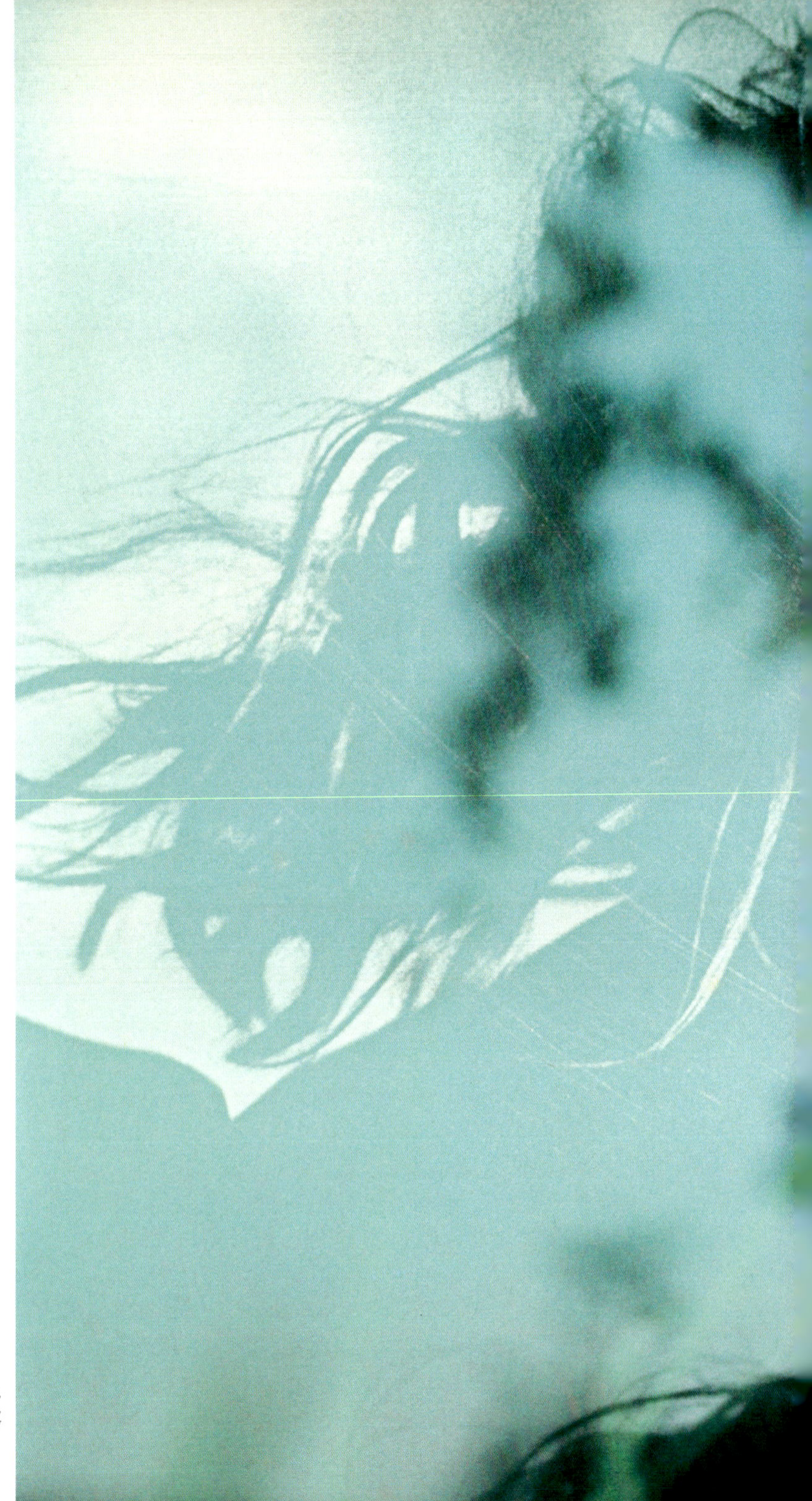

'The Word Is Unidentified',
September 1968,
by David Bailey

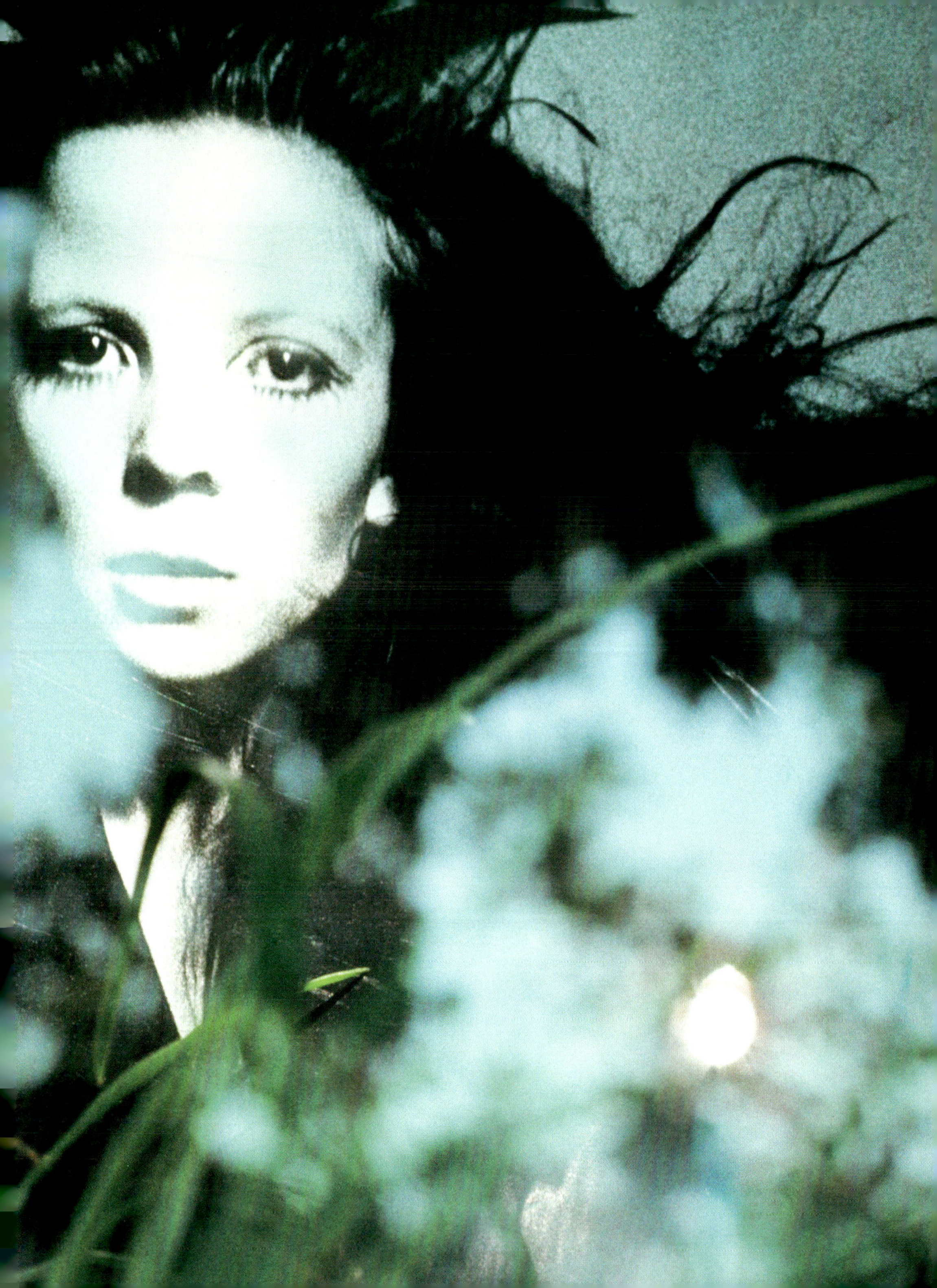

Sasha Pivovarova

'In Russia, we have proverb. Only bad soldiers don't want to be general.' Thus did Sasha Pivovarova from Moscow signal to American *Vogue* her intention to quit the other ranks for fast-track promotion. Supermodel status beckoned for the face of Prada ('that blank Prada look,' as one observer has called it, admiringly).

The serene blank look and elfin grace were put on hold for her most sustained moment with British *Vogue* – Tim Walker's 27-page epic 'White Nights', as meticulously planned as Napoleon's assault on Moscow but with more attention to detail. (Sasha revealed that she has read *War and Peace* at least twice, which is pre-production enough.) Walker suggested a two-week trip covering thousands of miles. (Red lights flashed and budgetary constraints kicked in at this point.) In the end, in the glowing white light of the midnight sun, on the Russian island of Eglovo in Lake Onega, Sasha was required, among other novelties, to sport 'swan's head' shoes and balance teacups on her head, as well as a gold plastic bowler hat. In so doing she revealed a playful side, unexpected from the Prada ice-maiden. Also unforeseen were the ministrations of the local priest. Glancing at Sasha, who was wearing a pleated lamé jacket in the evening light, he said approvingly: 'I am not sure what you are doing, but I like it.' However, the light-hearted trip was not without its moments of Chekhovian sorrow: two sisters sang old Russian folk songs, narratives telling of the death of traditional rural life. Moved greatly, Sasha wept.

Usually, Sasha presents a steelier aspect to the world, as her seven seasons of Prada campaigns show. She told one interviewer that the paucity of emotion in her face 'is inspired by the physical drama in silent films – it's cold and unreachable, like the stare of a sniper!'

Born in 1986 in Moscow, she was studying art history at the Russian State University for the Humanities before a photographer friend made a few exposures and sent them off to the modelling agency IMG (that is to say, straight to the top). Prada was her first stop.

With one eye on the distant future, Sasha has revealed an urge to create – a legacy perhaps from her studies and her childhood. She confessed to *Teen Vogue* that she played with coloured pencils while other girls played with dolls. She sketches all the time, with whatever might come to hand: charcoal, pencils, paint, itinerary papers, coffee, wine (although she abstains from the latter in favour of oolong tea). She has completed the illustrations for a book of Russian fairytales for Karl Lagerfeld. 'One gets the sense', said Jonathan Van Meter in *Vogue*, 'that, more than others, her life has been utterly transformed by modelling.'

Sasha Pivovarova (b. 1986, USSR)

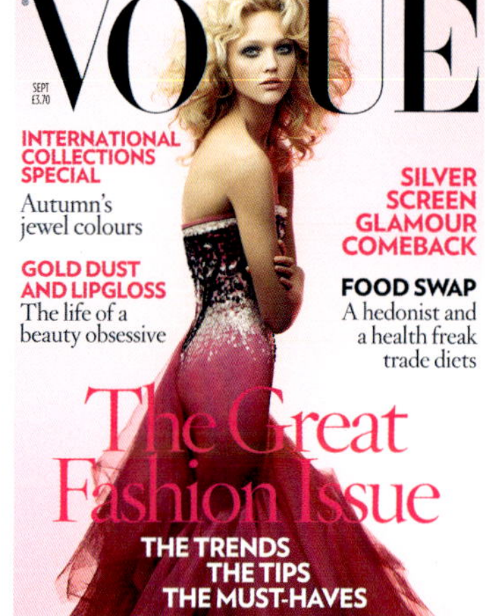

Above:
'The Great Fashion Issue', September 2007, by Craig McDean. Fashion by Dior

Opposite:
'Sasha', December 2007, by Mario Testino. Fashion by Vivienne Westwood

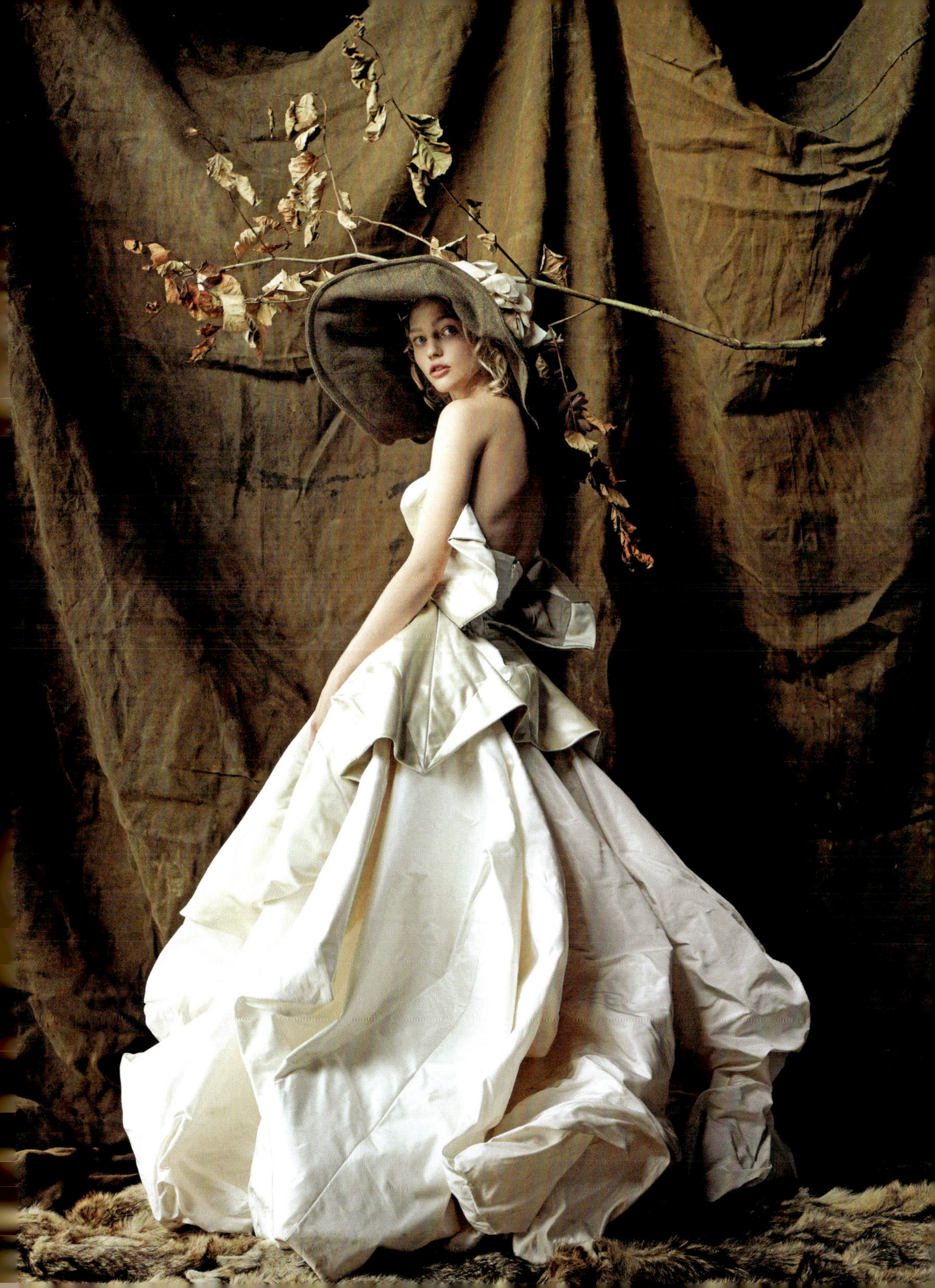

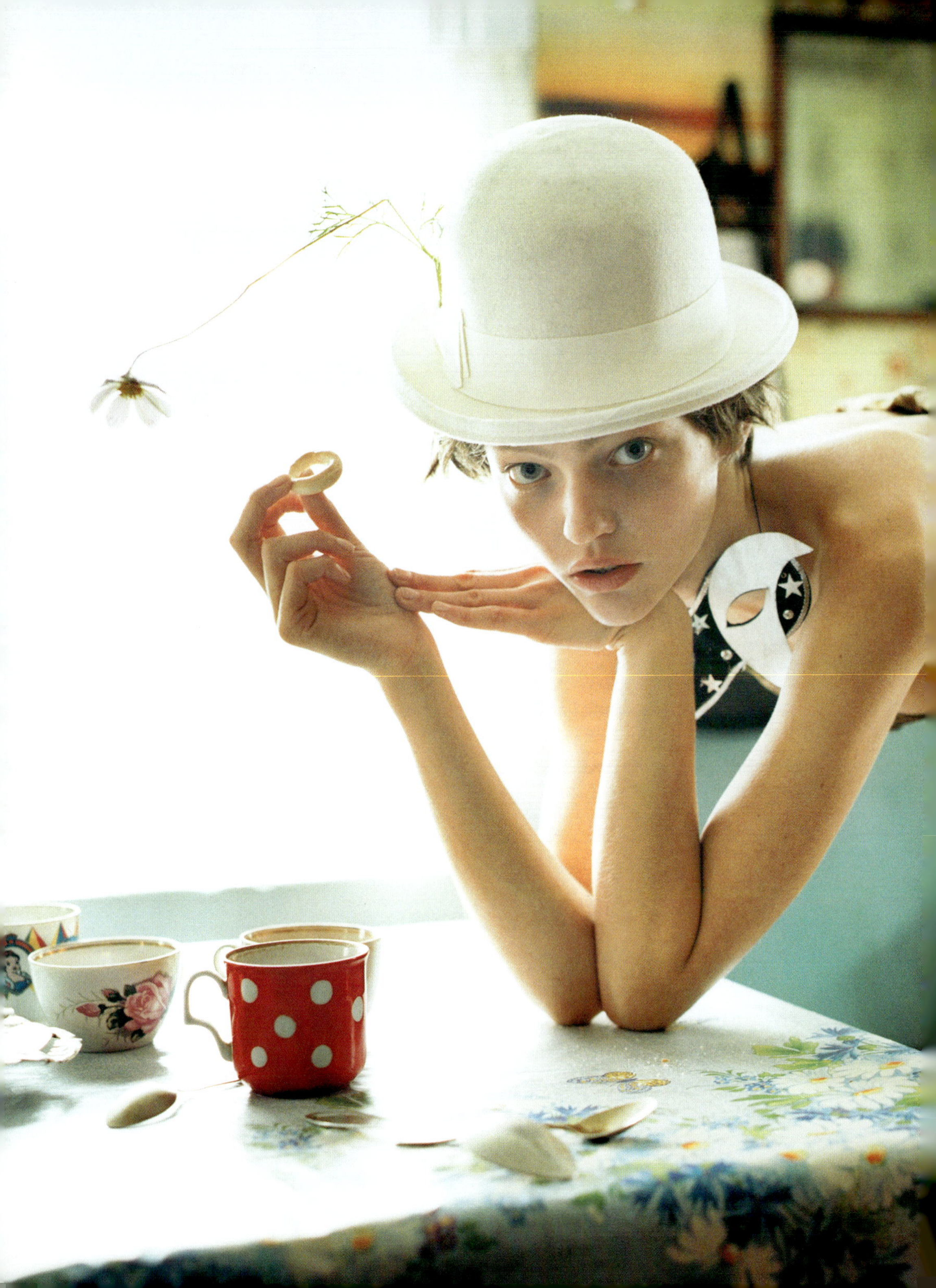

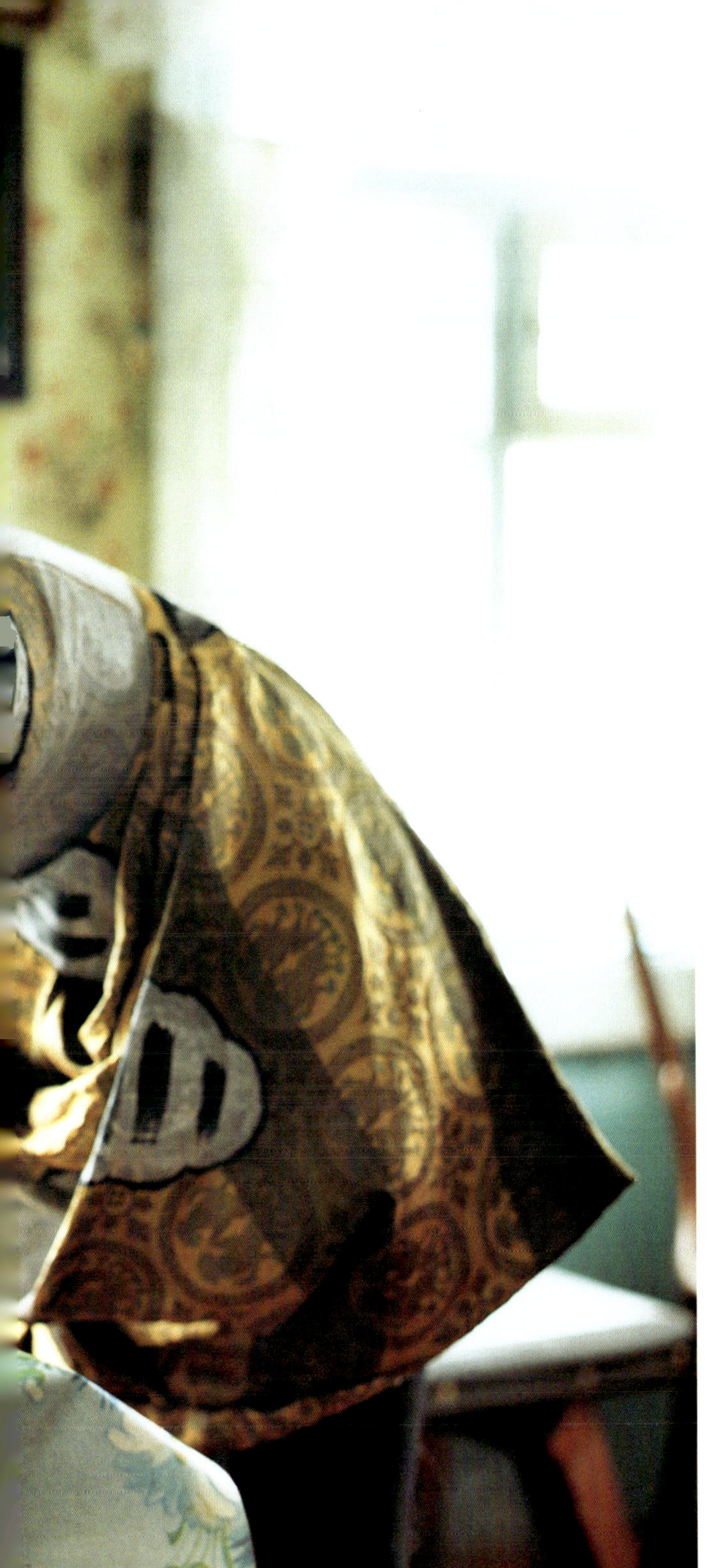

'White Nights',
January 2007,
by Tim Walker.
Fashion by Miu Miu

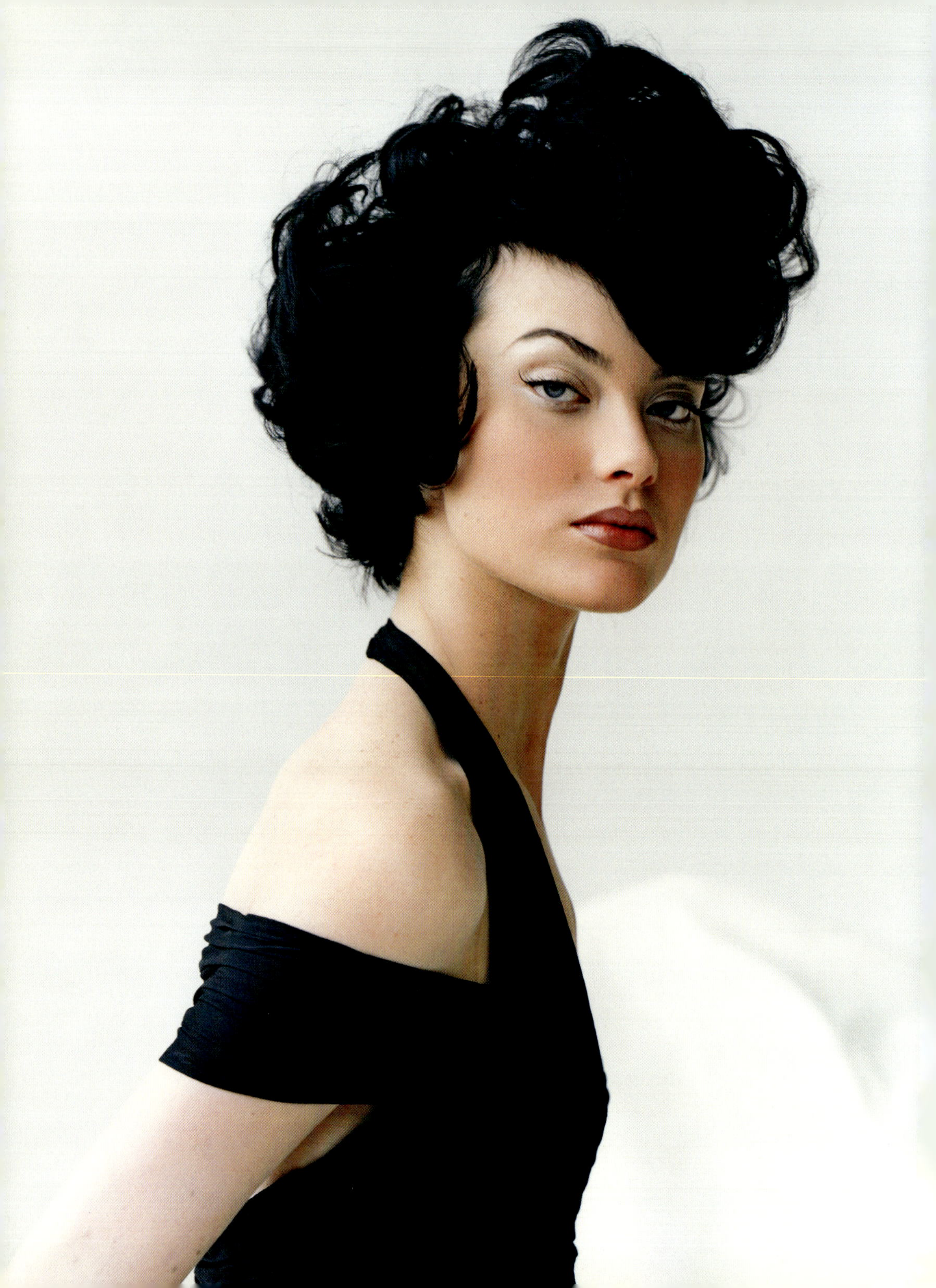

Shalom Harlow

In 1997, *Vogue* advised readers to look at almond-eyed Shalom Harlow while they could, for a career in Hollywood surely beckoned. Her debut that year in *In and Out*, a modern-day comedy of manners, was an eye-opening comic turn: she parodied a supermodel, obsessed with her diet, her boyfriend and, naturally, herself. *Vogue* lauded it as a screwball performance *par excellence*.

In the years that followed, she has carved out a career with roles large and not so large, with auteurs in small independents and with bigger names with bigger budgets. To each she brings the elegance and assurance that marked her out in her first incarnation as a star, back then in the Supermodel Mark II era – Shalom, Amber, Stella, Nadja and Kate were more approachable, more natural versions of their immediate predecessors (Linda, Christy, Naomi, Cindy). This second generation, *Vogue* observed, 'arrived too late to be intoxicated by the excesses of the 1980s'. Karl Lagerfeld revered their youth and unspoilt attitude: 'Of course, they are very young,' he told the magazine, 'very much like children… like an elf. There is a kind of vulnerability about them. They need protection.' Shalom was singled out by many for her catwalk presence, luminous skin and eyes that transfixed equally in the second and third dimensions.

In those now far-off days, Shalom and Amber were the best of friends, pictured together on the cover of three *Vogues* – Italian, British and American. 'Call them the new bohemians,' said *Vogue*. 'Amber and Shalom come from patchouli-soaked peace-and-love backgrounds. Both former Grateful Dead fans, they'd heard about each other before…'

On duty, neither particularly lived up to the 'Deadhead' stereotype, but an enthusiasm for music and movement is vital in the Harlow story, helping that rhythmic catwalk sway. She was discovered at a Cure concert in Toronto – her parents had fled there from post-revolutionary Grenada – and she studied ballet for a while, funding it from a paper round. And if modelling ever entered her young world, it was in the form of the original supermodels, whom she would later hold in the highest regard for starting it all ('She's my idol,' Harlow said of Linda Evangelista, 'she's a model's model') and who paved the way for her to take a different approach. 'The difference is our down-to-earthness,' she told *Vogue*. 'We make a conscious effort not to let the stardom go to our head.' She added, wistfully, 'I've sold my youth.'

Shalom has returned to modelling after a decade and a bit in the film industry, appearing in British *Vogue* in 2010 – big-haired but still gazelle-like – for a Douglas Sirk-style housewife-in-suburbia fantasy. Being older has brought a more balanced perspective to her *modus operandi*: 'I feel my beauty now, whereas before I couldn't recognise it.' And she believes she is far healthier now than then, telling *Vogue*'s Sarah Mower, 'I was too thin. I was working all the time. Spaghetti bolognese on planes…' Surgical enhancement is not at all on the horizon. 'For actresses, I can see that it's not easy to pass through your thirties and forties, but I admire the ones who have not had things done.'

Shalom Harlow (b. 1973, Canada)

Opposite:
'Couture Culture',
April 1995,
by Mario Testino.
Fashion by Valentino

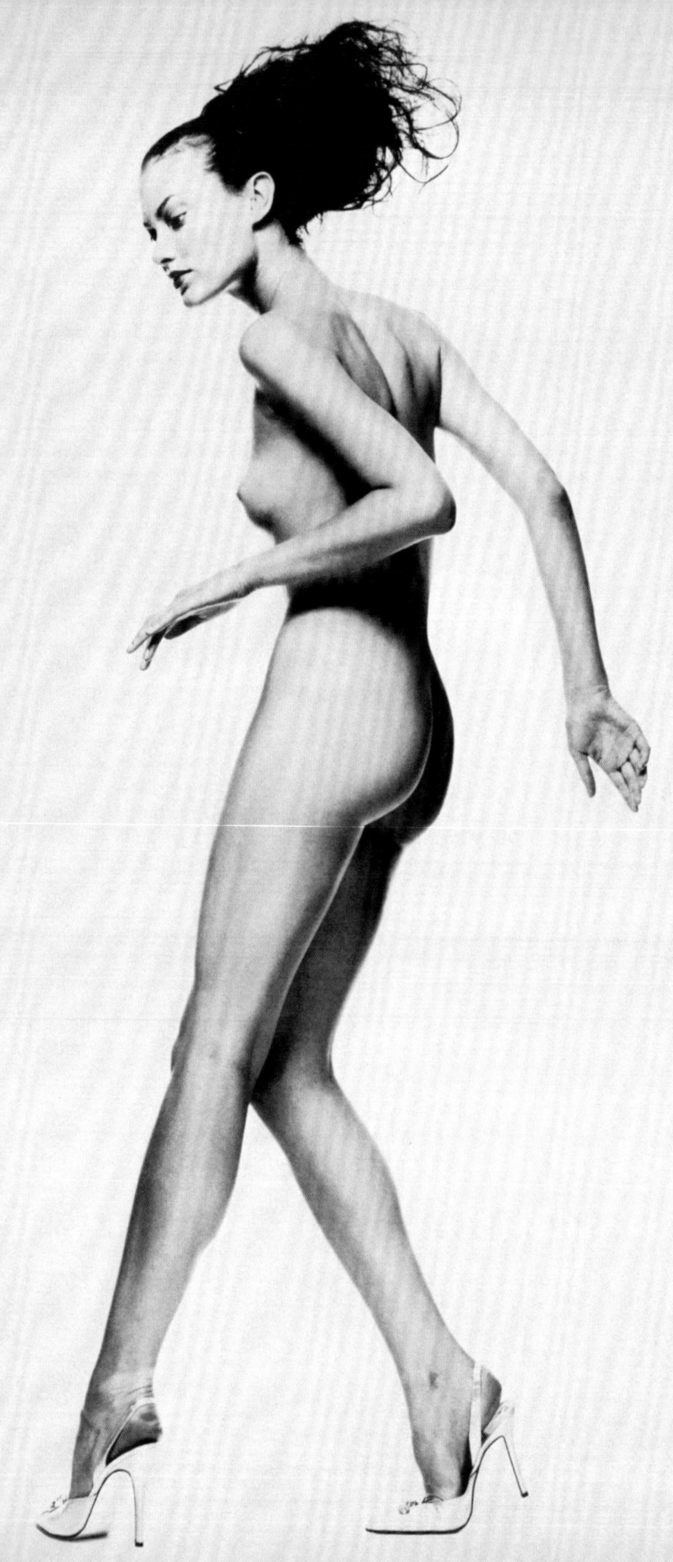

This page:
'The Couture', October 1995,
by Nick Knight.
Shoes by Atelier Versace

Opposite:
'Far from Heaven',
June 2010,
by Javier Vallhonrat.
Fashion by Dolce & Gabbana

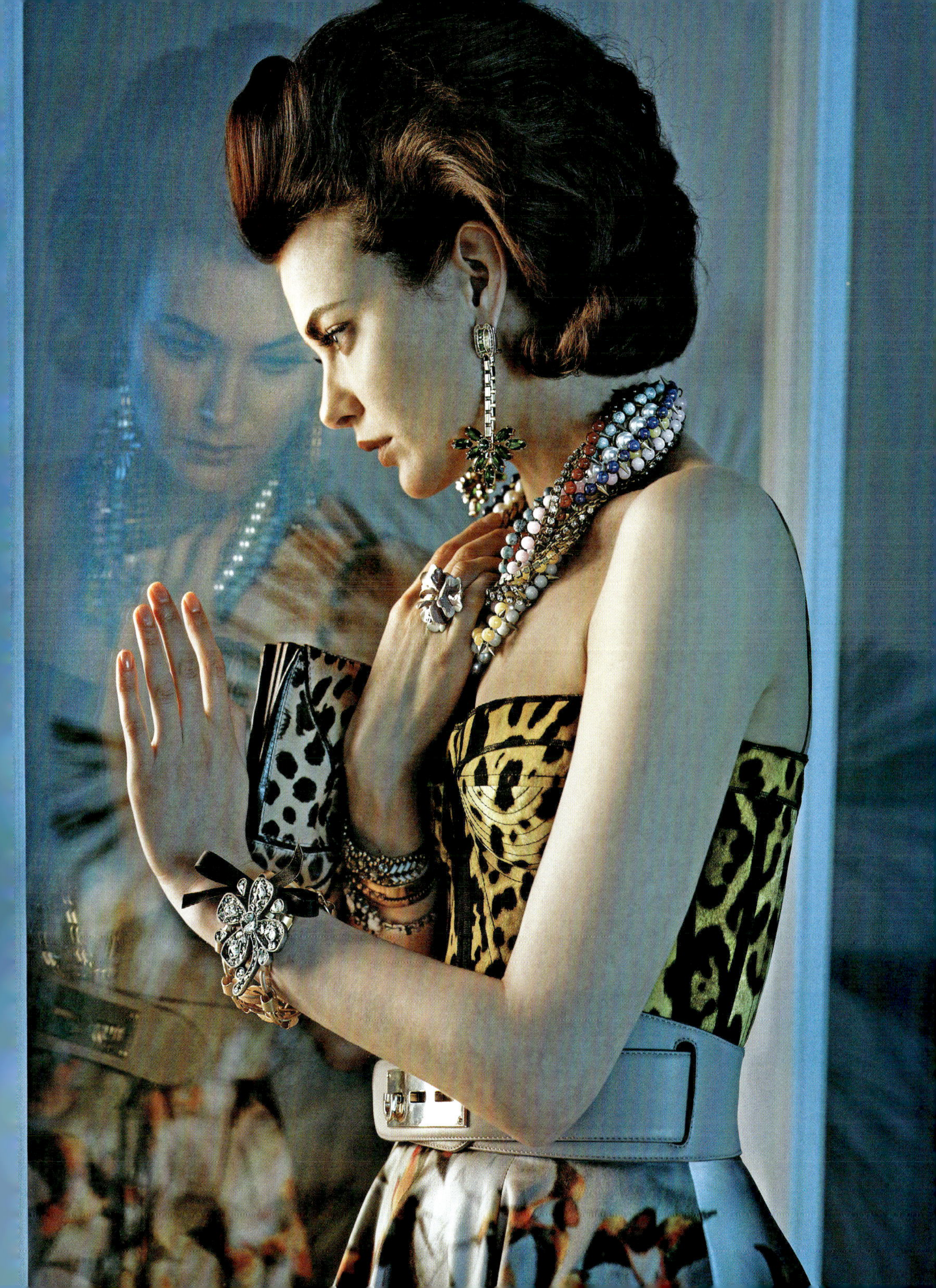

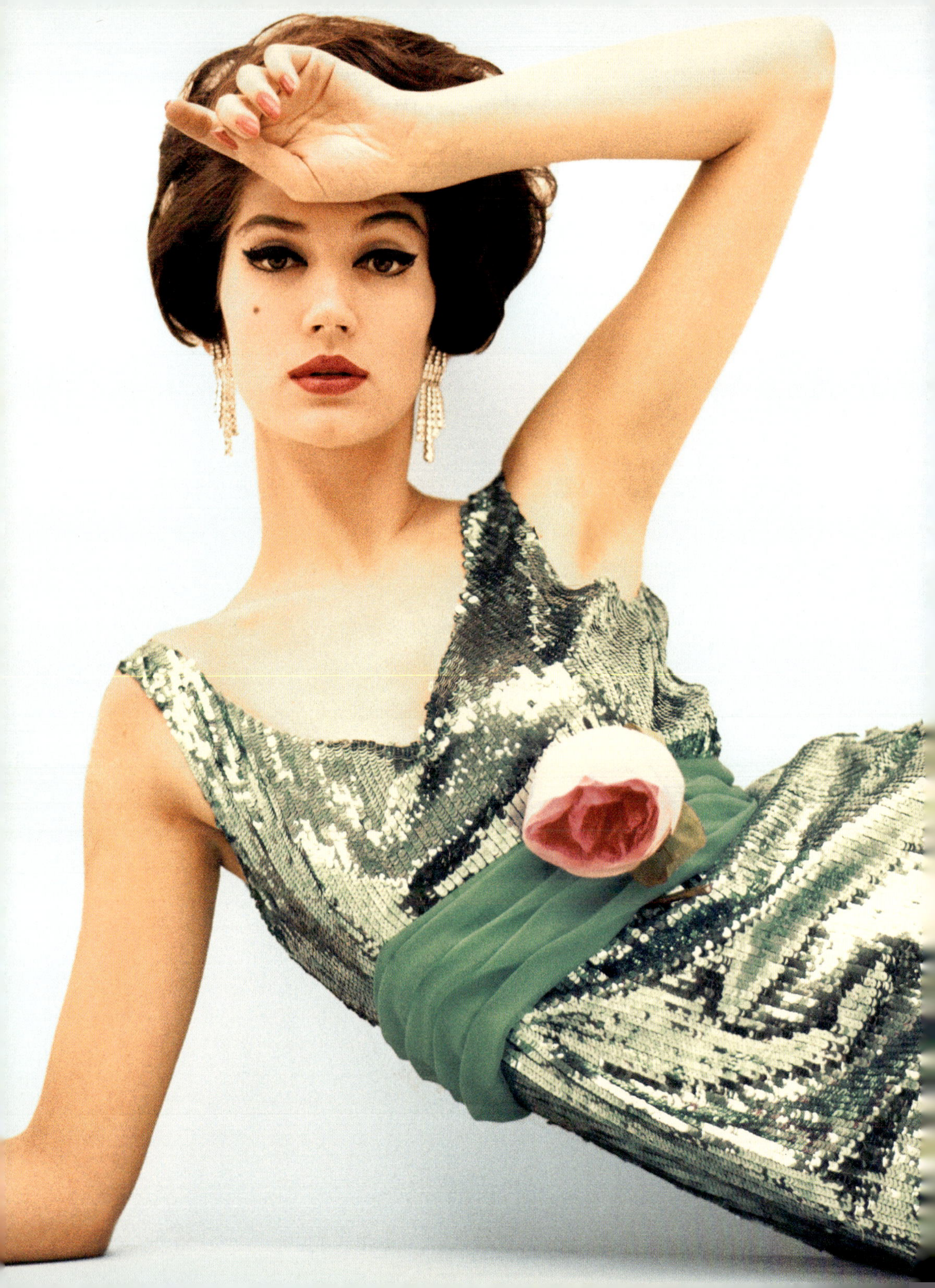

Simone d'Aillencourt

With her *vrai Parisienne* looks (including the obligatory beauty spot), Simone d'Aillencourt is best remembered for propelling herself along the early-morning banks of the Seine in a large Perspex bubble, like a hamster trapped inside a pet-shop novelty. This was not for enjoyment, but for the fashion photographs of Melvin Sokolsky at *Harper's Bazaar*. This *mise-en-scène* has been much copied, where possible, in capital cities across the globe. Simone was in the vanguard of the French model invasion of the 1950s. With their haughtiness and innate sense of chic, they broke through international barriers to become stars in Britain and the United States. Bettina had laid the trail earlier, and it's fair to say that Nicole de la Marge and the exotic Praline might have hogged the limelight, but two separate and fatal car crashes spelt the end of any dreams there. With Bettina having given up modelling for a romance with Aly Khan, the crown was Simone's to assume.

She was intrepid and hard-working. With her colleague Dorothy McGowan she was the star of William Klein's witty surrealist vignettes on the streets of Paris, New York and Rome, which outplayed his rivals in originality and verve. Klein's models usually refused to run and jump across the sidewalks, but stood silently in the road, like showroom mannequins dumped in the traffic. This frequently led to incidents from which Klein was often absent, as he might be some distance away from the action, armed with a powerful telephoto lens. One set saw Simone in an extravagant ballgown and long evening gloves in the middle of the Champs-Elysées with traffic squealing to a halt around her. The urgency of her strange gestures, those of a policeman quick on the scene and the steam rising from the Parisian streets gave the pictures a surreal and off-kilter appearance.

Simone had never intended to become a model. A stay in London, where she had come to improve her English, had prompted her in that direction – so many people had assumed she was an exotic French model that she felt she ought to oblige. She signed up at the Lucie Clayton Agency and it turned out she was a natural. In those days, models turned up at shoots expected to perform miracles with their hair and make-up. 'I don't think I'm pretty or beautiful, but I do love fashion and I could transform myself very quickly to suit whatever I was wearing,' she said later.

When modelling became less attractive for Simone, she opened her own agency, Models International, which blossomed. Her discoveries included Helmut Newton favourites Vibeke Knudson and Apollonia van Ravenstein. Following her success in Paris, Simone established an agency in Milan, World, which did not repeat its Parisian sister's success. Someone firebombed the building and its doors – or what was left of them – closed forever.

Simone d'Aillencourt (fl. 1956–1964)

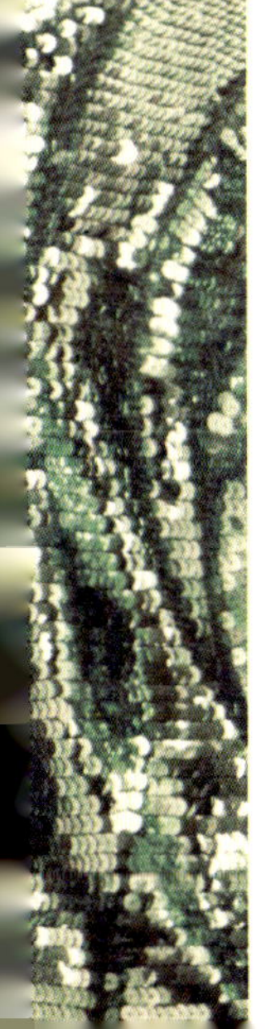

Left:
'Glamour Girl', September 1958, by Claude Virgin. Fashion by Frederick Starke

Stella Tennant

The granddaughter of the 10th Duke of Devonshire and fourth cousin, once removed, to the late Diana, Princess of Wales, Stella Tennant might on first glimpse appear to be a throwback to the days of the well-bred, impeccably behaved mannequin: stateliness, arched eyebrows, furled umbrellas, twinsets and tweed. However, Stella has striven never to be predictable or conventional, although the languid elegance of Barbara Goalen and the barely smiling demeanour of Anne Gunning can, at not much of a push, come naturally.

Her first pictures for *Vogue* showed a fierce independence of spirit and a tendency to the baroque. The magazine tagged it 'insouciant aristo-punk', for want of anything better. She had hair dyed jet-black and had recently pierced her own nose. This she accomplished while distractedly waiting on a station platform, betraying her heritage impeccably with an aristocratic disdain for inconveniences such as pain and personal comfort. She is also, as her grandmother pointed out, commendably no-nonsense. Her only comment after admiring Stella on the catwalk was: 'So good at lambing, you know.'

Despite having been cover girl of *Tatler* magazine several years before, Stella was discovered anew on a casting for a 'London Girls' shoot for Steven Meisel organised by *Vogue*'s talent scout nonpareil, Isabella Blow. 'She came off the train from Scotland smelling of goats,' exclaimed Blow in admiration. 'She reminded me of a farm animal' (again admiringly).

It was, however, her assistant, Plum Sykes, who called Tennant in – despite considering the nasal accoutrement unusual for *Vogue*. The prescient Sykes has noted that 'what really helped Stella is fashion's fickleness. What's considered weird one minute can be beautiful the next, while what is thought beautiful swiftly becomes boring'. Despite her imperious height – she stands just shy of 6ft tall – and her self-assured poise, Stella seemed unlikely to amount to anything other than a fleeting inner-city curiosity or decorative *éxotique*. *Vogue* put it with restraint: 'Stella challenges the conventions of what makes a great model.' She was perfect for an attitudinised stance against a monochromatic industrial background, but equally for a sumptuous tableau in celebration of the mystical, mythical orient. For the latter, she was, it must be said, the only leading model able to sport the season's most unusual accessory – a Gaultier silver nose-chain.

However, the nose-ring disappeared and the career took off. After all, *Vogue* noted, 'Stella would look chic wrapped in a shower curtain.' It did take a little time to coalesce, though. On location for *Vogue*, photographer Arthur Elgort attempted *sotto voce* to soften her innate superiority: 'Pretty, Stella, pretty.' But others admired the sparkle of novelty. 'When we first saw Stella,' said Loulou de la Falaise, muse to Yves Saint Laurent, 'we thought she was strange but fabulous and new.'

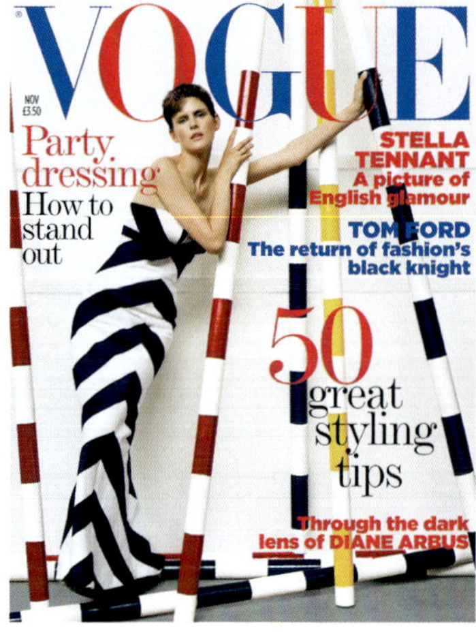

Tim Walker, who admires her spirit of adventure and her endless patience, told the writer Sarah Hay that 'When you're dealing with twee motifs, as I can, you need to combat that with grace and cool. If you watch Stella, the way she stands or crosses her legs and talks, every limb and bend in her body is graceful and cool without her trying, which is something that is very charming and you rarely come across that in life.'

Stella Tennant and her husband, David Lasnet, now live on an estate in the Scottish Borders with their four children. She once jokingly suggested to American *Vogue* that each step down the catwalk represented another acre for the farm. The pierced septum has not completely healed itself. 'Every now and then,' she revealed recently, 'I put a safety pin through it to freak the children out.'

Stella Tennant (b. 1970, UK)

Above:
'A Picture of English Glamour', November 2005, by Tim Walker. Fashion by Neil Cunningham

Opposite:
'In Her Own Style', January 1997, by Craig McDean

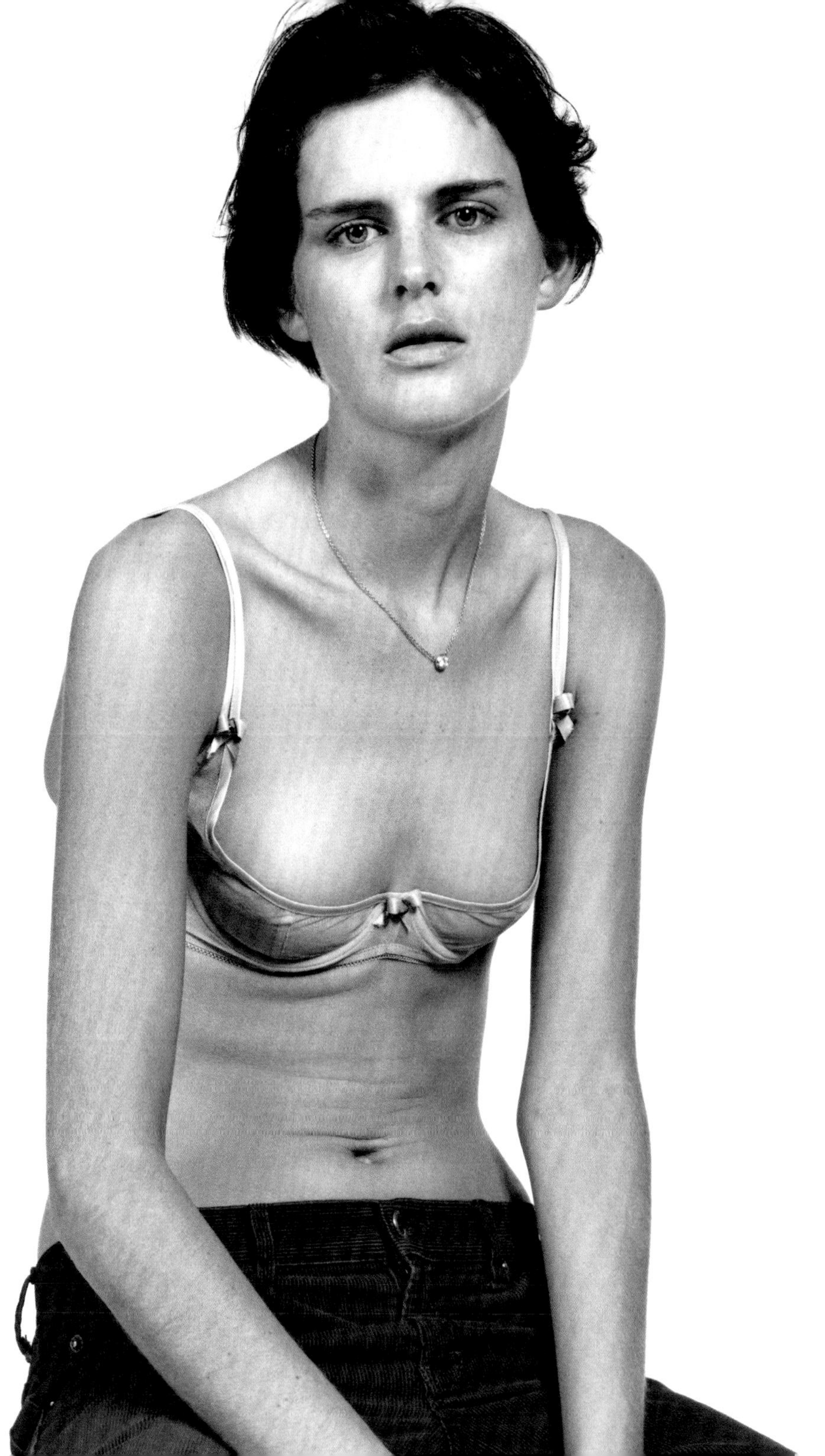

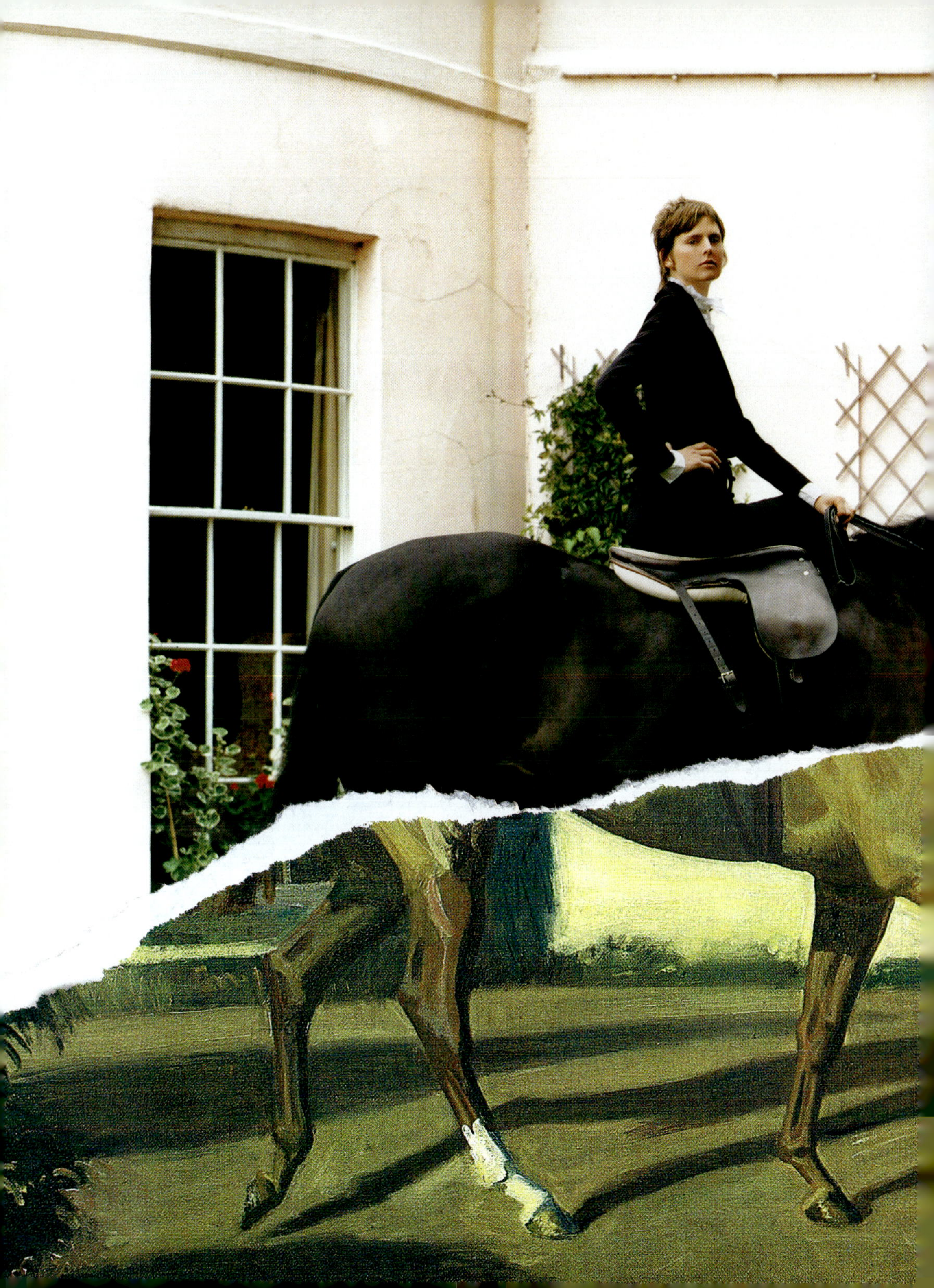

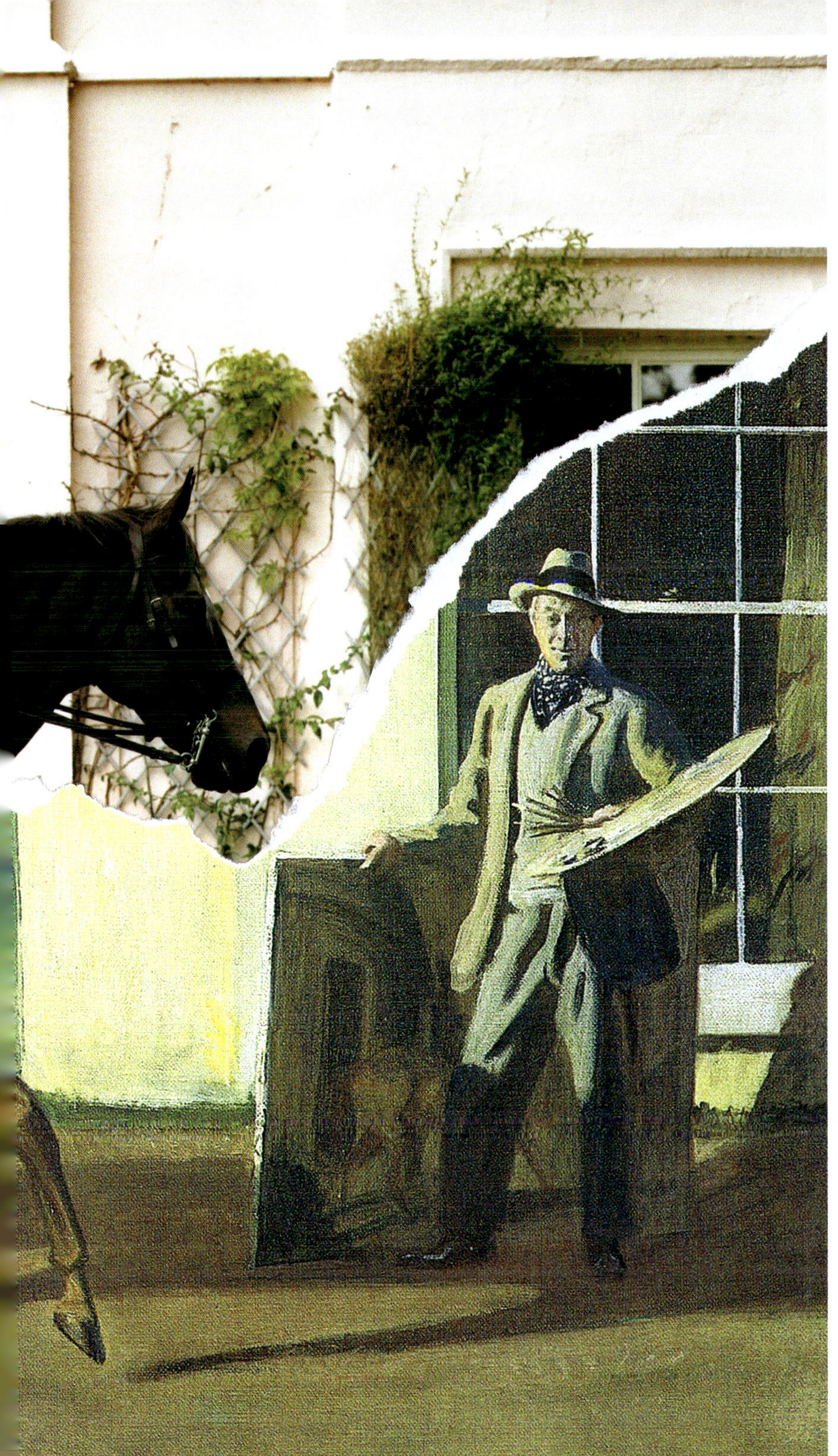

'Portrait of a Lady', November 2005, by Tim Walker. Fashion by Yves Saint Laurent

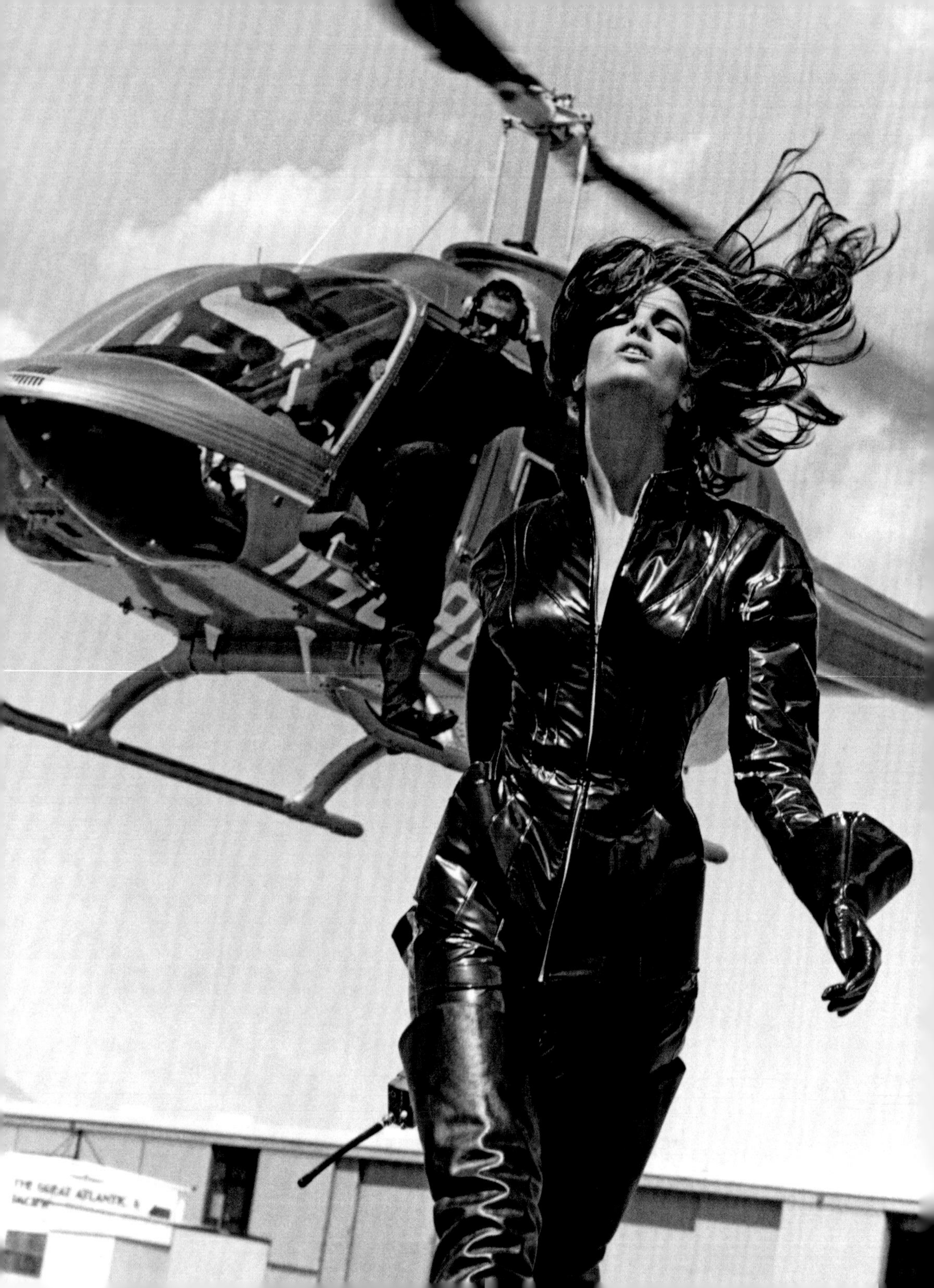

Stephanie Seymour

Over the past few decades, contemporary art and high fashion frequently collided, often in the work of the fashion photographer turned artist Juergen Teller. One memorable tableau featured a bikini-clad Stephanie Seymour lying astride Jeff Koons's *Puppy*, a $3 million, 43ft-high figure of a West Highland terrier constructed from hundreds of colourful herbaceous plants: pansies, begonias and carnations. It belonged to Seymour and her husband, multi-millionaire publishing magnate and polo enthusiast Peter Brant, and was reconstructed in the grounds of their Connecticut farm. It felt like mild ostentation and, since the marriage of Seymour and Brant is now over, Teller's photograph is a valediction of sorts for an era of flamboyance in both fashion and art.

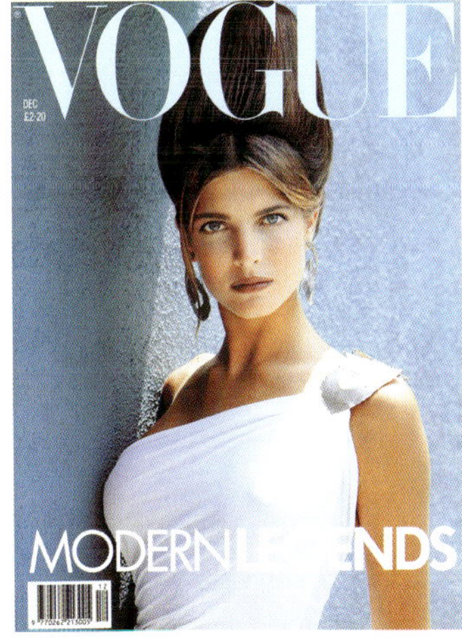

And frequently the excesses of the era, as far as the former was concerned, were delivered stylishly by the 'glamazon' Stephanie. Her cheekbones were sharp as knife blades; her legs seemed to reach her eyebrows, as more than one commentator noticed; her eyebrows themselves were like landing strips chiselled out of a mountainside; while her cleavage, another observed, 'you could park a Harley-Davidson in'.

At *Vogue* her best co-conspirator was Herb Ritts, for whom, ranged in front of his lens, her hair was coiffed into almost-impossible confections, from the pyramid to the puffball. Among the roles she played: a corsair in Vivienne Westwood corsets with rapier and jewel-encrusted eyepatch, and a catsuited Emma Peel supervixen, escaping from the surveillance of a menacing and low-flying helicopter.

She was a favourite, too, of Helmut Newton – for whom she would reprise similar roles – and Richard Avedon. The nudes she did for his Versace campaigns and catalogues have assumed the status of collectibles. But nothing else Seymour has done has taken on the mythic proportions of one particular shoot, a masterpiece of late-period Avedon and iconic of the model herself. As she recalled it: 'Avedon is such a character. He was teaching a photography course to some kids and I was the model… he said to me, "I think that everyone feels so comfortable showing their breasts all the time, but no one is showing their… you know." I said: "You're right, what is there to be ashamed of? I'll do it." We did it in front of the whole class…'

Born in San Diego, Stephanie entered modelling classes after starting out as the subject of her mother's photography class homework. She then entered an Elite agency-sponsored competition and became a regional finalist, though the title Look of the Year eluded her. A staple of Victoria's Secret mail-order catalogues and *Sports Illustrated* swimsuit specials, she was also sought after for *Vogue*'s summer issues.

In the early 1990s she assumed a rock-chick persona – tattoos, knuckleduster rings and fringed leather – after a well-documented liaison with rocker Axl Rose and appearances in several Guns N' Roses videos. It did not end well. 'It wasn't a happy time,' she revealed later, 'but I had great fun with my friends and because I was a single mother, I continued to work.'

Her marriage to Peter Brant ushered in something of a makeover and, as the writer Daisy Garnett noted, she resembled a Parisienne from the 1950s rather than the all-American lingerie girl she had once been, a Hamptons socialite perfectly at home at a Bridgehampton polo game. The marriage to Brant faltered after some 14 years, but not before they shared an enthusiasm for American contemporary art (Andy Warhol, Kenny Scharf and Jean-Michel Basquiat, as well as Koons). This in turn led to Brant financing artist Julian Schnabel's first film, *Basquiat* (1996), and the actor Ed Harris's directorial debut, *Pollock* (2000). In the latter, Stephanie played a small but pivotal role – decorously, and with the conviction she had always brought to her many previous roles, played out time and again in the pages of fashion magazines.

Stephanie Seymour (b. 1968, USA)

Opposite:
'The Avenging Spirit', August 1990, by Herb Ritts. Fashion by Thierry Mugler

Above:
'Modern Legends', December 1988, by Herb Ritts. Fashion by Giorgio di Sant'Angelo

Suzy Parker

Suzy Parker, flame-haired and with a temperament to match, was one of Horst's favourite models. 'The first time I ever photographed her, she couldn't keep still – I tried to organise the dress and the lights and the pose and she was all over the place. I just walked out.' After half an hour, a *Vogue* editor begged him to return. '[Suzy] had been crying and was still drying her tears. She looked like a scolded child, but pulled herself together bravely. And that was the start of our great friendship.' Suzy would in turn recall: 'When Horst exclaimed, as he often did, "How well she looks today!" he was referring not to me but to his odious little dachshund, Mabel.' When Suzy later became an actress, Horst joked that maybe she would do for the movies what she never did for him – hold still. 'She was livid and didn't talk to me for years…'

It all started for the youngest of the four Texan Parker sisters around 1948, when the oldest, Dorian Leigh – then among America's highest-paid models – decided to move to a new agency, insisting as a precondition that her young sister join too. The Ford agency agreed readily, sight unseen – and never regretted it, as in time Suzy became a bigger name than Dorian. 'Frankly, to get Dorian Leigh, I would have taken on Gargantua…' recalled Eileen Ford.

It was the first decent thing Dorian had done for her sister. (On Suzy's birth, Dorian, who was 15 years older, had suggested the names Cecilia Renée Ann – which, when allied to Parker, would have given her obscene initials.) Under her sister's benign patronage Suzy, who at 15 was already 5ft 10in tall, became a star quickly. An early favourite of Richard Avedon, years later Suzy would declare that the 'only joy I ever got out of modelling was with Dick'. Avedon confided to Dorian: 'I don't know if I can work with someone so beautiful. There may not be enough I can do to create something of my own.' However, the pair went on location to Paris in 1950 and the resulting pictures proved a turning point in Suzy's career.

From now on, for several seasons, the dynamic Suzy was a fixture in Paris. French *Vogue*'s prêt-a-porter issue of 1953 underscored this by announcing simply 'Collections – Suzy Parker!' The model, one commentator pointed out, was suddenly more important than the clothes.

One person for whom this did not pass by unnoticed was Coco Chanel. The pair's deep friendship was pivotal in Chanel's decision to re-open her dormant *maison* in 1954. At around the same time, having kick-started a legend into a second life, Suzy decided on one for herself: photography. She secured an apprenticeship with Henri Cartier-Bresson, although her bubbly disposition proved incompatible with the master's asceticism. She was underwhelming here, so she kept on modelling, a reliable standby for a whole generation of photographers who would call on her when things got tricky. 'I have knocked myself out,' she once declared. 'The reason I am the best-paid model is because I am the *best* model.'

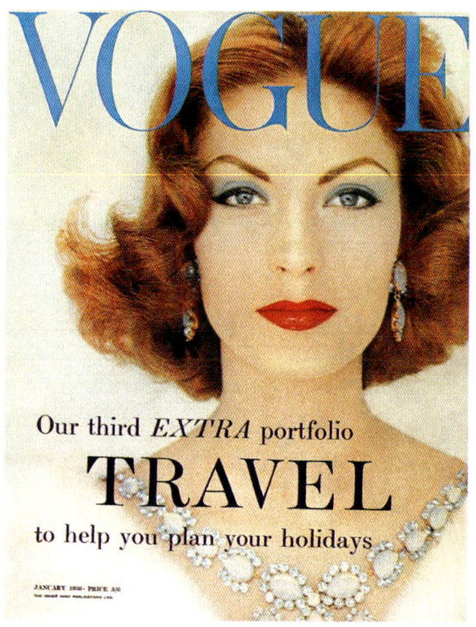

The marriage of Grace Kelly to Prince Rainier of Monaco led to a vacancy, and Hollywood duly came calling. A cameo in *Funny Face* (1957) proved she could do it for at least five minutes, and *Kiss Them for Me* (also 1957), a Cary Grant and Jayne Mansfield vehicle, proved she could shine. More followed. Suzy married her leading man from *Circle of Deception* (1960), Bradford Dillman, and gave it all up for motherhood, cordon-bleu cookery and the occasional domestic vignette for *Vogue*. ('By day she wears easy, unfitted suits with casual throwaway chic, discarding an old Chanel suit as soon as she gets a new one…') A happy ending for the russet-haired youngest sister, who had never really believed she had very much to offer. But, as *Vanity Fair* put it, 'everyone fell for Suzy'.

Suzy Parker (b. Cecilia Parker, 1932, USA; d. 2003)

Above:
'The Great New Fake Jewels', January 1958, by Leombruno-Bodi. Jewellery by Miriam Haskell

Opposite
'The Fashion – Reading from South to North', December 1953, by John Rawlings. Fashion by Emilio Pucci

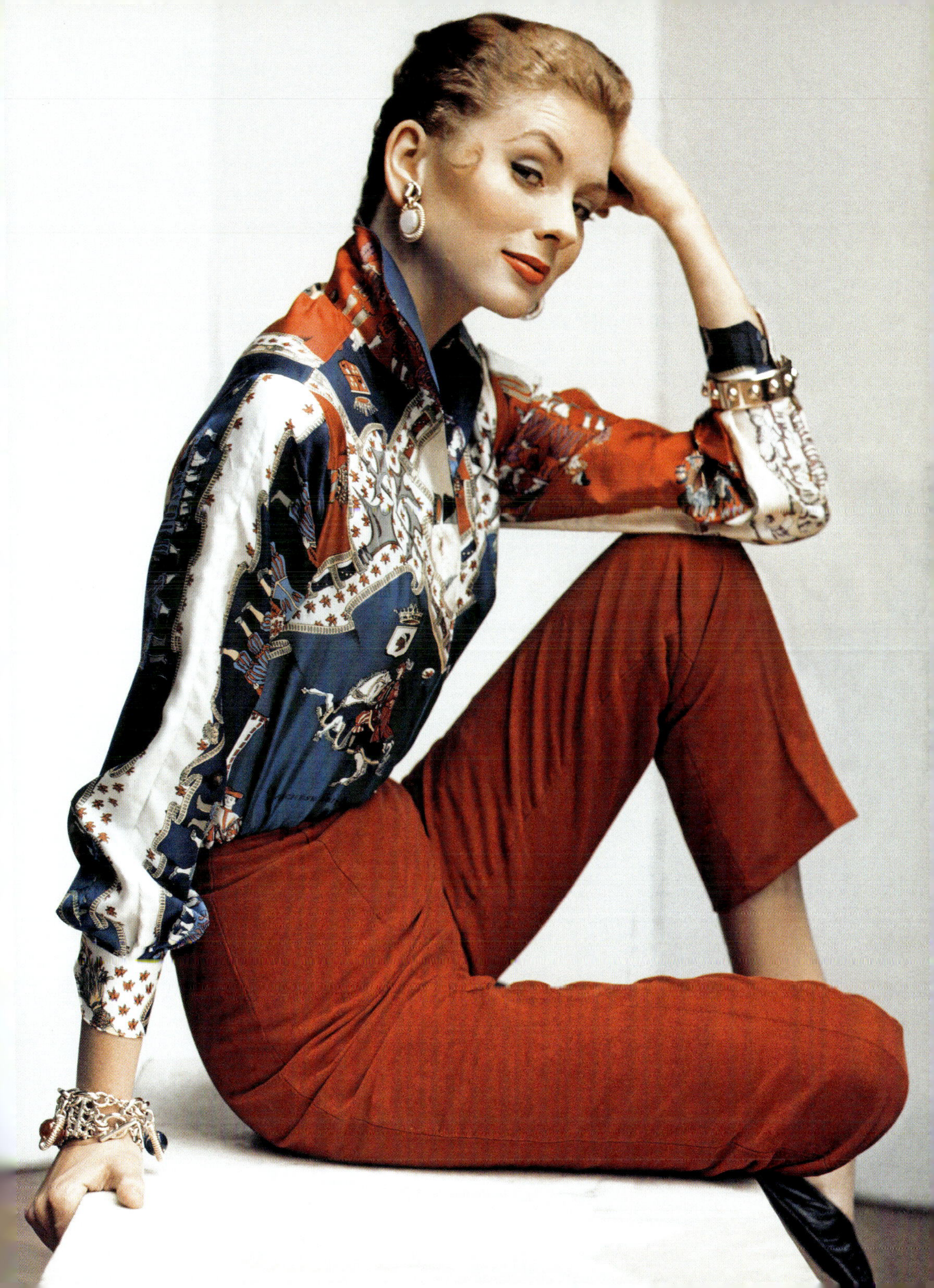

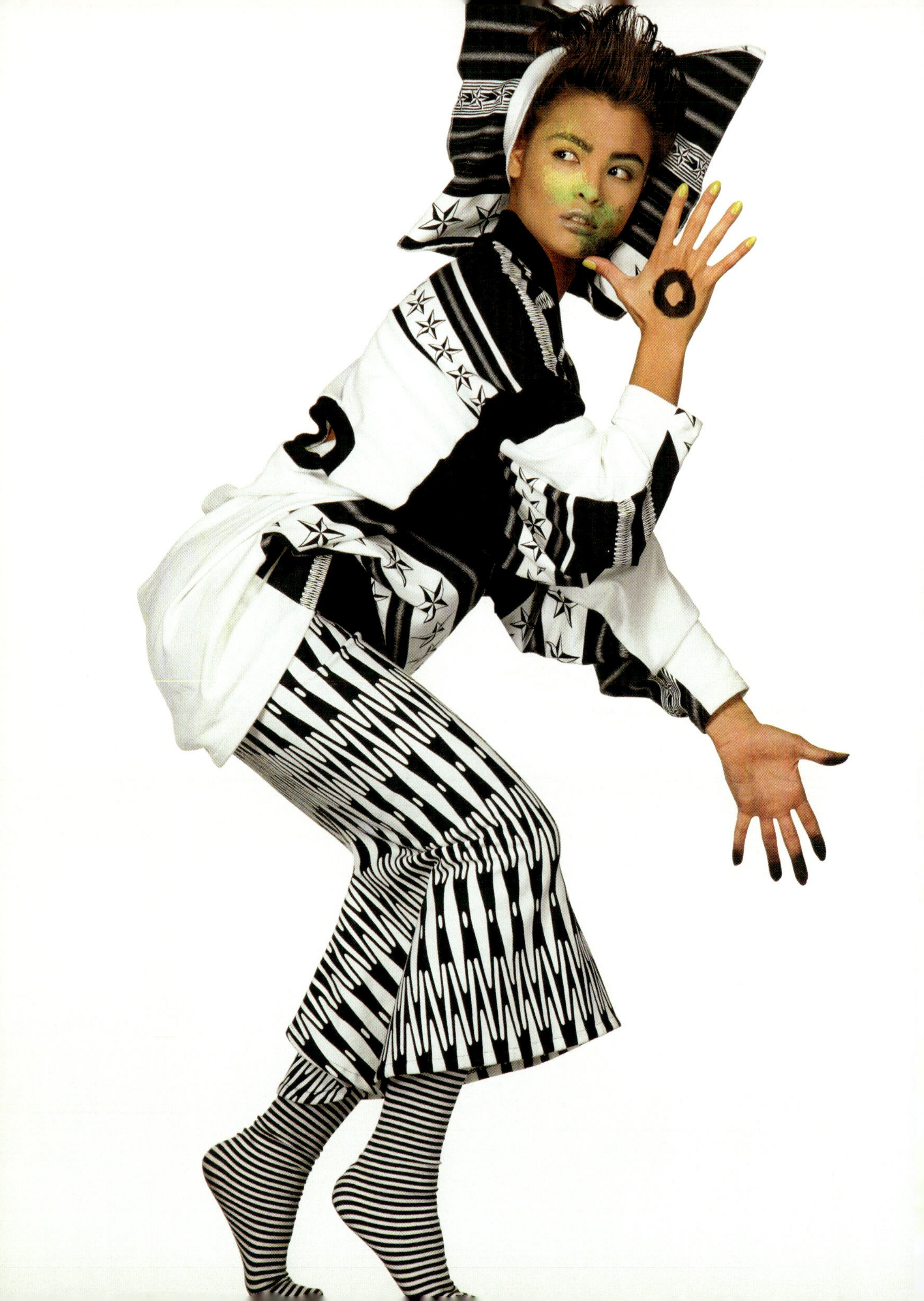

Talisa Soto

Picked out because she reminded him of 'a young Marlon Brando', Talisa Soto was discovered by the photographer Bruce Weber. She could regularly be found as a pioneering Nebraskan settler in one of his homages to America's frontiersman past. 'Working with Bruce was a unique and eye-opening experience,' she says. 'Bruce was a movie director at heart. I always felt we were creating a mini independent film, instead of working on a typical photo shoot. I will forever be grateful for his huge role in launching my successful modelling career.'

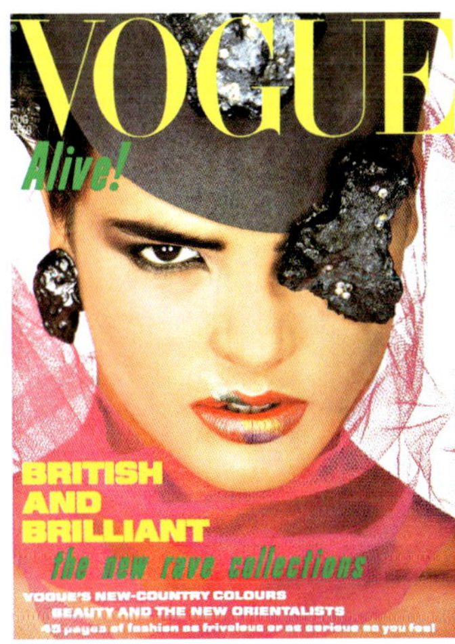

Weber's fashion stories were epic in scale (and ambition), taken customarily against the expansive skyline and the vastness of the American landscape. 'It was always almost filmic, in a way,' confirmed Weber. 'We had a script and an idea of the pictures and Grace [Coddington] would dress people up as characters. And casting it was a huge process… On our shoots we were like one big, extended family and I think we brought to the pictures the life a family brings to all its members. I suppose we were like a repertory company out on the road together.' They were, as someone else once put it, thank-you notes to people for being beautiful.

'If you're weak in this world, forget it, you might as well stay in bed,' Talisa told *Vogue* with conviction. Born in Brooklyn, of Puerto Rican descent, Talisa (real name Miriam) moved with her parents to Northampton, Massachusetts, where she honed her determination and her work ethic. Her first modelling job, at age 15, was in Paris with Weber. She also collaborated with Albert Watson on one of *Vogue*'s most unusual covers of the 1980s. A few years after strikingly applied make-up had become *de rigueur*, courtesy of the New Romantic youth movement, *Vogue* produced its own eye-catching approximation involving pink netting from John Lewis, and brooches fashioned out of diamanté-studded rocks.

Soto gave up modelling in the late 1980s and left New York for acting lessons in Los Angeles. Paul Morrissey cast her in his *Spike of Bensonhurst*: 'Paul wanted me as a mysterious, observant shadow everywhere, but my part got bigger and bigger…' She capitalised on this and achieved greater fame as a Bond girl: Lupe Lamora, the Latin American spitfire of *Licence to Kill*. The all-action arena of *Vogue* was good training ground. 'One of my all-time favourite pictures from the couture,' remembered Grace Coddington in her book *Grace*, 'is one that Bruce got after a long night of waiting for a Givenchy dress to arrive. Just as we were about to collapse, 15-year-old Talisa climbed into a purple charmeuse gown, grabbed a performing poodle we had rented, and balanced it on one hand…'

Talisa Soto (b. Miriam Soto, 1967, USA)

Opposite:
'The New Rave', August 1984, by Albert Watson. Fashion by Bodymap

Above:
'Alive!', August 1984, by Albert Watson. Fashion by Fred Spurr

Tatjana Patitz

'You can lose track of yourself in this business,' the German-born, Swedish-raised amazon Tatjana Patitz told *Vogue*, as her escalating career threatened to get out of hand, 'and you mustn't take yourself too seriously. You never know when your time might be over.' At the time of saying it, there was no immediate danger of either happening. Tatjana was self-deprecating, but magazines took her and her colleagues extremely seriously indeed.

'Every five years or so,' *Vogue* announced, 'a handful of young women at the peak of their profession seem to encapsulate the look of the time...' The pages of the magazine were never going to be big enough to contain the soaring ambitions of the first wave of supermodels, of which Tatjana was one-fifth. She and Cindy, Christy, Naomi and Linda launched their own make-up ranges and lingerie lines, were the faces behind perfumes and wristwatches, co-owned restaurants, dated boxers and pop stars, made appearances in films (usually playing beautiful models), were chat-show staples and were among the highest-earning young women of their generation. The minutiae of their social lives were picked over by the tabloid press, their utterances given sibylline significance.

This was in spite of *Vogue's* first impression, which saw Tatjana as 'slightly odd-looking' while at the same time praising her 'uncosmeticised womanliness, new and important in the 1980s'. It also noticed a ruthless attitude to work and an unequivocal approach to modelling as a career, not necessarily a novelty but something not seen for a while. Nothing was ever too much trouble; the supermodels would push themselves to the limit in pursuit of perfection, to the point of terminal ennui, pain or irascibility. For Tatjana, on location with Herb Ritts, any suffering was worth the result: 'We were in the desert. It was pretty hot and she was wearing wool,' recalled *Vogue* fashion editor Sarajane Hoare. Tatjana was the least concerned by the slog: 'I like photographers who don't go out on the safe side, who are willing to go one step further. That's when I get a kick out of this job...'

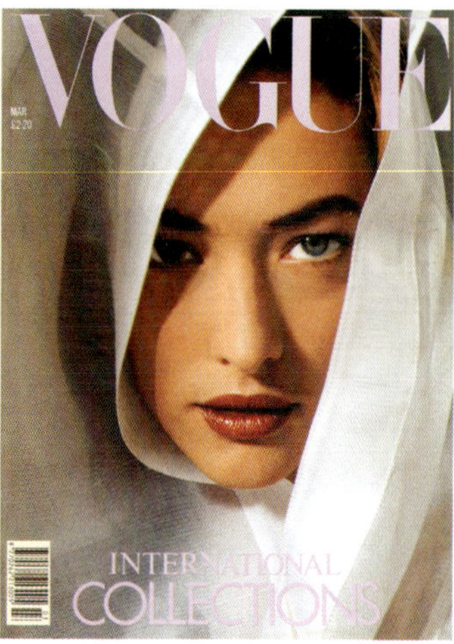

At just shy of 6ft, Teutonically self-composed, and dominating any room she cared to walk into, Tatjana was the biggest beast in a seething jungle; *Vogue* amplified the comparison by fixating on her lynx-like eyes, impossibly blue and 'curved around her temples like a cat's'. The gaze has mesmerised fellow German Peter Lindbergh, whose pictures first brought her to wider attention, and particularly Ritts, for whom she acted out any role he threw at her: stranded mermaid on black sand; fleeting sprite on forest floor; nearly naked nereid beneath tumbling waterfall; surfer girl; plainswoman; Cossack.

While admiring her astonishing presence, *Vogue*'s Kate Phelan recalled: 'She'll just sit there with a cigarette, her hand over half her face, and it's perfect. Then, when she's had enough, she'll just turn away; she won't look at the photographer any more. She decides when the shoot is over.'

Tatjana Patitz (b. 1966, West Germany)

Above:
'International Collections', March 1989, by Sante d'Orazio. Fashion by Isaac Mizrahi

Opposite:
'Callas-thenics', July 1988, by Herb Ritts. Fashion by Azzedine Alaïa

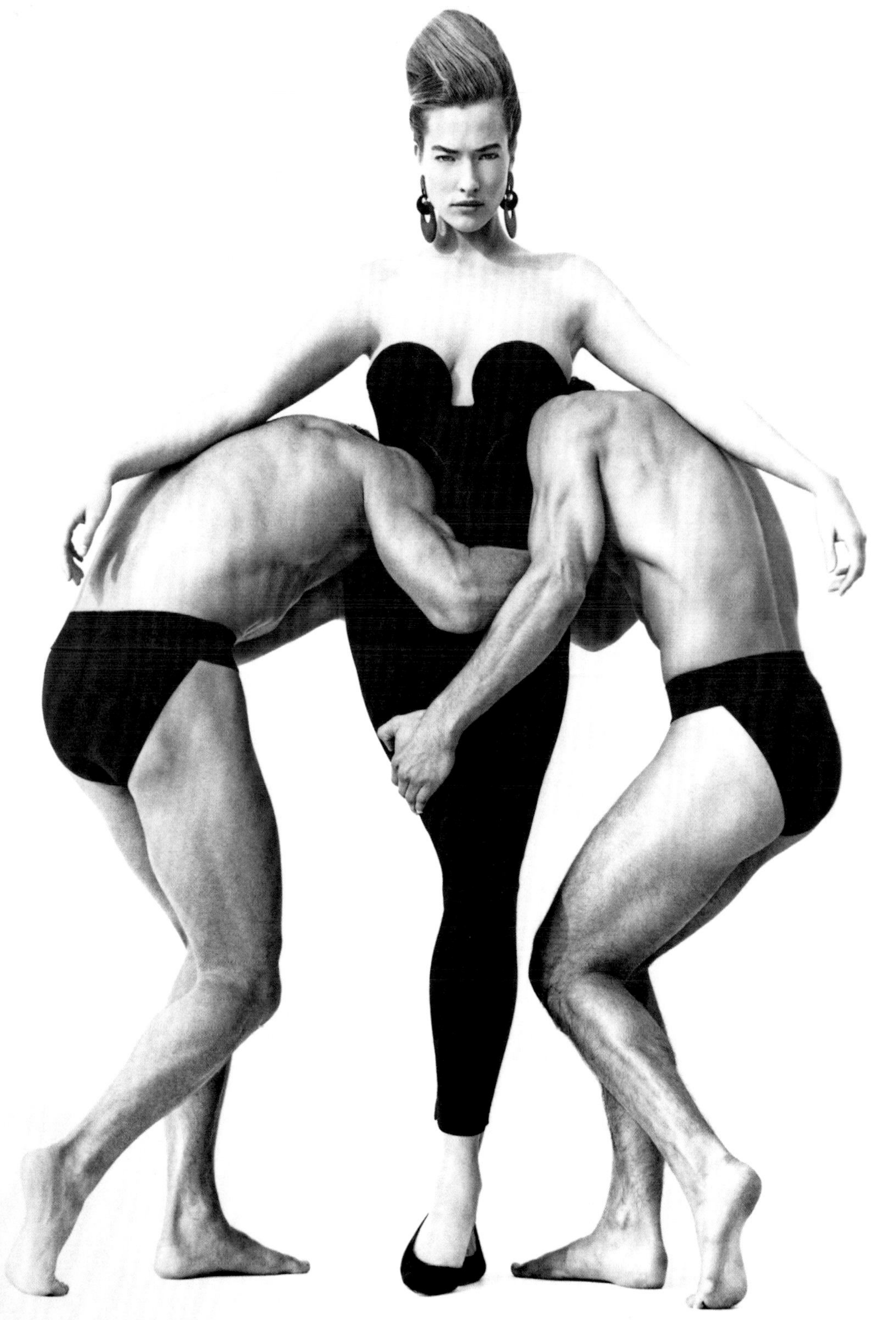

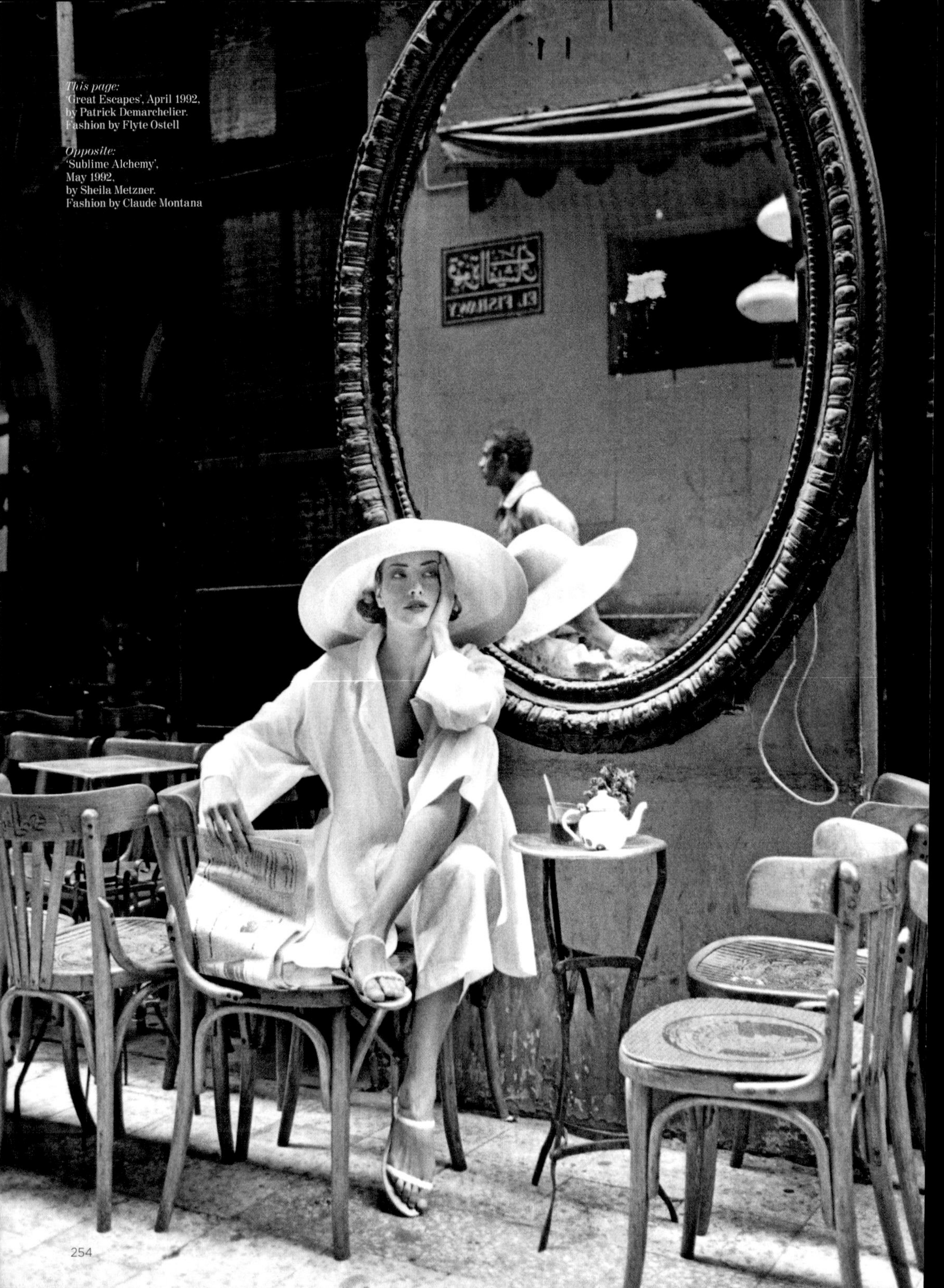

This page:
'Great Escapes', April 1992,
by Patrick Demarchelier.
Fashion by Flyte Ostell

Opposite:
'Sublime Alchemy',
May 1992,
by Sheila Metzner.
Fashion by Claude Montana